Obstetric Intensive Care Manual

Notice

Obstetric Intensive Care Manual

Third Edition

Editor

Michael R. Foley, MD

Clinical Professor, Department of Obstetrics/Gynecology
University of Arizona School of Medicine
at the Arizona Health Sciences Center
Tucson, Arizona
Chief Medical Officer
Scottsdale Healthcare System
Scottsdale, Arizona

Assistant Editors

Thomas H. Strong, Jr., MD

Director, Maternal-Fetal Medicine
Banner Thunderbird Samaritan Medical Center
Glendale, Arizona
Clinical Professor, Department of Obstetrics/Gynecology
University of Arizona School of Medicine
at the Arizona Health Sciences Center
Tucson, Arizona
Associate Director, Phoenix Perinatal Associates
Phoenix, Arizona

Thomas J. Garite, MD

Professor Emeritus, Obstetrics and Gynecology
University of California, Irvine
Director of Research and Education for Obstetrix
Pediatrix Medical Group
Editor-in-Chief, American Journal of Obstetrics and Gynecology
Steamboat Springs, Colorado

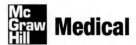

New York   Chicago   San Francisco   Lisbon   London   Madrid   Mexico City
Milan   New Delhi   San Juan   Seoul   Singapore   Sydney   Toronto

Obstetric Intensive Care Manual, Third Edition

1 2 3 4 5 6 7 8 9 0   DOC/DOC   14 13 12 11 10

ISBN 978-0-07-163772-5
MHID 0-07-163772-9

This book was set in Times Roman by Glyph International.
The editors were Alyssa K. Fried and Peter J. Boyle.
The production supervisor was Catherine H. Saggese.
Project management was provided by Anupriya Tyagi, Glyph International.
The designer was Mary McKeon; the cover art director was Anthony Landi and the designer Ty Nowicki.
Image: Tim Platt/Getty Images.
RR Donnelley was printer and binder.

This book is printed on acid-free paper.

Library of Congress Cataloging-in-Publication Data

Obstetric intensive care manual / editor, Michael R. Foley ; assistant editors,
    Thomas H. Strong Jr., Thomas J. Garite. — 3rd ed.
        p. ; cm.
    Includes bibliographical references and index.
    ISBN-13: 978-0-07-163772-5 (hardcover : alk. paper)
    ISBN-10: 0-07-163772-9 (hardcover : alk. paper)   1. Obstetrical emergencies.   I. Foley,
    Michael R.   II. Strong, Thomas H.   III. Garite, Thomas J.
    [DNLM: 1. Intensive Care—methods.   2. Pregnancy Complications—therapy.
    3. Emergencies.   4. Pregnancy.   WQ 240]
    RG571.O266 2011
    618.2′025—dc22
                                                                2010028041

McGraw-Hill books are available at special quantity discounts to use as premiums and sales promotions, or for use in corporate training programs. To contact a representative please e-mail us at bulksales@mcgraw-hill.com.

To Lisa, Bonnie, Molly, and Michael for their unending loving support.
To Bette and Ray for giving me this opportunity.

—Michael R. Foley

For Rebekah and Trey, my life's reason and reward.

—Thomas H. Strong, Jr.

To my mentors, Roger Freeman and Ted Quilligan, and to Fred Zuspan, who we sorely miss.
Thank you for setting the example for how best to serve the specialty by improving care and
outcomes for women and children and for how to treat patients,
students, and colleagues along the way.

—Thomas J. Garite

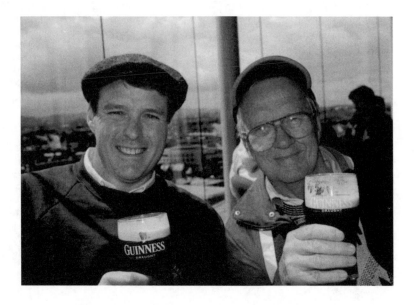

This third edition is dedicated to my dad, Raymond T. Foley.

Contents

Contributors

Tamerou Asrat, MD
Clinical Associate Professor
Department of Obstetrics and Gynecology
University of California at Irvine
Irvine, California
Chapter 13

Michael A. Belfort, MBBCH, MD, PhD
Professor, Department of Obstetrics and Gynecology
University of Utah School of Medicine
Salt Lake City, Utah
Director of Perinatal Research
Director of Fetal Therapy
HCA Healthcare
Nashville, Tennessee
Chapter 10

Paul Berkowitz, MD
Medical Director, Inpatient Services
Department of Psychiatry
Desert Vista Behavioral Health Center
Mesa, Arizona
Chapter 21

Linda R. Chambliss, MD, MPH
Perinatology Department
St. Joseph's Hospital and Medical Center
Phoenix, Arizona
Chapter 26

William H. Clewell, MD
Director, Fetal Medicine and Surgery
Phoenix Perinatal Associates
Phoenix, Arizona
Clinical Professor, Obstetrics and Gynecology
University of Arizona College of Medicine
Tucson, Arizona
Chapter 16

Lisa A. Dado, MD
Valley Anesthesiology Consultant
Phoenix Children's Hospital
Phoenix, Arizona
Chapter 20

Gary A. Dildy III, MD
Attending Perinatologist
Maternal Fetal Medicine Center
St. Mark's Hospital
Salt Lake City, Utah
Director of Maternal-Fetal Medicine
MountainStar Division
Hospital Corporation of America
Nashville, Tennessee
Professor Adjunct
Department of Obstetrics and Gynecology
Louisiana State University School of Medicine
New Orleans, Louisiana
Chapter 14

John P. Elliott, MD
Director, Division of Maternal Fetal Medicine
Banner Good Samaritan Medical Center
Associate Director, Maternal Fetal Medicine
Phoenix Perinatal Associates
Phoenix, Arizona
Chapter 19

Michael R. Foley, MD, CMO
Clinical Professor, Department of Obstetrics and Gynecology
University of Arizona School of Medicine at the Arizona
  Health Sciences Center
Tucson, Arizona
Chief Medical Officer
Scottsdale Healthcare System
Scottsdale, Arizona
Chapter 11

Karrie E. Francois, MD
Amomi Pregnancy and Wellness Spa
Perinatal Medical Director, Scottsdale Healthcare
Scottsdale, Arizona
Clinical Assistant Professor
University of Arizona,
Phoenix, Arizona
and A.T. Still University
Mesa, Arizona
Chapter 3

Thomas J. Garite, MD
Professor Emeritus, Obstetrics and Gynecology
University of California at Irvine
Director of Research and Education for Obstetrix
Pediatrix Medical Group
Editor-in-Chief, American Journal of Obstetrics
* and Gynecology*
Steamboat Springs, Colorado
Chapter 22

Alfredo F. Gei, MD
Director, Division of Maternal-Fetal Medicine
Department of Obstetrics and Gynecology
Methodist Hospital
Houston, Texas
Chapters 12 and 23

Cornelia R. Graves MD
Medical Director, Tennessee Maternal Fetal Medicine
Director, Perinatal Services, Baptist Hospital
Clinical Professor, Vanderbilt University
Nashville, Tennessee
Chapter 25

Ravindu P. Gunatilake, MD
Maternal-Fetal Medicine Fellow
Department of Obstetrics and Gynecology
Duke University Hospital
Durham, North Carolina
Chapter 11

Christina S. Han, MD
Clinical Instructor
Department of Obstetrics, Gynecology, and
* Reproductive Sciences*
Yale University School of Medicine
New Haven, Connecticut
Chapter 7

Cathleen M. Harris, MD, MPH
Amomi Pregnancy Wellness
Scottsdale, Arizona
Chapter 18

William C. Mabie, MD
GHS Professor of Clinical Obstetrics and Gynecology
University of South Carolina School of
* Medicine-Greenville*
Greenville Hospital System University Medical Center
Greenville, South Carolina
Chapter 1

Stephanie R. Martin, DO
Department Chairman
Maternal-Fetal Medicine
Memorial Health System
Colorado Springs, Colorado
Chapters 2 and 8

Jennifer McNulty, MD
Associate Clinical Professor
Department of Obstetrics and Gynecology
Division of Maternal Fetal Medicine
University of California at Irvine
Staff Perinatologist
Long Beach Memorial Women's Hospital
Long Beach, California
Chapter 15

Keith S. Meredith, MD
Regional Vice President
Mountain Region
Pediatrix/Obstetrix Medical Group
Phoenix, Arizona
Chapter 24

Marlin D. Mills, MD
Phoenix Perinatal Associates
Phoenix, Arizona
Chapter 21

Robert A. Myers, MD
Director, Inpatient HIV Services
Maricopa Medical Center
Phoenix, Arizona
Chapter 26

Michael P. Nageotte, MD
Executive Careline Director
Long Beach Memorial Hospital
Long Beach, California
Professor, Department of Obstetrics and Gynecology
University of California at Irvine
Irvine, California
Chapter 13

Michael J. Paidas, MD
Associate Professor
Co-Director, Yale Women and Children's Center
*   for Blood Disorders*
Co-Director, National Hemophilia Foundation—Baxter
*   Clinical Fellowship Program at Yale*
Division of Maternal-Fetal Medicine
Department of Obstetrics, Gynecology, and
*   Reproductive Sciences*
Yale University School of Medicine
New Haven, Connecticut
Chapter 7

Pranav Patel, MD
Neonatal Medicine
Phoenix Perinatal Associates
Phoenix, Arizona
Chapter 24

Jordan H. Perlow, MD
Associate Director, Maternal-Fetal Medicine
Banner Good Samaritan Medical Center
Partner, Phoenix Perinatal Associates
Obstetrix Medical Group of Phoenix
Phoenix, Arizona
Chapter 6

Robert A. Raschke, MD
Medical Director Critical Care Medicine
Banner Good Samaritan Medical Center
Professor of Clinical Medicine
University of Arizona College of Medicine
Phoenix, Arizona
Chapter 17

George R. Saade, MD
Division Chief, Maternal-Fetal Medicine
Professor, Obstetrics and Gynecology
Department of Obstetrics and Gynecology
University of Texas Medical Branch
Galveston, Texas
Chapter 9

Philip Samuels, MD
Associate Professor, Obstetrics and Gynecology
Ohio State University College of Medicine and
*   Public Health*
Residency Program Director
Ohio State University/Mt. Carmel Health Program in
*   Obstetrics and Gynecology*
Columbus, Ohio
Chapter 4

Baha M. Sibai, MD
Professor and Chair
Department of Obstetrics and Gynecology
University of Cincinnati College of Medicine
Cincinnati, Ohio
Chapter 5

Robert M. Silver, MD
Department of Obstetrics and Gynecology
University of Utah School of Medicine
Salt Lake City, Utah
Chapter 27

Irene P. Stafford, MD
Assistant Instructor
Department of Obstetrics and Gynecology
University of Texas Southwestern Medical Center
Dallas, Texas
Chapter 14

Thomas H. Strong, Jr., MD
Director, Maternal-Fetal Medicine
Banner Thunderbird Samaritan Medical Center
Glendale, Arizona
Clinical Professor, Obstetrics and Gynecology
University of Arizona School of Medicine
  at the Arizona Health Sciences Center
Tucson, Arizona
Associate Director, Phoenix Perinatal Associates
Phoenix, Arizona

Victor R. Suarez, MD
Division of Maternal-Fetal Medicine
Department of Obstetrics and Gynecology
Advocate Christ Medical Center
Oak Lawn, Illinois
Chapters 12 and 23

Foreword *to the Third Edition*

Questions and Answers

We all have questions. Over the years, when I saw patients in consultation, I would always ask, "How can we help you?", followed by, "What questions do you have? I want to be sure we answer them before you leave." I would also encourage my patients to bring a written list of their questions. I emphasized this because I found that patients would often come to see me, and, in the midst of giving their history and having their physical examination, the important questions they had on their mind were forgotten. I wanted to be sure they didn't find themselves traveling home with unanswered questions. Today, patients often come to us extremely well prepared. In many instances, they have already answered their questions through extensive research including a review of the articles we have published! Yet, they still do have questions.

Some of these obstetrical patients will require intensive care. The question is not, "Will this happen?" The question is, "When will this happen?" For most of us, these significant complications occur infrequently in our practice, and so we find ourselves not as well prepared to face these difficult situations. The questions then might be, "What do *we* do now?", "What's the best treatment?", "What do *we* do next?" Note that I have used the word *we* because patients needing intensive care must be managed by a team, including the obstetrician, maternal-fetal medicine specialist, critical care nurse, obstetrical nurse, intensivist, respiratory therapist, and in some instances, the hematologist, infectious disease specialist, and the endocrinologist. Only through collaboration as a team, sharing the knowledge and experience we all have had, can these patients be treated most effectively. We must also remember that these critical situations may happen in the antepartum, intrapartum, or postpartum periods.

Now, in this third edition of the *Obstetric Intensive Care Manual*, Dr. Mike Foley and his colleagues have answered our questions. This book is presented in a very practical manual, providing a hands-on approach to our patients.

Whether we work in a major academic medical center with large intensive care units or in a small rural hospital, this manual will serve as an important resource for all of us. Dr. Foley and his collaborators present information on more frequently seen emergencies including obstetric hemorrhage, hypertensive crises, and cardiac disease as well as others that we see less frequently including the anaphylactoid syndrome of pregnancy (amniotic fluid embolism), thyroid storm, and psychiatric disorders. Again, all are presented in a very practical style that makes the translation from the written word to action easy to undertake.

Finally, I want to add how honored I am to write this foreword for the third edition. The foreword for the second edition was written by my dear friend Dr. Fred Zuspan. Throughout my career, Dr. Zuspan or "Z" and his inseparable partner, Dr. Ted Quilligan or "Q" were my valued mentors. Dr. Z was my predecessor as chair of obstetrics and gynecology at Ohio State. I was thrilled a number of years ago when the Society for Maternal-Fetal Medicine asked me to present the SMFM Achievement Award to Dr. Z and Dr. Q. Dr. Z passed away this year, and our colleagues, our patients, and our students lost a beloved friend and leader. It was my honor when Dr. Foley trained as a resident and fellow in maternal-fetal medicine at the Ohio State University Medical Center to serve as his mentor. Dr. Z did as well. Mike was an outstanding resident and fellow, and I am so proud to see the contributions he has made not only to academic medicine but to his community. This book is one of his most important contributions, and I know that you, your team, and most importantly your patients will benefit from its wisdom.

Steven G. Gabbe, MD
Senior Vice President for Health Sciences
Chief Executive Officer
The Ohio State University Medical Center
Columbus, Ohio

Foreword *to the Second Edition*

The *Obstetric Intensive Care Manual,* developed by Drs. Michael Foley and Thomas Strong, Jr., 6 years ago, was a best seller. McGraw-Hill is now publishing this new edition.

The second edition has many new features and enlists an additional senior editor, Dr. Thomas Garite, a recognized expert in maternal-fetal medicine and the editor-in-chief of the *American Journal of Obstetrics and Gynecology.* A number of distinguished clinicians and academicians also have been asked to contribute chapters in their specific areas of expertise, bringing an expanded knowledge base to this second edition: George Saade (Galveston, Texas), Michael Belfort (Provo, Utah), Karrie Francois (Phoenix, Arizona), Stephanie Martin (Phoenix, Arizona), Charles Lockwood (New Haven, Connecticut), Baha Sibai (Cincinnati, Ohio), Alfredo Gei (Galveston, Texas), Mike Nageotte (Long Beach, California), Jennifer McNulty (Long Beach, California), Cathleen Harris (Phoenix, Arizona), Keith Meredith (Phoenix, Arizona), Connie Graves (Nashville, Tennessee), and Bob Silver (Salt Lake City, Utah).

Before these new authors came on board, the first manual was thoroughly evaluated by being "field tested" by fellows, residents, and practicing physicians. This field-testing led to additional topics and revisions for this new edition. The principal questions for such a revision are: What is needed in a manual that can be stuck in a pocket and is most useful in deciding on the care of the critically ill patient? Will you take care of the patient or refer the patient to another care center?

The anxiety of caring for the critically ill patient is tremendous. Some of this is predicated on escalating malpractice costs. No matter what you do for these patients the end results may leave something to be desired. Sometimes there is no place to send critically ill patients and the burden of responsibility is on your shoulders, and this manual will not only provide you with scholarly information but will help you be a "hands on" physician. You can begin working with the patient now and make a referral or get further help later.

It is hoped that this handbook will be in the hands of all obstetric caregivers. If you care for obstetric patients, you cannot predict emergencies, but this manual will better prepare you for the emergencies and the complexities that arise in obstetric intensive care.

This new manual contains 27 different chapters about the pregnant patient who encounters an emergency or an urgent problem with her pregnancy. This book will help the practitioner make proper choices for care of the patient. "Hands on" is the basis of medicine and where it all starts; you can go from there with your mental algorithm on what to do. This manual will assist you in your thinking.

Good luck in learning this complicated topic of intensive care and enjoy your education.

Frederick P. Zuspan, MD
Professor and Chairman Emeritus
Department of Obstetrics and Gynecology
The Ohio State University College of Medicine
Columbus, Ohio
Editor-in-Chief Emeritus
American Journal of Obstetrics and Gynecology

Thank you to Dr. Zuspan for being our mentor! We are all extremely indebted to his unparalleled contributions to the field of maternal-fetal medicine. Dr. Zuspan passed away in the summer of 2009. He is missed by all of us. . . .

Michael R. Foley, MD
Thomas H. Strong, Jr., MD
Thomas J. Garite, MD

Preface

Most, if not all, practitioners in the field of obstetrics will undoubtedly, at some point in their career, willingly or otherwise, find themselves caring for a critically ill parturient. Unfortunately, but quite predictably due to the nature of our business, we are often unprepared to deal with these rare, emergent complexities at a moment's notice. We are not afforded the luxury of having the time to page through a comprehensive textbook in order to review the problem at hand. What is needed, when we find ourselves "up to our eyebrows in alligators," is a handy, brief, pragmatic source that provides a short review of pathophysiology and diagnostic methods while placing a primary focus on "what to do and how often" type management.

The third edition of the *Obstetric Intensive Care Manual* has evolved from "in the trenches" type testing. What worked well was expanded, what was missing was added, and what did not work well was remodeled. I am extremely indebted to Drs. Strong and Garite for their fabulous editorial assistance during the preparation of this third edition. As always, I am grateful to my mentors Dr. Frederick P. Zuspan and Dr. Steven G. Gabbe, and my colleagues at Phoenix Perinatal Associates–Obstetrix Medical Group of Phoenix, Scottsdale Healthcare, and the OB/GYN Residents at Banner Good Samaritan in Phoenix, Arizona, for their guidance and friendship over the years in preparation for "real life" practical obstetric care delivery. Thank you to all the outstanding contributing authors, past and present, for making this book a valuable asset to obstetric care providers worldwide.

To know what you do not know is the best.
To pretend to know when you do not know is disease.
—*Lao Tzu*

As educators and caregivers, we should strive to capably manage and understand the true essence of "disease."

Michael R. Foley, MD
Scottsdale, Arizona

Acknowledgments

Drs. Foley, Strong, and Garite are extremely indebted to Susan Weisman for her outstanding editorial assistance during the preparation of this book. We all appreciate her good humor, wit, and graciousness.

Basic Hemodynamic Monitoring for the Obstetric Care Provider

• William C. Mabie

Pulmonary artery catheterization has been around for a long time. Werner T O Forssmann performed the first human cardiac catheterization on himself as an intern in 1929. In 1953, Sven Ivar Seldinger published his technique for arterial cannulation over a guidewire. Werner T O Forssmann, Andre F Cournand, and Dickinson W Richards won the Nobel Prize for the development of heart catheterization and for discoveries in cardiovascular physiology in 1956. In 1970, Drs H J C Swan and William Ganz introduced their flow-directed pulmonary artery catheter (PAC).

Like fetal heart rate monitoring, PAC monitoring was introduced despite a lack of prospective clinical trials demonstrating efficacy or improved patient outcome. It made sense to transfer technology from the cardiac catheterization lab to the bedside. By understanding the disease process, one could tailor therapy to the individual patient. Initially used to guide therapy of acute myocardial infarction, its use grew more widespread during the evolution of the intensive care unit (ICU).

In the last few years there has been a reappraisal of the PAC, and it is falling out of vogue. This has occurred because recent randomized trials have shown that, even though it is relatively safe, PAC monitoring provides no benefit in mortality and it increases length of stay, cost, and morbidity.[1-4] It has been argued that use of the PAC is a marker for a more aggressive and morbid style of care.[5] There is no firm explanation for the apparent lack of effectiveness of the PAC, but several possibilities have been suggested: (1) It is only a monitoring device. If no effective therapy exists for the abnormalities detected, no discernable benefit can be shown. (2) Physicians and nurses do not know how to reliably acquire and interpret the data. (3) There is no consensus about management based on the hemodynamic data. (4) The data are not relevant to the clinical questions (eg, volume status). The wedge pressure does not reflect left ventricular preload in the setting of diminished left ventricular compliance (eg, ischemia), high juxtacardiac pressure (eg, positive end-expiratory pressure), or right heart overload due to pulmonary embolism. (5) Once the pathophysiology of a disease process is understood, you take that knowledge to the next patient, and there is less potential to demonstrate a benefit from invasive monitoring.

Nevertheless, more than half of this chapter is devoted to invasive hemodynamic monitoring. This is because PAC monitoring remains a large part of the critical care curriculum. It illustrates how the pathophysiology of cardiogenic shock, severe preeclampsia/eclampsia, septic shock, and acute respiratory distress syndrome (ARDS) was unraveled. Fluid, inotropic, and afterload therapy are still based on clinical investigations which employed the PAC. Finally, though it may one day soon be relegated to a footnote in medical history, there are still a lot of pulmonary artery catheters being sold.[6]

■ INDICATIONS FOR INVASIVE HEMODYNAMIC MONITORING

Studies supporting the use of the Swan-Ganz catheter emphasize its ability to provide information that history, physical examination, and chest x-ray cannot supply. However, the benefits of this intervention on patient outcome have never been demonstrated in any subset of patients (eg, general ICU, ARDS, shock, sepsis, heart failure, or major surgery). Although there does not need to be a moratorium on its use, and it is reasonable to choose to use PAC monitoring to answer a specific clinical question (eg, etiology of hypoperfusion or the response to therapy), there is no evidence-based list of conditions that may require PA catheterization. The decision to place a Swan-Ganz catheter should be made on a case-by-case basis after carefully weighing the risks and benefits.

Following are definitions of some hemodynamic terms.

Wedge Pressure: Also known as the pulmonary artery occlusion pressure (PAOP), wedge pressure is a measure of left ventricular preload. The pulmonary artery wedge pressure is obtained with a balloon-tipped catheter advanced into a branch of the pulmonary artery until the vessel is occluded, forming a free communication through the pulmonary capillaries and veins to the left atrium. A true wedge position is in a lung zone where both pulmonary artery and pulmonary venous pressures exceed alveolar pressure (West Zone 3).

Preload: Initial stretch of the myocardial fiber at end diastole. Clinically, the preload to the right and left ventricles (end-diastolic pressures) is assessed by the central venous pressure and wedge pressure, respectively.

Afterload: Reflected by both the wall tension of the ventricle during ejection and the resistance to forward flow in the form of vascular resistance (vasoconstriction). The pulmonary vascular resistance (PVR) and the systemic vascular resistance (SVR) are the primary afterloads for the right and left ventricles, respectively, in a normal heart.

Contractility: The inherent force and velocity of myocardial contraction when preload and afterload are held constant.[7]

Inserting the Swan-Ganz Catheter

The Swan-Ganz catheter is most commonly inserted through the internal jugular vein or the subclavian vein. It may also be inserted through the basilic vein in the arm or the femoral vein. Several commercial trays containing the necessary equipment are available for central venous cannulation using the Seldinger technique. The procedure is performed under continuous electrocardiographic monitoring. The equipment needed for inserting the Swan-Ganz catheter is shown in Fig 1-1. The technique for venous cannulation and passing the catheter through the heart will not be described here.

Hemodynamic Waveforms

The right atrial pressure tracing (Fig 1-2A) consists of three distinct waves *a*, *c*, and *v*. The *a* wave is a small wave due to atrial systole. The declining pressure that immediately follows the *a* wave is called the *X* descent. The *c* wave may or may not appear as a distinct wave. It reflects the increase in right atrial pressure produced by closure of the tricuspid valve. The negative wave following the *c* wave is called the *X'* descent. The *v* wave is caused by right atrial filling and concomitant right ventricular systole, which causes the leaflets of the closed tricuspid valve to bulge back into the right atrium. The *Y* descent immediately follows the *v* wave. The pressure changes produced by the *a*, *c*, and *v* waves are usually within 3 to 4 mm Hg of each other so that the mean pressure is taken. The normal resting mean right atrial pressure is 1 to 7 mm Hg. Elevated right atrial pressures may occur in the following conditions: right ventricular failure, tricuspid stenosis and regurgitation, cardiac tamponade, constrictive pericarditis, pulmonary hypertension, chronic left ventricular failure, and volume overload.

The phases of systole and diastole in the right ventricular pressure tracing can be divided into seven events (Fig 1-2B). Systolic events include (1) isovolumetric contraction, (2) rapid ejection, and (3) reduced ejection. Diastolic events include (4) isovolumetric relaxation, (5) early diastole, (6) atrial systole, and (7) end diastole.

The pulmonary artery pressure tracing is seen in Fig. 1-2C. There is a sharp rise in pressure followed by a decline in pressure as the volume decreases. When the right ventricular pressure falls below the level of the pulmonary artery pressure, the pulmonary valve snaps shut. This sudden closure of the valve leaflets causes the dicrotic notch in the pulmonary artery pressure tracing. Normal pulmonary artery systolic pressure is 20 to 30 mm Hg. Normal end-diastolic pressure is 8 to 12 mm Hg. Elevated pulmonary artery pressures are seen in pulmonary disease, primary pulmonary hypertension, mitral stenosis or regurgitation, left ventricular failure, and intracardiac left-to-right shunts. Hypoxia increases pulmonary vascular resistance and pulmonary artery pressure.

When a small branch of the pulmonary artery is occluded by inflation of the balloon on the Swan-Ganz catheter, the pressure tracing reflects left atrial pressure. The waveform looks similar to the right atrial pressure tracing described in Fig 1-2A. The *a* wave of the wedge pressure is produced by left atrial contraction followed by the *X* descent (Fig 1-2D). The *c* wave is produced by

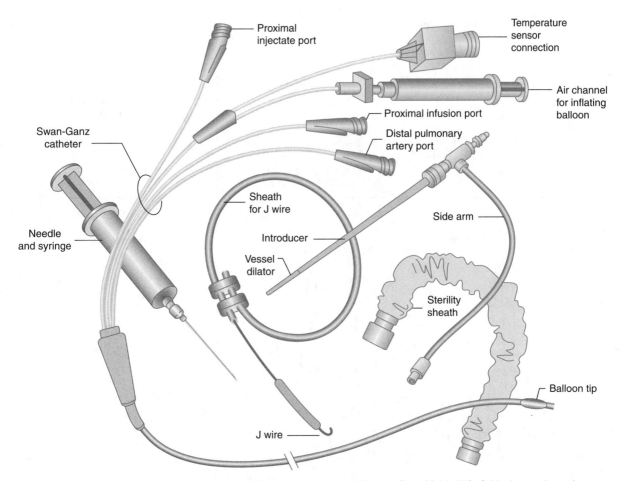

FIGURE 1-1. Equipment needed for inserting the Swan-Ganz catheter. (*Source*: From Mabie WC: Critical care obstetrics. In: Gabbe SG, Niebyl JR, Simpson JL (eds), *Obstetrics: Normal and Problem Pregnancies*, 3rd edn., New York: Churchill Livingston, 1996; Chapter 18, pp. 533-559.)

closure of the mitral valve, but is usually not seen. The *v* wave is produced by filling of the left atrium and bulging back of the mitral valve during ventricular systole. The decline following the *v* wave is called the *Y* descent. The normal resting mean wedge pressure is 6 to 12 mm Hg. Elevated wedge pressure is seen in left ventricular failure, mitral stenosis or regurgitation, cardiac tamponade, constrictive pericarditis, and volume overload.[8]

■ DETERMINING THE HEMODYNAMIC PROFILE

Thermodilution cardiac output is determined using the Fick principle in which a known quantity and concentration of a detectable marker travels a known distance to a point where its concentration is measured. From this information,

the quantity of blood passing the reference point can be calculated. With thermodilution cardiac output, temperature is the marker; and it is given as a bolus of saline through the proximal central venous port of the Swan-Ganz catheter. The change in temperature is measured approximately 30 cm downstream at a thermistor near the tip. Cardiac output is measured using five (10 cc) injections of iced or room temperature saline. Highest and lowest values are discarded with the mean of the three remaining values recorded. The value for the first injection is usually high because of heat gained by the injectate in cooling the catheter. In general, the greater the difference in temperature between the saline bolus and the blood, the more accurate the cardiac output determination. Instead of requiring a bolus of saline, the continuous cardiac output Swan-Ganz catheter has a copper coil proximal to the

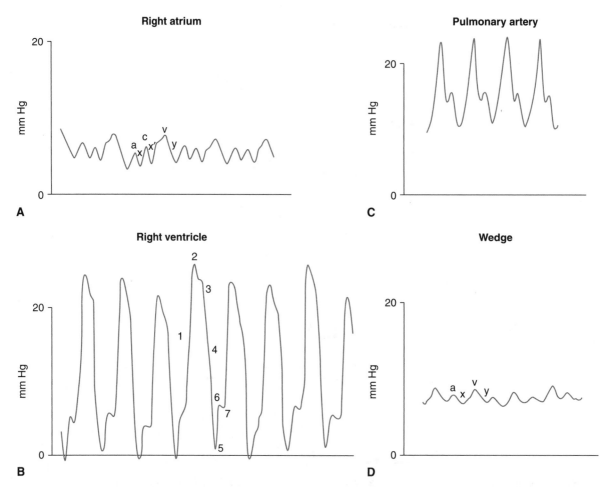

FIGURE 1-2. (A-D) Pulmonary artery catheter placement. Waveforms and normal pressures. (*Source:* Daily EK, Schroeder JP: *Hemodynamic Waveforms: Exercises in Identification and Analysis.* St. Louis: CV Mosby, 1983.)

thermistor which heats the blood passing by it by a few hundredths of a degree centigrade. The heated blood travels a known distance to the thermistor where the change in temperature is measured. This technique does not result in a continuous cardiac output measurement, but it is repeated every 10 sec so that for practical purposes it is continuous. The following measured hemodynamic variables are then used to calculate the rest of the hemodynamic profile: heart rate, blood pressure, pulmonary artery pressure, pulmonary artery wedge pressure, central venous pressure, cardiac output, and patient's height and weight. The derived variables include cardiac index, stroke volume and index, systemic vascular resistance and index, pulmonary vascular resistance and index, and left and right ventricular stroke work and indices (Table 1-1 provides formulas).

Oxygen Transport

Arterial oxygen content (CaO_2) is the sum of the oxygen bound to hemoglobin and that dissolved in plasma as described by the equation:

$$CaO_2 = (Hgb \times 1.36 \times SaO_2) + (PaO_2 \times 0.003)$$

where 1.36 is the amount (in milliliters) of oxygen bound to 1 g of hemoglobin (Hgb); SaO_2 is the arterial oxygen saturation; and 0.003 is the solubility coefficient of oxygen in human plasma. If SaO_2 is 1.0 or 100 percent saturated, Hgb is 15 g/dL, and PaO_2 is 100 mm Hg, then

$$CaO_2 = (15 \times 1.36 \times 1.0) + (100 \times 0.003)$$
$$= 20 + 0.3$$
$$= 20 \text{ mL/dL}$$

■ **TABLE 1-1.** Derived Hemodynamic Parameters

Parameter	Abbreviation	Formula	Units
Pulse pressure	PP	BP syst − BP diast	mm Hg
Mean arterial pressure	MAP	BP diast + 1/3PP	mm Hg
Cardiac index	CI	$\dfrac{CO}{BSA}$	L/min/m^2
Stroke volume	SV	$\dfrac{CO \times 1000}{HR}$	mL
Stroke index	SI	$\dfrac{SV}{BSA}$	mL/beat/m^2
Systemic vascular resistance	SVR	$\dfrac{MAP - CVP}{CO} \times 80$	dyn/s/cm^{-5}
Systemic vascular resistance index	SVRI	SVR × BSA	dyn/s/cm^{-5}/m^2
Pulmonary vascular resistance	PVR	$\dfrac{\overline{PAP} - PCWP}{CO} \times 80$	dyn/s/cm^{-5}
Pulmonary vascular resistance index	PVRI	PVR × BSA	dyn/s/cm^{-5}/m^2
Left ventricular stroke work	LVSW	SV × MAP × 0.136	g/m
Left ventricular stroke work index	LVSWI	$\dfrac{LVSW}{BSA}$	g/m/m^2
Right ventricular stroke work	RVSW	SV × $\overline{PAP}$ × 0.136	g/m
Right ventricular stroke work index	RVSWI	$\dfrac{RVSW}{BSA}$	g/m/m^2

Key: BP syst, systolic blood pressure; BP diast, diastolic blood pressure; CO, cardiac output; HR, heart rate; BSA, body surface area; $\overline{PAP}$ mean pulmonary artery pressure; PCWP, pulmonary capillary wedge pressure.[7]

The amount of oxygen dissolved in the plasma usually does not make a significant contribution to CaO_2.

Mixed venous blood gives an estimate of the balance between oxygen supply and demand. For example, in low cardiac output states with a high rate of peripheral oxygen extraction, mixed venous oxygen tension (PvO_2) is low. Normal PvO_2 ranges from 35 to 45 mm Hg and mixed venous oxygen saturation (SvO_2) ranges from 0.68 to 0.76. Clinical concern for tissue hypoxia arises when the PvO_2 falls below 30 mm Hg and/or the SvO_2 falls by 5% to 10% over 3 to 5 minutes or to a value below 0.60. Mixed venous oxygen content is measured on blood drawn from the pulmonary artery rather than from the superior vena cava, inferior vena cava, or the right atrium. This is necessary because oxygen saturation in the inferior vena cava is higher than in the superior vena cava. Drainage of coronary sinus blood into the right atrium contaminates that chamber with markedly desaturated blood owing to the high myocardial oxygen extraction rate. After blood from the three sources passes through the right ventricle into the pulmonary artery it is thoroughly mixed resulting in a true "mixed venous" sample.

Mixed venous oxygen content is calculated as follows:

$$CvO_2 = (Hgb \times 1.36 \times SvO_2) + (PvO_2 \times 0.003)$$

If $Hgb = 15$ g, $SvO_2 = 0.75$, and $PvO_2 = 40$ mm Hg, then

$$CvO_2 = (15 \times 1.36 \times 0.75) + (40 \times 0.003)$$
$$= 15 + 0.12$$
$$= 15 \text{ mL/dL}$$

The arterial-venous oxygen content difference is described by the equation:

$$A\text{-}Vo_2 = Cao_2 - Cvo_2$$

Substituting the above calculations,

$$A\text{-}Vo_2 = 20 - 15 = 5 \text{ mL } O_2/dL$$

The normal range of the arterial-venous oxygen content difference is 3.5 to 5.0 mL/dL. Oxygen delivery (Do_2) is the product of arterial oxygen content (Cao_2) and cardiac output (CO) as expressed by the equation

$$Do_2 = CO \times Cao_2 \times 10$$

If cardiac output equals 5 L/min, then

$$Do_2 = 5 \times 20 \times 10 = 1000 \text{ mL/min}$$

Oxygen delivery is normally about 1000 mL/min. Oxygen consumption is the amount of oxygen that diffuses into the tissues and is expressed by the equation:

$$Vo_2 = CO \times (Cao_2 - Cvo_2) \times 10$$
$$= 5 \times 5 \times 10 = 250 \text{ mL/min}$$

Oxygen consumption is normally about 250 mL/min.

Oxygen delivery and consumption can also be indexed to body surface area. Normal values for the oxygen delivery index are 400 to 550 mL/min/m² and for the oxygen consumption index are 110 to 150 mL/min/m².

Low Svo_2 and Pvo_2 may indicate the presence of shock; however, in two settings these parameters may be artificially elevated. Patients with cirrhosis have arteriovenous shunting throughout the body, so that the oxygen carried in the blood is unavailable for metabolism in the tissues at the capillary level. In the case of septic shock, there may be arteriovenous shunting as in cirrhosis or there may be a metabolic defect such that the oxygen and substrate are there, but the cells do not pick it up.

A second concern pertaining to studies of the relationship between oxygen delivery and consumption relates to the concept of mathematical coupling. The same variables are used in calculating both oxygen delivery and consumption causing movement in the same direction. This concern has been substantiated by studies using different techniques for measuring oxygen delivery and consumption.[9]

Shoemaker et al[10] popularized the concept of supranormal oxygen delivery in resuscitation from shock using aggressive volume expansion with crystalloid, colloid, and blood and inotropic support with dobutamine. The therapeutic goals were a cardiac index above 4.5 L/min/m²,

oxygen delivery index above 600 mL/min/m², and oxygen consumption index above 170 mL/min/m². Other studies have shown that it is difficult to achieve such physiologic goals, and that such therapy is associated with no benefit or with increased morbidity and mortality.[11] Although Shoemaker et al were treating high-risk general surgical patients and many of the negative studies treated a more heterogeneous population, the inconsistent results indicate that there is a little role for maximizing oxygen delivery.

Oxyhemoglobin Dissociation Curve

Some familiarity with the oxyhemoglobin dissociation curve is necessary to understand oxygen transport and the influence of shifts in the curve. Acidosis, increased red cell 2,3-diphosphoglycerate (DPG), and fever shift the curve to the right, thus reducing the hemoglobin affinity for oxygen and increasing oxygen unloading in the tissues. Alkalosis, reduced red cell 2,3-DPG, and hypothermia cause the curve to shift to the left with the opposite effects on tissue oxygenation. As seen in Fig 1-3, hemoglobin is 50% saturated (P_{50}) at a Pao_2 of 27 mm Hg. A Pao_2 of 60 mm Hg correlates with an oxygen saturation of about 90%.

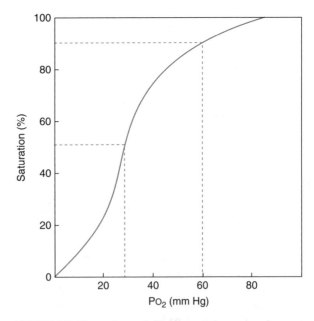

FIGURE 1-3. The oxyhemoglobin dissociation curve of normal blood. Hemoglobin is 50% saturated at a Pao_2 of 27 mm Hg. A Pao_2 of 60 mm Hg correlates with an oxygen saturation of about 90%. (*Source:* From Mabie WC: Critical care obstetrics. In: Gabbe SG, Niebyl JR, Simpson JL (eds), Obstetrics: Normal and Problem Pregnancies, 3rd edn., New York: *Churchill Livingston*, 1996; Chapter 18, pp. 533-559.)

Therefore, little is gained in oxygen saturation by increasing PaO_2 much higher than 60 mm Hg. On the other hand, if PaO_2 is less than 60 mm Hg, small changes in PaO_2 result in large changes in oxygen saturation. A PaO_2 less than 20 mm Hg is incompatible with life.[7]

■ HEMODYNAMIC SUPPORT

Cardiac output is determined by four factors: (1) preload, (2) afterload, (3) heart rate, and (4) contractility. Hemodynamic therapy directed at each of these factors is summarized in Table 1-2. According to the Frank-Starling principle, the force of striated muscle contraction varies directly with the initial muscle length. The relationship between myocardial fiber length and fiber shortening can be graphically described by the curve in Fig 1-4. Fiber length can best be equated with preload or filling volume of the ventricle. To allow clinical estimation of preload the pressure correlate of the filling volume is used, that is, right or left ventricular end-diastolic pressure. Varying compliance will alter the pressure-volume relationship. For example, a poorly compliant left ventricle resulting from myocardial hypertrophy or ischemia requires higher intracavitary pressure to achieve a specific end-diastolic volume or fiber stretch.

Afterload is defined as the wall tension of the ventricle during ejection. This is best reflected by the systolic blood pressure. In the absence of aortic or pulmonary stenosis, vascular resistance in the appropriate bed—systemic or pulmonary—will determine the afterload for that side of the heart. The effect of afterload on ventricular output is shown in Fig 1-5.

Heart rate has a marked effect on cardiac output (ie, cardiac output = heart rate × stroke volume). Increases in heart rate are accomplished at the expense of diastolic filling time, systolic emptying time being rate independent. Marked increases in heart rate may lead to circulatory depression when they cause myocardial ischemia or when reduced diastolic filling or loss of atrial "kick" prevent adequate ventricular preload. As a general rule, a heart rate that exceeds the difference of 220 and the patient's age in years reduces cardiac output and myocardial perfusion.

Contractility is defined as the force of ventricular contraction when preload and afterload are held constant. An increase in contractility is associated with an increase in stroke volume despite no change in preload. Factors that affect contractility include sympathetic impulses, catecholamines, acid-base and electrolyte disturbances, ischemia, loss of myocardium, hypoxia, and drugs or toxins. A third heart sound, distant heart sounds, and a narrow pulse pressure suggest impaired contractility. Radionuclide ventriculograms and two-dimensional (2D) echocardiography allow determination of ventricular size and contractile state. Effects of altered myocardial contractility on cardiac output at a given preload are shown in Fig 1-6.

Figure 1-7 uses the Starling curves to summarize the effects of increases and decreases of preload, afterload, and contractility on ventricular function. The therapeutic rationale for supporting the cardiovascular system based on the Frank-Starling relationship is illustrated in Fig 1-8.

The primary adjustment to improve low cardiac output is to optimize preload using volume administration. Because of the lack of correlation between measurements

■ TABLE 1-2. Hemodynamic Therapy

Decreased preload	Decreased afterload	Heart rate	Contractility	Increased preload	Increased afterload
Crystalloid	Volume	Usually not	Dopamine	Diuretics	Arterial dilators
Colloid	Vasopressors	treated unless	Dobutamine	Furosemide	Hydralazine
Blood	Phenylephrine	complete heart	Epinephrine	Ethacrynic acid	Nifedipine
	Inotropic	block treated	Digoxin	Bumetanide	Nicardipine
	vasopressors	with pacemaker	Intra-aortic	Venodilators	Mixed A-V dilator
	Norepinephrine		balloon pump	Furosemide	Nitroprusside
	Epinephrine		Biventricular	Morphine	Venous dilator
	Vasopressin		assist device	Nirtroglycerin	Nitroglycerin
					Alpha-beta blocker
					Labetalolol

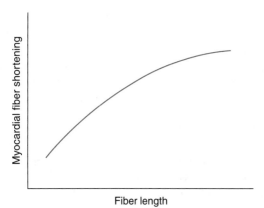

FIGURE 1-4. Starling curve relating myocardial fiber length to fiber shortening. (*Source*: Rosenthal MH: Intrapartum intensive care management of the cardiac patient. *Clin Obstet Gynecol* 1981;24:789-807.)

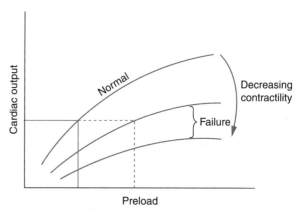

FIGURE 1-6. Cardiac function curves demonstrating downward displacement secondary to decreased contractility and failure. Dotted line represents increased preload demands in failure. (*Source*: Rosenthal MH: Intrapartum intensive care management of the cardiac patient. *Clin Obstet Gynecol* 1981;24:789-807.)

on the right and left sides of the heart in patients with significant cardiopulmonary disease, pulmonary capillary wedge pressure (PCWP) is monitored to optimize left ventricular preload and to avoid pulmonary edema. If blood pressure and cardiac output do not respond to fluids (eg, PCWP of approximately 15 mm Hg), then a positive inotropic agent may be needed to increase myocardial contractility. Dopamine is the drug of choice in most situations. It is utilized because its activity is modified at different doses. At 2 to 3 mcg/kg/min, renal and splanchnic vasodilatation occur. Positive inotropy occurs up to 10 mcg/kg/min. Vasoconstriction predominates

over 10 mcg/kg/min. These dose ranges reflect a predominance of action only. There is a great deal of overlap and individuality of response. The usual therapeutic range for dopamine in clinical practice is 3 to 20 mcg/kg/min. When the requirement exceeds this, a more potent inotropic vasopressor such as norepinephrine is substituted at a dose of 1 to 30 mcg/min. If the systolic blood pressure is quite low (<70 mm Hg) after fluid resuscitation, norepinephrine is the drug of first choice.

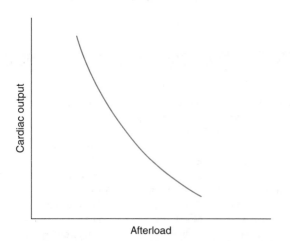

FIGURE 1-5. Relationship of afterload to cardiac output at a constant preload. (*Source*: Rosenthal MH: Intrapartum intensive care management of the cardiac patient. *Clin Obstet Gynecol* 1981;24:789-807.)

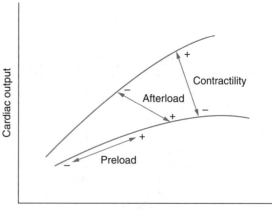

FIGURE 1-7. Alteration in Starling curve of ventricular function caused by increases and decreases in preload, afterload, and contractility. (*Source*: Rosenthal MH: Intrapartum intensive care management of the cardiac patient. *Clin Obstet Gynecol* 1981;24:789-807.)

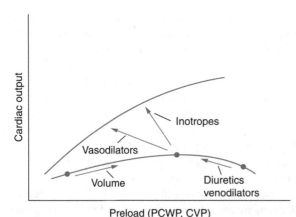

FIGURE 1-8. Treatment approaches for altered hemodynamic states based on Starling's law of the heart. PCWP, pulmonary capillary wedge pressure; CVP, central venous pressure. (*Source*: Rosenthal MH: Intrapartum intensive care management of the cardiac patient. *Clin Obstet Gynecol* 1981;24:789-807.)

Afterload may be manipulated with vasodilators in cardiac failure or in low cardiac output states secondary to severe hypertension. Vasodilators have varying effects on arterial and venous resistances. Nitroglycerin, predominantly a venodilator, may cause a greater reduction in preload than in afterload. Nitroprusside, an equal arterial and venular vasodilator, may be preferred; however, marked decreases in systemic vascular resistance result in hypotension, poor perfusion, and myocardial ischemia. The use of a vasodilator requires careful observation of the adequacy of intravascular volume and the net effect on cardiac output.[12]

Hemodynamics of Normal Pregnancy

Table 1-3 summarizes the invasive hemodynamic findings in normal pregnancy as determined by Clark et al.[13] Ten normal primiparous patients between 36 and 38 weeks gestation underwent pulmonary artery catheterization, arterial line placement, and central hemodynamic assessment in the left lateral recumbent position. Studies were repeated in the same patients between 11 and 13 weeks postpartum. Mean arterial pressure, central venous pressure, and pulmonary artery wedge pressure remained unchanged during pregnancy. Cardiac output increased about 40% owing to an increase in both heart rate and stroke volume. Systemic and pulmonary vascular resistances fell.

■ ALTERNATIVES TO PULMONARY ARTERY CATHETERIZATION

Current thinking emphasizes that there is no single best monitoring device to guide management of the critically ill patient. Multiple parameters have to be examined to get the whole picture. For example, history and physical, vital signs, mental status, capillary refill, intake and output, oxygen saturation, laboratory values, chest x-ray, and electrocardiogram.

Some of the recently investigated noninvasive tests include estimating the central venous pressure (CVP) at the bedside and assessing "volume responsiveness" using pulse pressure variation during the respiratory cycle or passive leg raising to produce a temporary autotransfusion.

Vinayak et al[14] showed that external jugular vein examination correlates with the catheter- measured CVP and reliably categorizes patients with low ($\leq$5 cm H_2O), normal (6-9 cm H_2O), or high ($\geq$10 cm H_2O) CVPs.

There has been considerable study of arterial pressure waveforms (eg, radial artery catheter) as an indicator of intravascular volume and response of the cardiac output to a fluid challenge. During inspiration, pressure around the heart falls and venous return increases. This leads to an

■ TABLE 1-3. Hemodynamic Values in Healthy Nonpregnant, Pregnant, and Postpartum Subjects				
Parameters	Units	Nonpregnant	36-38 weeks gestation	Postpartum
Heart rate	beats/min	60-100	83 $\pm$ 10	71 $\pm$10
Mean arterial pressure	mm Hg	90-110	90.3 $\pm$ 5.8	86.4 $\pm$ 7.5
Central venous pressure	mm Hg	1-7	3.6 $\pm$ 2.5	3.7 $\pm$ 2.6
Pulmonary artery wedge pressure	mm Hg	6-12	7.5 $\pm$ 1.8	6.3 $\pm$ 2.1
Cardiac output	L/min	4.3-6.0	6.2 $\pm$ 1.0	4.3 $\pm$ 0.9
Stroke volume	mL/beat	57-71	74.7	60.6
Systemic vascular resistance	dyn/s/cm^{-5}	900-1400	1210 $\pm$ 266	1530 $\pm$ 520
Pulmonary vascular resistance	dyn/s/cm^{-5}	<250	78 $\pm$ 22	119 $\pm$ 47

increase in stroke volume and pulse pressure. The changes in pulse pressure are greater when the ventricle is operating on the steep rather than the flat portion of the Frank-Starling curve. These swings in pulse pressure correlate with relative hypovolemia or "preload reserve." Empiric investigation has shown that when there is greater than 13% increase in pulse pressure during the respiratory cycle, patients are highly likely to respond to a 500 mL fluid challenge. On the other hand, if the change in pulse pressure during respiration is less than 13%, the patient is hypervolemic and unlikely to respond to a fluid challenge.[15]

Passive leg raising has been studied in critically ill ventilated patients to predict which hemodynamically unstable patients will increase their systemic blood flow in response to volume expansion. Fluid loading in a non-volume-responsive patient delays definitive therapy and may be detrimental. Using an automatic bed elevation technique to raise the lower limbs and an esophageal Doppler to measure aortic blood flow, Monnet et al[16] showed that an increase in aortic blood flow of greater than or equal to 10% with passive leg raising reliably predicts volume responsiveness.

In the most recent trial evaluating resuscitation in septic shock, PAC monitoring was not used.[17] Rather patients were randomized to routine care or early goal-directed therapy targeting arterial blood pressure, right atrial pressure, urine output, and right atrial oxygen saturation as a surrogate for mixed-venous oxygen saturation. The study utilized a CVP catheter that incorporated an oxygen saturation sensor.

Bedside Ultrasound

A big reason for the decline in use of the PAC is that technology has passed it by.[18,19] Most intensivists would rather have a bedside echocardiogram than a PAC-derived hemodynamic profile to evaluate a critically ill patient. Alternatively, the information derived from the two technologies may be complimentary. Ultrasound technology is not exclusive to the radiologist or cardiologist. Just as ultrasound has been incorporated into OB/GYN training and practice, so it has in general surgery and critical care. The FAST (focused assessment by sonography in trauma) examination has largely replaced diagnostic peritoneal lavage. Surgeons use portable, hand-held, ultrasound devices as an extension of the physical examination to image the gallbladder, liver, pancreas, spleen, and urinary bladder.

In the ICU, much of the early work was done with transesophageal echocardiography (TEE). TEE was used in the operating room for cardiovascular monitoring, and its use migrated to the ICU. It is useful for the evaluation of suspected aortic dissection, prosthetic heart valves, source of cardiac emboli, detection of intracardiac shunt, and unexplained hypotension. However, TEE has its limitations. It provides limited views of some areas of the heart and great vessels. It requires topical anesthesia and sedation. Serious complications occur in less than 0.5% of patients, primarily injury to the GI tract. There are contraindications such as esophageal pathology, upper GI bleeding, and atlantoaxial disease.

Transthoracic echocardiography (TTE) is not associated with any significant risk to the patient. Satisfactory images can be obtained 85% to 90% of the time. Still, TEE might be required for aortic dissection, endocarditis, prosthetic valves, severe obesity, emphysema, and mechanical ventilation.

General indications for performance of a TTE in the ICU are hemodynamic instability (ventricular failure, hypovolemia, pulmonary embolism, valvular dysfunction, tamponade, complication of cardiothoracic surgery), infective endocarditis, aortic dissection, unexplained hypoxemia, and source of emboli. Bedside ultrasonography may also be used for central line placement and drainage of pleural effusions or intra-abdominal fluid collections.[18,19] Bedside TTE has been shown to compare favorably to PAC monitoring in critically ill obstetric patients. [20]

Global systolic function of the heart can be assessed by fractional shortening and ejection fraction. Fractional shortening is determined by an M-mode "ice pick" view through the heart.

$$\text{Fractional shortening} = \frac{\text{End-diastolic dimension} - \text{End-systolic dimension}}{\text{End-diastolic dimension}}$$

Normal fractional shortening is 30% to 42%. Ejection fraction represents stroke volume, and its determination requires left ventricular volume measurement. Most echocardiographic units measure volume by digitizing the left ventricular endocardial surface. Simpson's method is used to estimate ventricular volume from two orthogonal apical views.

$$\text{Ejection fraction} = \frac{\text{End-diastolic volume} - \text{End-systolic volume}}{\text{End-diastolic volume}}$$

Normal ejection fraction is 50% to 75%.

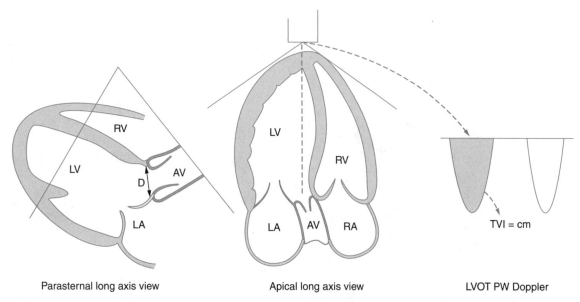

Parasternal long axis view   Apical long axis view   LVOT PW Doppler

FIGURE 1-9. Schematic of the calculation of stroke volume from the LVOT area and the TVI. LVOT, left ventricular outflow tract; TVI, time velocity integral; PW, pulsed wave. (*Source:* Oh JH, Seward JB, Tajik AJ. The Echo Manual. Boston, Little, Brown, and company, 1994 p56.)

Cardiac output is most commonly determined by 2D- and Doppler **echocardiography** (Fig 1-9). Left ventricular outflow tract (LVOT) area is calculated by measuring the aortic valve diameter at the annulus in the parasternal long axis view. The time velocity integral (TVI) is measured from the apical long axis view by placing the pulsed wave Doppler sample volume between the aortic valve leaflets. TVI (cm) is the area under the velocity curve and is equal to the sum of the velocities (cm/sec) during the ejection time (sec). TVI can be easily determined by the built-in calculation package in the ultrasound unit. TVI multiplied by the valve area equals the stoke volume. Stroke volume multiplied by heart rate equals cardiac output.[21]

In the critical care setting global ventricular function can be assessed qualitatively by visual inspection alone. An experienced clinician can look at the size of the cardiac chambers and the myocardial "squeeze" and make a functional diagnosis. The ability to repeat a bedside echocardiogram is vital to assessing the efficacy of therapy.

Volume status can be assessed by left ventricular cavity size (eg, left ventricular cavity obliteration in systole usually means severe hypovolemia) or by vena cava collapsibility.

Right ventricular dysfunction can be assessed. Massive pulmonary embolism produces right ventricular dilatation, a septal shift compromising the left ventricular cavity,

and high-velocity tricuspid regurgitation. These findings may guide fluid and inotropic therapy or thrombolysis.[18]

Tricuspid regurgitation velocity reflects the pressure difference between the right ventricle and the right atrium (Fig 1-10). Pulmonary artery systolic pressure can be estimated by measuring the tricuspid regurgitation velocity with pulsed Doppler and using the simplified Bernoulli equation to calculate the pressure gradient across the valve. Pressure gradient = $4 \times$ (velocity)^2. For example, if the tricuspid regurgitation velocity is 4 m/sec, the pressure drop across the tricuspid valve during systole is $4 \times 4^2 =$ 64 mm Hg. If the right atrial pressure is estimated to be 10 mm Hg, then right ventricular systolic pressure is 64 + 10 = 74 mm Hg. This is compatible with fairly severe, long-standing, pulmonary hypertension.[21]

Additional information that can be rapidly obtained using beside echocardiography includes cardiac chamber size and wall thickness, regional wall motion abnormalities (eg, acute myocardial infarction), valvular stenosis or insufficiency, diastolic function, and presence of a pericardial effusion or tamponade.

In summary, bedside ultrasonography is becoming an indispensable tool in the management of critically ill patients. However, the acquisition and interpretation of images are highly dependent on the skill of the operator.[18,19]

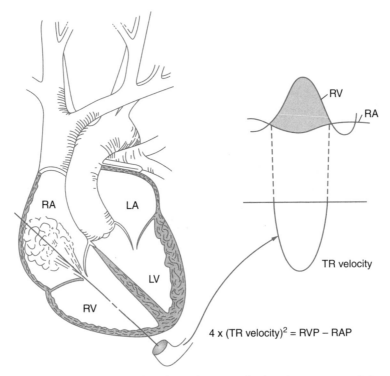

FIGURE 1-10. Schematic of the heart demonstrating how to measure systolic right ventricular pressure from the peak velocity of tricuspid regurgitation. (*Source*: Oh JH, Seward JB, Tajik AJ. The Echo Manual. Boston, Little, Brown, and company, 1994 p179.)

REFERENCES

1. Harvey W, Harrison DS, Linger M, et al. Assessment of the clinical effectiveness of pulmonary artery catheters in management of patients in intensive care (PAC-Man): a randomized controlled trial. *Lancet.* 2005;366:472-477.

2. Shah MR, Hasselblad V, Stevenson LW, et al. Impact of the pulmonary artery catheter in critically ill patients. Meta-analysis of randomized clinical trials. *JAMA.* 2005;294:1664-1670.

3. The ESCAPE Investigators and ESCAPE Study Coordinators. Evaluation study of congestive heart failure and pulmonary artery catheterization effectiveness. *JAMA.* 2005;294:1625-1633.

4. The National Heart, Lung, and Blood Institute Acute Respiratory Distress Syndrome (ARDS) Clinical Trials Network. Pulmonary-artery versus central venous catheter to guide treatment of acute lung injury. *N Engl J Med.* 2006;354:2213-2224.

5. Connors AF Jr, Speroff T, Dawson NV, et al. The effectiveness of right heart catheterization in the initial care of critically ill patients. *JAMA.* 1996;276:889-897.

6. Wiener RS, Welch HG. Trends in the use of the pulmonary artery catheter in the United States, 1993-2004. *JAMA.* 2007;298:423-429.

7. Mabie WC. Critical care obstetrics. In: Gabbe SG, Niebyl JR, Simpson JL, eds. *Obstetrics: Normal and Problem Pregnancies.* 3rd ed. New York: Churchill Livingston; 1996: 533-559 (chapter 18).

8. Daily EK, Schroeder JP. *Hemodynamic Waveforms: Exercises in Identification and Analysis.* St. Louis, MO: CV Mosby; 1983.

9. Snyder JV. Oxygen transport: The model and reality. In: Snyder JV, Pinsky MR, eds. *Oxygen Transport in the Critically Ill.* Chicago, IL: Year Book Medical Publishers; 1987: 3-15.

10. Shoemaker WC, Appel PL, Kram HB, et al. Prospective trial of supranormal values of survivors as therapeutic goals in high-risk surgical patients. *Chest.* 1988;94:1176-1186.

11. Hayes MA, Timmins AC, Yau EHS, et al. Elevation of systemic oxygen delivery in the treatment of critically ill patients. *N Engl J Med.* 1994;330:1717-1722.

12. Rosenthal MH: Intrapartum intensive care management of the cardiac patient. *Clin Obstet Gynecol.* 1981;24: 789-807.

13. Clark SL, Cotton DB, Lee W, et al. Central hemodynamic assessment of normal term pregnancy. *Am J Obstet Gynecol.* 1989;161:1439-1442.

14. Vinayak AG, Levitt J, Gehlbach B, et al. Usefulness of the external jugular vein examination in detecting abnormal central venous pressure in critically ill patients. *Arch Intern Med.* 2006;166: 2132-2137.

15. Michard F, Boussat S, Chemla D, et al. Relation between respiratory changes in arterial pulse pressure and fluid responsiveness in septic patients with acute circulatory failure. *Am J Respir Crit Care Med.* 2000;162:134-138.

16. Monnet X, Rienzo M, Osman D, et al. Passive leg raising predicts fluid responsiveness in the critically ill. *Crit Care Med.* 2006;34:1402-1407.

17. Rivers E, Nguyen B, Havstad S, et al. Early goal-directed therapy in the treatment of severe sepsis and septic shock. *N Engl J Med.* 2001;345:1368-1377.

18. Beaulieu Y, Marik PE. Beside ultrasonogrpahy in the ICU. Part 1. *Chest.* 2005;128 :881-895.

19. Beaulieu Y, Marik PE. Beside ultrasonogrpahy in the ICU. Part 2. *Chest.* 2005;128:1766-1781.

20. Belfort MA, Rokey R, Saade GR, Moise KJ. Rapid echocardiographic assessment of left and right heart hemodynamics in critically ill obstetric patients. *Am J Obstet Gynecol.* 1994;171:884-892.

21. Oh JK, Seward JB, Tajik AJ. *The Echo Manual.* Boston, MA: Little, Brown and Company; 1994.

CHAPTER 2

Transfusion of Blood Components and Derivatives in the Obstetric Intensive Care Patient

• *Stephanie R. Martin*

Obstetric hemorrhage remains one of the leading causes of maternal death in the United States, often necessitating the transfusion of blood products as a life saving measure. More commonly, the practitioner encounters less acute situations and must decide which blood products, if any, are appropriate for the patient. In this chapter, we will address the blood products currently available for transfusion, the indications for their use, and potential risks. We will also discuss alternatives and techniques to avoid transfusion, including available colloid solutions, use of the "autologous transfusion device," and acute normovolemic hemodilution (ANH).

In modern obstetric practice, transfusion of whole blood is uncommon. Typically, whole blood is separated into its components (red blood cells, platelets, fibrinogen, and other clotting factors) and stored. Blood component therapy allows treatment of specific derangements in the patient's blood. The potential benefits of administering blood products must be weighed against the potential risks, both short- and long term.

■ RISKS OF TRANSFUSION

Transfusion risks are typically categorized into infectious and noninfectious complications. Adverse events are reported to complicate approximately 10% of the 14.2 million red cell units administered annually in the United States. Fortunately, less than 0.5% of these are serious reactions. Nevertheless, death related to transfusion may be significantly underreported.[1] Patient concerns regarding transfusion risks have traditionally focused on the spread of viral infectious diseases. However 40% to 50% of deaths related to transfusion result from ABO incompatibility, transfusion-related acute lung injury, and bacterial contamination of platelets.[2]

Infectious Transfusion Risks

Improvements in screening strategies for prospective donors and testing of donated blood products have significantly reduced the likelihood of viral infection from contaminated blood. In the United States, each unit of donated blood is tested for hepatitis B surface antigen and core antibody, hepatitis C antibody, HIV and HTLV (human T-cell leukemia virus) types 1 and 2 antibodies, West Nile virus, and syphilis. Nucleic acid testing is also performed for HIV-1 and hepatitis C as it detects viral genome before an antibody response develops. Table 2-1 outlines infectious risks from transfusion and their estimated frequency. Composite risk for HIV, hepatitis B and C,

■ TABLE 2-1. Infectious Risks from Transfusion and Their Estimated Frequency[3,4]	
Hepatitis B	1 in 100,000 - 1 in 400,000
Hepatitis C	1 in 1.6 million - 1 in 3.1 million
HIV 1 and 2	1 in 1.4 million - 1 in 4.7 million
HTLV 1 and 2	1 in 500,000 - 1 in 3 million
Bacterial contamination PRBCs	1 in 28,000 - 1 in 143,000
Bacterial contamination platelets	1 in 2,000 - 1 in 8,000

and HTLV infection from transfusion is estimated at less than 1 in 30,000.

Other infectious diseases can be transmitted through blood products but are not universally screened by direct testing of the blood product. Rather, screening of the individual donor is performed by a detailed questionnaire designed to identify persons at risk for harboring specific diseases. Some examples of these diseases include cytomegalovirus, Chagas disease, babesiosis, malaria, Creutzfeldt-Jakob disease, hepatitis A, Lyme disease, Epstein-Barr virus, and human herpes viruses. Alarmingly, 1 to 2 in 100 donations test positive for hepatitis G virus, SEN virus, and transfusion-transmitted virus. The significance of these viruses remains to be determined.[5]

Clinically significant cytomegalovirus (CMV) infections usually occur in immunocompromised patients. However, a small but significant portion of persons in the population has never been exposed to CMV and has no natural immunity to it. While CMV infection in the adult is usually a benign, subclinical process, primary maternal infection confers a 40% risk of in-utero transmission and can have devastating effects. Therefore, CMV seronegative, leukoreduced blood products should be administered to the seronegative pregnant patient.

Bacterial contamination of blood products, particularly platelets, accounts for 17% to 22% of infectious deaths related to transfusion, making this one of the leading causes.[6]

Noninfectious Transfusion Risks

Noninfectious transfusion risks are more common than infectious risks and are often under-recognized and underreported. Noninfectious risks of transfusion can be further categorized as hemolytic and nonhemolytic in nature.

Hemolytic Transfusion Reactions

Acute Hemolytic Transfusion Reaction

Over 250 red cell antigens have been identified, any of which can lead to a hemolytic transfusion reaction when administered to incompatible recipients. Testing of blood type, antibody screen, and crossmatch are performed to avoid transfusion of incompatible blood. Approximately 0.2% to 0.6% of the general population is sensitized.[7] Acute hemolytic reactions occur with exposure to incompatible ABO types at a rate of 1 in 12,000 to 19,000 units transfused. Clinically, the patient develops sudden onset of fever, chills, flank and back pain, circulatory collapse, and microangiopathic thromboses. This type of reaction is most commonly the result of error.

Delayed Hemolytic Transfusion Reaction

Delayed hemolytic reactions occur as a result of exposure to incompatible human leukocyte antigen (HLA) and complicate 1 in 1000 to 1 in 9000 red cell transfusions.[8] HLAs are present on all cells except mature red blood cells. HLA alloimmunization occurs in response to a prior exposure to incompatible blood or from prior pregnancy. Because these antigens are present on tissues apart from red cells, the hemolytic reaction occurs extravascularly and is less severe than reactions to incompatible red cell antigens.

Nonhemolytic Transfusion Reactions

The nonhemolytic transfusion reaction is much more common (1 in 100). Usually characterized by febrile or urticarial reactions, more serious reactions such as transfusion-related lung injury and graft-versus-host disease can also develop.

Transfusion-Related Acute Lung Injury

Transfusion-related acute lung injury (TRALI) complicates at least 1 in 5000 transfusions with a 6% risk of mortality and is believed to be the most common cause of mortality related to transfusion.[9] TRALI is defined as noncardiogenic pulmonary edema developing within 6 hours of initiating transfusion of blood products. Clinically, patients develop sudden onset of respiratory distress, pulmonary edema, fever, and hypotension. The etiology remains unclear; however, available evidence suggests that certain patients may be susceptible to inflammatory substances and antibodies in the blood product as a result of illness or surgery. The response to these substances leads to capillary damage and permeability which results in sudden onset of pulmonary edema. Treatment is primarily supportive and may require ventilatory support. Unlike acute respiratory distress syndrome (ARDS), TRALI typically resolves rapidly and is less likely to be fatal. It is important to consider TRALI in the differential diagnosis of acute pulmonary edema and avoid use of diuretics as it may worsen outcomes.[10,11]

Febrile Reactions

Fever associated with the administration of leukoreduced blood products occurs in 0.1% to 1% people annually and is more common if the product is not leukoreduced.[12] The febrile response is hypothesized to be the result of cytokine release from white blood cells in the blood product. Utilization of leukoreduced blood products and prophylactic antipyretic therapy dramatically decreases the likelihood of a febrile reaction.[13]

Allergic Reactions

Allergic reactions manifest primarily as urticaria, itching, flushing, rash, or angioedema without fever. These types of responses are common and can be quite severe, including anaphylaxis. Antihistamines can be administered prophylactically. With minor reactions, intravenous antihistamines may allow completion of the transfusion. More severe reactions require cessation of the transfusion.

Alloimmunization can result in platelet antibodies which may prevent therapeutic response in the thrombocytopenic patient who receives platelet transfusion. Rarely, graft-versus-host disease can occur following transfusion of some blood components (platelets, white blood cells, etc) into an immunocompromised individual.

Transfusion-Associated Graft-Versus-Host Disease

This rare complication of transfusion primarily affects immunosuppressed individuals and carries a high mortality rate (>90%). Irradiation of blood products may eliminate this risk.[14]

Miscellaneous Complications

Massive transfusion, defined as replacement of the blood volume in 24 hours or administration of more than 10 units

in a few hours, carries particular risks to the patient. The citrate component in stored blood products binds with calcium and this leads to hypocalcemia when administered in large amounts. Alkalosis is also common following massive transfusion, as is hypothermia, potassium disturbances, and decreased 2,3-DPG. Warming the infused blood and maintaining normothermia of the patient can minimize some of these effects. Monitoring acid-base balance and potassium and calcium levels is essential in the setting of massive transfusion. Coagulation defects are also common when patients receive large amounts of blood products; therefore, monitoring and correction of clotting status are warranted.

Transfusion-Related Immunomodulation

The transfusion of blood products does appear to suppress the host immune system with both beneficial and detrimental effects. Patients receiving transfusions have lower rates of renal transplant rejection and improvement in certain autoimmune disease activity, that is, rheumatoid arthritis.[15] However, more recent studies suggest that patients, particularly surgical and trauma, patients, receiving blood transfusions have increased rates of mortality, postoperative infections and multiorgan system failure.[16-19] This has prompted an ongoing reevaluation of the thresholds for transfusion in critically ill and surgical patients.

■ THRESHOLD FOR TRANSFUSION

Red cell transfusions are performed primarily with the intent to improve oxygen delivery. Recent data suggest that the benefit of transfusion may not be self-evident in the critically ill or surgical patient without active hemorrhage. In a large study of critically ill patients, lowering the transfusion goal from 10 g/dL to 7 g/L with a transfusion trigger of 7 g/dL failed to show benefit from more liberal transfusion. Younger (<55 years) and less critically ill patients, however, had a survival benefit in the restrictive transfusion group. This approach has also been supported in a pediatric critically ill population, but has not been studied in pregnant women.[20-22] The exact threshold for transfusion in a hemodynamically stable patient without evidence of active bleeding remains to be defined. Table 2-2 summarizes expected clinical findings with increasing blood loss.

Those blood products that are most commonly used in pregnancy are generally subdivided into cellular or plasma components (Table 2-3).

■ TABLE 2-2. Clinical Staging of Hemorrhagic Shock by Volume of Blood Loss

Severity of shock	Volume (mL)[a]	Findings	Blood loss (%)
None	None	Up to 20	Up to 900
Mild	Tachycardia (<100 beats/min)	20-25	1200-1500
	Mild hypotension		
	Peripheral vasoconstriction		
Moderate	Tachycardia (100-120 beats/min)	30-35	1800-2100
	Hypotension (80-100 mm Hg)		
	Restlessness		
	Oliguria		
Severe	Tachycardia (>120 beats/min)	>35	>2400
	Hypotension (<60 mm Hg)		
	Altered consciousness		
	Anuria		

[a]Based on an average blood volume of 6000 mL at 30 weeks' gestation.
Reproduced, with permission, from Creasy and Resnick's Maternal Fetal Medicine

■ TABLE 2-3. Blood Components

Component	Contents	Indications	Volume (mL)	Shelf life	Expected effect
PRBCs	Red cells, some plasma, few WBCs	Correct anemia	300	42 d	Increase Hct 3% per unit, Hgb 1 g/U
Leukocyte-poor blood	RBCs, some plasma, few WBCs	Correct anemia, reduce febrile reactions	250	21-24 d	Increase Hct 3% per unit, Hgb 1 g/U
Platelets	Platelets, some plasma, RBCs, few WBCs	Bleeding due to thrombocytopenia	50	Up to 5 d	Increase total platelet count 7500/mm^3/U
Fresh frozen plasma	Fibrinogen, plasma, clotting factors V, XI, XII	Treatment of coagulation disorders	250	2 h thawed, 12 mo frozen	Increase total fibrinogen 10-15 mg/dL/U
Cryoprecipitate	Fibrinogen, factors V, VIII, XIII, von Willebrand factor	Hemophilia A, von Willebrand disease, fibrinogen deficiency	40	4-6 h thawed	Increase total fibrinogen 10-15 mg/dL/U

■ CELLULAR COMPONENTS

Red Blood Cells

- Most patients requiring replacement of red blood cells should receive packed red blood cells (PRBCs).
- One unit of PRBCs contains roughly 250 mL of RBCs, 50 mL of plasma, and has a hematocrit of approximately 80%. The decreased plasma volume of packed cells minimizes the risk of fluid overload.
- Transfusion of 1 unit of PRBCs into a 70-kg person will usually increase the hemoglobin level by 1 g/dL.
- Like whole blood, PRBCs have a shelf life of approximately 6 weeks when stored at 1 to 6°C.

- Frozen RBCs can be stored at −70°C for years, but the freezing process destroys white blood cells (WBCs) which may be present in the unit of blood.
- When WBCs have been removed from a unit of blood, the blood is considered to be "leukocyte-poor" and poses lower risk of febrile transfusion reactions.
- The precise threshold for transfusion is not known, particularly in gravidas. Patients who are actively hemorrhaging and displaying cardiovascular instability or evidence of fetal compromise should be considered as candidates for RBC transfusion.

Autologous Blood

Autologous transfusion is the collection and reinfusion of the patient's own RBCs. Therefore, donor and recipient are identical. Exclusive or supplemental use of autologous blood should reduce many transfusion-related complications and is particularly useful for the patient with multiple antibodies. In both pregnant and nonpregnant patients, perioperative autologous blood donation has been demonstrated to reduce the likelihood of receiving allogeneic blood products.[23-25] Autologous blood donation appears to be a safe procedure during pregnancy.[26,27] However, the use of autologous blood does not eliminate risk to the patient. Concerns remain regarding bacterial contamination of stored blood and human error. The indications for transfusing donated blood should be the same as for allogeneic blood. The American Association of Blood Bank standards do not permit the rollover of unused autologous units into the general blood supply as the donors are not considered "volunteers." Unused units will be discarded.

Patients with an active seizure disorder or significant cardiopulmonary disease are not candidates for autologous blood donation.

The guidelines for autologous blood donation during pregnancy are as follows:

- A minimum predonation hemoglobin of 11 g/dL.
- Because RBCs may be refrigerated in liquid form for only 6 weeks, initiation of autologous blood donation generally occurs no earlier than 6 weeks before their anticipated use. The last donation should be planned at least 2 weeks before the estimated date of delivery.
- One week should elapse between donations.
- Autologous blood should be used selectively. The unnecessary transfusion of autologous blood increases

the risk of circulatory overload, exposure to bacterial contamination, and human error.
- Due to the special logistics of autologous blood, autologous donor candidates should be aware that this technique is more costly than allogeneic transfusions and may not be covered by their health insurer.
- Patients should be aware that autologous blood donation does not completely eliminate the possibility of allogeneic transfusion.

Preoperative donation may also lead to anemia and an increased risk for postoperative transfusion. Consideration should therefore be given to maximizing the hemoglobin with supplemental iron, erythropoietin, folate, and vitamin B_{12}.

Platelet Concentrates

Platelets for infusion can be prepared either by separation from whole blood of multiple donors and pooled together into a single unit, or by apheresis of platelets from a single donor. The apheresis method results a unit equivalent to 4 to 6 pooled units from whole blood.[28] Platelets can be stored for 5 days.

Platelet concentrates are indicated for the treatment of hemorrhage due to thrombocytopenia or platelet dysfunction (thrombocytopathia). The cause of thrombocytopenia or thrombocytopathia must be determined. For example, in the presence of immune thrombocytopenic purpura (ITP), where platelets are destroyed via an antibody-mediated process, corticosteroids rather than platelets probably represent the best therapy. Additionally, patients taking aspirin preparations can experience potentially serious bleeding despite normal platelet counts. When ordering a platelet transfusion, the following should be considered:

- In the pregnant patient, thrombocytopenia is considered to be present when the platelet count falls below 100,000/mm³. Bleeding following major surgery or trauma rarely occurs when the platelet count is 50,000/mm³ or greater, assuming normal platelet function. When the platelet count ranges from 20,000 to 50,000/mm³, bleeding with major surgery or trauma can occasionally occur. Platelet transfusion may be performed prophylactically in nonbleeding patients with platelet counts of 10,000 to 20,000 platelets/mm³ or less.[28] When the platelet count falls to 10,000/mm³, bleeding with trauma or surgery is more likely. Spontaneous bleeding can occur once the platelet count drops below 10,000/mm³.

- Among patients receiving massive transfusions within a short period of time, dilutional thrombocytopenia can occur. Following replacement of one blood volume, 35% to 40% of a patient's platelets usually remain. Ideally, platelet replacement therapy in the setting of massive hemorrhage should be guided by platelet count results.
- One unit of apheresis platelets contains, on average, 4.2×10^{11} platelets, an amount roughly equivalent to 4 to 6 pooled units. Therefore, an average platelet concentrate (pooled or apheresis) will increase the platelet count in a 75-kg patient by approximately 7000 to 10,000 platelets/mm³ 1 hour post transfusion.[28] Therefore, the platelet count can be assessed immediately following completion of the transfusion.
- Platelet concentrates contain sufficient numbers of serum-bound RBCs to cause alloimmunization to red cell antigens. Therefore, the possibility of Rh immunization by red cells should be considered in Rh-negative female recipients.
- Platelet transfusion is contraindicated in thrombotic thrombocytopenic purpura (TTP) and will be ineffective in the setting of increased platelet destruction (heparin-induced thrombocytopenia, idiopathic thrombocytopenic purpura).

■ PLASMA COMPONENTS

Fresh-Frozen Plasma

Fresh-frozen plasma (FFP) is plasma extracted from whole blood or plasma apheresis within 6 hours of collection and then frozen. A typical unit of FFP contains 250 mL of fluid and 700 mg of fibrinogen, as well as all plasma proteins and clotting factors. FFP is indicated to correct deficiencies of multiple clotting factors in bleeding patients. Clotting factor deficiencies can arise from liver disease, vitamin K deficiency, massive hemorrhage, or disseminated intravascular coagulation. FFP may also be used for specific factor deficiencies (factors II, V, VII, IX, X, and XI) when specific component therapy is not available, and can provide rapid reversal of warfarin. Warfarin causes a deficiency of the vitamin K–dependent factors (II, VII, IX, and X). While vitamin K will eventually reverse this deficiency, FFP can affect a more rapid recovery.

- One unit of FFP will typically increase the fibrinogen level by approximately 10 to15 mg/dL. When FFP is indicated, 15 mL/kg is a reasonable guideline for the initiation of FFP therapy (target serum fibrinogen level is ~100 mg/dL).
- It should be kept in mind that 20 to 30 minutes are required to thaw FFP in the blood bank.
- Anti-ABO antibodies are not removed from FFP, therefore ABO compatibility should be considered.
- When only Factor VIII, von Willebrand factor, or fibrinogen is needed, cryoprecipitate is a more appropriate therapeutic choice. Inappropriate uses of FFP include use of this blood component for volume expansion or as a nutritional supplement.

Cryoprecipitate

Cryoprecipitate is extracted from thawed FFP. The product is a cold insoluble fraction of FFP which precipitates under these conditions. Cryoprecipitate is rich in factor VIII (80-120 units) and fibrinogen (200 mg) and also contains von Willebrand factor and factor XIII. One unit of cryoprecipitate will raise the fibrinogen level by the same amount as 1 unit of FFP (10-15 mg/dL). However, as 1 unit of cryoprecipitate consists of only 40 mL of fluid, it more efficiently raises the fibrinogen level than does a 250 mL unit of FFP. Indications for the use of cryoprecipitate include the treatment of von Willebrand disease, factor VIII deficiency, and fibrinogen deficiency as may occur in the setting of hemorrhage. ABO compatibility is not an issue with cryoprecipitate administration.[29]

■ COLLOID SOLUTIONS

Intravenous fluids containing particles that will not pass through a semipermeable membrane and are larger than 10,000 Da are known as colloids. Compared to crystalloid solutions, colloids are more expensive, less readily available, and may be associated with anaphylactoid reactions. Colloids tend to produce greater elevations in colloid oncotic pressure than crystalloids. They also produce greater increases in plasma volume and deplete extracellular fluid. Patients receiving a colloid solution must be adequately prehydrated with crystalloids. The properties of the available colloid solutions are outlined in Table 2-4.

Albumin

Albumin solutions may rapidly restore intravascular volume, especially if serum albumin levels are less than 2 g/dL. Use should be limited to patients with decreased plasma

■ TABLE 2-4. Colloid Infusions			
Colloid	Dose (mL)	Crystalloid volume expansion equivalent	Estimated duration of effect (h)
Albumin			
5% solution	500-700	Similar to crystalloid	24
25% solution	100-200	3.5 times crystalloid	24
Hetastarch (Hespan or Hextend)	500-1000	Similar to crystalloid	24-36
Dextran (70)	500	1050 mL over 2 h	24

volume and adequate extracellular volume. Albumin is available in concentrations of 5% or 25%. Five percent solutions are generally limited to patients with burns or peritonitis and have limited use in an acute situation. When 25 g of albumin are infused, intravascular volume will increase by roughly 450 mL over 60 minutes as a result of the considerable oncotic activity of albumin. However, the benefits are only transient and may result in complications such as pulmonary edema, if administered excessively. Supplemental albumin is rapidly redistributed throughout the extracellular space, disappearing from the circulation at a rate of up to 8% per hour. In the setting of shock or sepsis, the rate can approach 30% per hour.

Dextran

Dextran is a glucose polymer solution available with polymers having mean molecular weights of 40,000 (dextran 40) or 70,000 (dextran 70). A 6% dextran 70 solution is used for indications similar to those of 5% albumin. Dextran 40 is rarely used for acute volume expansion. A 500 mL infusion of dextran produces intravascular volume expansion of 1050 mL over 2 hours and improves capillary blood flow by reducing viscosity and red cell aggregation. As with albumin, the effects of dextran are temporary and may be associated with pulmonary edema if used too aggressively. Both forms are degraded into glucose.

In doses exceeding 20 mL/kg/24 h, dextran may also interfere with platelet function by impeding clotting factor activation and by binding with fibrin to produce less stable clots. Anaphylactoid reactions complicate 1 in 3300 dextran infusions. Interference with laboratory crossmatching of blood has also been described. Therefore, blood typing and crossmatching should be performed prior to its administration.

Hetastarch

Hydroxymethyl starch is a synthetic molecule available as a 6% solution in normal saline (Hespan). Like albumin and dextran, it possesses considerable oncotic activity and can induce intravascular fluid expansion. However, hetastarch increases colloid oncotic pressure more effectively than albumin and lasts 24 to 36 hours. The recommended dose is 20 mL/kg/24 h. Hetastarch may also prolong prothrombin and partial thromboplastin times, decrease platelet counts, and reduce clot tensile strength. Therefore, it should be used cautiously in patients who may have a coagulopathy. Hetastarch may also artifactually increase serum amylase levels. Hextend is a newer hetastarch 6% solution in a physiologic electrolyte solution. It may offer an advantage over Hespan in that the lower molecular weight may be associated with less risk for coagulation abnormalities.

■ CELL SALVAGE

The immediate recycling of blood lost during surgery or following trauma has become an accepted treatment modality. Autologous blood, collected preoperatively or intraoperatively, offers a variety of advantages over allogeneic blood. As a perfectly compatible source, unstored autologous blood essentially eliminates the risk of viral disease transmission or isoimmunization. However, the use of intraoperative cell salvage in obstetrics has raised some potential concerns. The primary concern involves the theoretic risk of inducing amniotic fluid embolism by transfusing blood contaminated with amniotic fluid. This concern has limited the widespread implementation of cell salvage in obstetrics.

Cell salvage technology appears to effectively remove contaminants from the salvaged blood.[30-32] Hundreds of reports have been published documenting successful use of intraoperative cell salvage in obstetrics.[33,34] This safety record has prompted The American College of Obstetricians and Gynecologists and others to recommend consideration of this technology for patients at risk for intraoperative hemorrhage.[35]

Once the operating field is cleared of amniotic fluid, the suction device is changed and the blood is collected into the Cell Saver. The Cell Saver can provide a unit of blood with a hematocrit of 50% in approximately 3 minutes. In patients where blood loss is anticipated to be excessive, more than one Cell Saver may be employed.

■ ACUTE NORMOVOLEMIC HEMODILUTION

Patients at risk for significant intraoperative hemorrhage, as in the setting of anticipated invasive placentation, may be candidates for acute normovolemic hemodilution (ANH). Immediately preoperatively, blood is collected from the patient into special storage bags containing an anticoagulant obtained from the blood bank. At the same time, the patient is given large amounts of crystalloid and/or colloid in a 3:1 ratio, resulting in a dilutional decrease in maternal hematocrit. Blood lost intraoperatively is therefore more dilute. After blood loss is under control (or at the discretion of the surgeon), the patient's blood is reinfused, resulting in an increase in hematocrit. Other potential advantages include preservation of clotting factors and a decreased likelihood of allogeneic transfusion and its associated morbidities.

No adverse fetal effects have been described with this process.[36-38] However, patients who might not tolerate an acute decrease in hematocrit are not candidates for ANH, as are those who are already anemic or have coronary artery disease, pulmonary disease, renal or hepatic insufficiency, or evidence of fetal compromise. There is no role for ANH in the setting of acute hemorrhage.

■ MASSIVE TRANSFUSION

Massive transfusion is most commonly defined as the need to administer 10 units of PRBC in a 24-hour period. This correlates with massive hemorrhage defined as loss of greater than 50% of the patient's blood volume.[39] In the nonobstetric literature, mortality rates of 30% to 70% are reported with massive transfusion.[40] Anticipation and correction of coagulopathy, acidosis, and hypothermia are essential in the management of the massively hemorrhaging patient. Effective resuscitation should include adequate intravenous access, including central and arterial line

placement, maintenance of core temperature above 35°C, utilization of blood warmers, and correction of hypocalcemia and hyperkalemia, in addition to the timely administration of crystalloid and component therapy.

Accreditation of Level I Trauma centers by the American College of Surgeons requires the development of a massive transfusion protocol. Key components include a method for rapid communication between the relevant departments in addition to establishing the type and amount of blood products to be delivered and administered. Controversy continues regarding the most appropriate guidelines for massive transfusion, particularly the appropriate ratio of FFP to PRBCs. Emerging data from military combat resuscitations support higher ratios of 1:1. The civilian data are less clear; FFP:PRBCs of 1:1.5 to 1:2 are common. A recent publication demonstrated a mortality reduction in the nonobstetric trauma population following implementation of a massive transfusion protocol. This reduction was attributed to improved communication and more efficient administration of blood products. After protocol implementation, mortality decreased by 58%, and time to first documented transfusion of PRBCs decreased 39%. A summary of the protocol utilized in this publication is summarized in Fig 2-1.[40] Management principles are outlined in Table 2-5.

■ TABLE 2-5. Massive Transfusion Management Principles

Manage airway and breathing.
Evaluate and address cause of hemorrhage.
Establish two large bore peripheral intravenous lines.
Consider central line and arterial line placement.
Administer crystalloid (1-2 L) initially.
Initiate massive transfusion protocol, if available.
Administer PRBCs, FFP, and platelets in a timely fashion.
　　Ratio FFP:PRBCs 1:1.5 - 1:1.8
Maintain core temperature >35°C.
Monitor CBC, PT, PTT, fibrinogen every 30 min.
Correct hypocalcemia.
Correct hyperkalemia.
Correct acidosis (pH = 7.4, normal base deficit, normal lactate).
Continue product replacement until:
　　Hemodynamically stable
　　Platelet count >50,000
　　INR <1.5

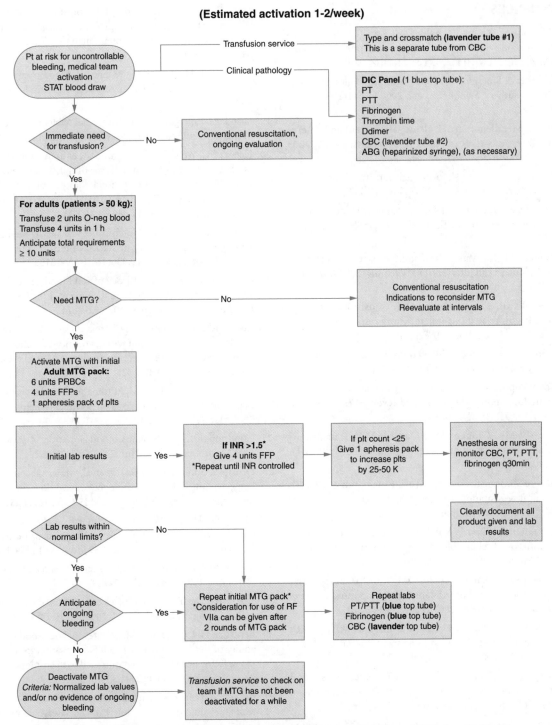

FIGURE 2-1. Sample massive transfusion guideline. (*Reproduced, with permission, from Riskin DJ, Tsai TC, Riskin L, et al. Massive transfusion protocols: the role of aggressive resuscitation versus product ratio in mortality reduction. J Am Coll Surg. 2009 Aug;209[2]:198-205.*)

REFERENCES

1. Despotis GJ, Zhang L, Lublin DM. Transfusion risks and transfusion-related pro-inflammatory responses. *Hematol Oncol Clin North Am.* 2007 Feb;21(1):147-161.

2. Shander A. Emerging risks and outcomes of blood transfusion in surgery. *Semin Hematol.* 2004 Jan;41(1)(suppl 1): 117-124.

3. Busch MP, Kleinman SH, Nemo GJ. Current and emerging infectious risks of blood transfusions. *JAMA.* 2003 Feb 26;289(8):959-962.

4. Dodd RY. Current risk for transfusion transmitted infections. *Curr Opin Hematol.* 2007 Nov;14(6):671-676.

5. Shander A. Emerging risks and outcomes of blood transfusion in surgery. *Semin Hematol.* 2004 Jan;41(1)(suppl 1): 117-124.

6. Wagner SJ. Transfusion-transmitted bacterial infection: risks, sources and interventions. *Vox Sang.* 2004 Apr;86(3): 157-163.

7. Despotis GJ, Zhang L, Lublin DM. Transfusion risks and transfusion-related pro-inflammatory responses. *Hematol Oncol Clin North Am.* 2007 Feb;21(1):147-161.

8. Goodnough LT. Risks of blood transfusion. *Anesthesiol Clin North America.* 2005 Jun;23(2):241-252, v.

9. Toy P, Popovsky MA, Abraham E, et al. Transfusion-related acute lung injury: definition and review. *Crit Care Med.* 2005 Apr;33(4):721-726.

10. Looney MR, Gropper MA, Matthay MA. Transfusion-related acute lung injury: A review. *Chest.* 2004 Jul;126(1): 249-258.

11. Moore SB. Transfusion-related acute lung injury (TRALI): Clinical presentation, treatment, and prognosis. *Crit Care Med.* 2006 May;34(Suppl 5):114S-117S.

12. Kleinman S, Chan P, Robillard P. Risks associated with transfusion of cellular blood components in Canada. *Transfus Med Rev.* 2003 Apr;17(2):120-162.

13. Despotis GJ, Zhang L, Lublin DM. Transfusion risks and transfusion-related pro-inflammatory responses. *Hematol Oncol Clin North Am.* 2007 Feb;21(1):147-161.

14. Kleinman S, Chan P, Robillard P. Risks associated with transfusion of cellular blood components in Canada. *Transfus Med Rev.* 2003 Apr;17(2):120-162.

15. Despotis GJ, Zhang L, Lublin DM. Transfusion risks and transfusion-related pro-inflammatory responses. *Hematol Oncol Clin North Am.* 2007 Feb;21(1):147-161.

16. Busch MP, Kleinman SH, Nemo GJ. Current and emerging infectious risks of blood transfusions. *JAMA.* 2003 Feb 26;289(8):959-962.

17. Hill GE, Frawley WH, Griffith KE, Forestner JE, Minei JP. Allogeneic blood transfusion increases the risk of postoperative bacterial infection: a meta-analysis. *J Trauma.* 2003 May;54(5):908-914.

18. Landers DF, Hill GE, Wong KC, Fox IJ. Blood transfusion-induced immunomodulation. *Anesth Analg.* 1996 Jan;82(1): 187-204.

19. Shander A. Emerging risks and outcomes of blood transfusion in surgery. *Semin Hematol.* 2004 Jan;41(1) (suppl 1): 117-124.

20. Hebert PC, Wells G, Blajchman MA, et al. A multicenter, randomized, controlled clinical trial of transfusion requirements in critical care. Transfusion Requirements in Critical Care Investigators, Canadian Critical Care Trials Group. *N Engl J Med.* 1999 Feb 11;340(6):409-417.

21. Lacroix J, Hebert PC, Hutchison JS, et al. Transfusion strategies for patients in pediatric intensive care units. *N Engl J Med.* 2007 Apr 19;356(16):1609-1619.

22. Marik PE, Corwin HL. Efficacy of red blood cell transfusion in the critically ill: a systematic review of the literature. *Crit Care Med.* 2008 Sep;36(9):2667-2674.

23. Bouchard D, Marcheix B, Al-Shamary S, et al. Preoperative autologous blood donation reduces the need for allogeneic blood products: a prospective randomized study. *Can J Surg.* 2008 Dec;51(6):422-427.

24. Yamada T, Mori H, Ueki M. Autologous blood transfusion in patients with placenta previa. *Acta Obstet Gynecol Scand.* 2005 Mar;84(3):255-259.

25. Goodnough LT. Autologous blood donation. *Anesthesiol Clin North America.* 2005 Jun;23(2):263-270, vi.

26. Droste S, Sorensen T, Price T, et al. Maternal and fetal hemodynamic effects of autologous blood donation during pregnancy. *Am J Obstet Gynecol.* 1992 Jul;167(1):89-93.

27. McVay PA, Hoag RW, Hoag MS, Toy PT. Safety and use of autologous blood donation during the third trimester of pregnancy. *Am J Obstet Gynecol.* 1989 Jun;160(6):1479-1486.

28. Slichter SJ. Platelet transfusion therapy. *Hematol Oncol Clin North Am.* 2007 Aug;21(4):697-729, vii.

29. Yazer MH. The blood bank "black box" debunked: pretransfusion testing explained. *CMAJ.* 2006 Jan 3;174(1):29-32.

30 Bernstein HH, Rosenblatt MA, Gettes M, Lockwood C. The ability of the Haemonetics 4 Cell Saver System to remove tissue factor from blood contaminated with amniotic fluid. *Anesth Analg.* 1997 Oct;85(4):831-833.

31. Catling SJ, Williams S, Fielding AM. Cell salvage in obstetrics: an evaluation of the ability of cell salvage combined with leucocyte depletion filtration to remove amniotic fluid from operative blood loss at caesarean section. *Int J Obstet Anesth.* 1999 Apr;8(2):79-84.

32. Waters JH, Biscotti C, Potter PS, Phillipson E. Amniotic fluid removal during cell salvage in the cesarean section patient. *Anesthesiology.* 2000 Jun;92(6):1531-1536.

33. Rebarber A, Lonser R, Jackson S, Copel JA, Sipes S. The safety of intraoperative autologous blood collection and autotransfusion during cesarean section. *Am J Obstet Gynecol.* 1998 Sep;179(3, pt 1):715-720.

34. Weiskopf RB. Erythrocyte salvage during cesarean section. *Anesthesiology.* 2000 Jun;92(6):1519-1522.

35. Postpartum Hemorrhage. The American College of Obstetricians and Gynecologists Practice Bulletin No. 76. American College of Obstetricians and Gynecologists. *Obstet Gynecol.* 2006;108:1039-1047.

36. Grange CS, Douglas MJ, Adams TJ, Wadsworth LD. The use of acute hemodilution in parturients undergoing cesarean section. *Am J Obstet Gynecol.* 1998 Jan;178(1, pt 1):156-160.

37. Rebarber A, Lonser R, Jackson S, Copel JA, Sipes S. The safety of intraoperative autologous blood collection and autotransfusion during cesarean section. *Am J Obstet Gynecol.* 1998 Sep;179(3, pt 1):715-720.

38. Shander A, Rijhwani TS. Acute normovolemic hemodilution. *Transfusion.* 2004 Dec;44(Suppl 12):26S-34S.

39. Malone DL, Hess JR, Fingerhut A. Massive transfusion practices around the globe and a suggestion for a common massive transfusion protocol. *J Trauma.* 2006 Jun;60(Suppl 6): 91S-96S.

40. Riskin DJ, Tsai TC, Riskin L, et al. Massive transfusion protocols: the role of aggressive resuscitation versus product ratio in mortality reduction. *J Am Coll Surg.* 2009 Aug;209(2): 198-205.

Postpartum Hemorrhage

• *Karrie Francois*

Postpartum hemorrhage remains one of the leading causes of maternal morbidity and mortality throughout the world.[1,2] In order to manage postpartum hemorrhage effectively, the obstetrician must have a thorough understanding of normal delivery–related blood loss, physiologic responses to hemorrhage, the most common etiologies of postpartum hemorrhage, and appropriate therapeutic interventions.

■ NORMAL BLOOD LOSS

Normal delivery–related blood loss depends upon delivery type. The average blood loss for a vaginal delivery, cesarean delivery, and cesarean hysterectomy is 500, 1000, and 1500 cc, respectively.[3-5] These values are often underestimated and unappreciated clinically due to the significant blood volume expansion that accompanies pregnancy.

Postpartum hemorrhage has been defined in published literature.[4-6] Definitions have included subjective assessments greater than the standard norms, a 10% decline in hematocrit, and need for blood transfusion. Because of these varied definitions, the exact incidence of postpartum hemorrhage is difficult to determine; however, rough estimates suggest that postpartum hemorrhage complicates 1% to 5% of all deliveries.[7]

■ PHYSIOLOGIC RESPONSE TO HEMORRHAGE

The pregnant patient is able to adapt to hemorrhage more effectively than her nonpregnant counterpart due to hemodynamic changes that accompany pregnancy. These changes include increased red cell mass, increased plasma volume, and increased cardiac output. In the early phases of hemorrhage, the body compensates by raising systemic vascular resistance in order to maintain blood pressure and perfusion to vital organs. However, as bleeding continues, further vasoconstriction is impossible resulting in drops in blood pressure, cardiac output, and end-organ perfusion.[3,8] Table 3-1 classifies the physiologic responses that occur with various stages of hemorrhage. It is important for the obstetrician to recognize these responses since the quantity of blood loss that occurs during a postpartum hemorrhage is often underestimated as stated previously.

■ ETIOLOGIES OF POSTPARTUM HEMORRHAGE

The etiologies of postpartum hemorrhage can be categorized as primary—those occurring within 24 hours of delivery—and secondary—those occurring from 24 hours until 6 weeks after delivery.[9] Table 3-2 lists the most common causes of primary and secondary postpartum hemorrhage. Since the obstetrician is faced with primary postpartum hemorrhage more often than secondary, the remainder of this chapter will focus on its risk factors and therapy.

Uterine Atony

Uterine atony, or the inability of the uterine myometrium to contract effectively, is the most common cause of primary postpartum hemorrhage. At term, blood flow through the placental site averages 600 cc/min.[10] After placental delivery, the uterus controls bleeding by contracting its myometrial fibers in a tourniquet fashion around the spiral arterioles. If inadequate uterine contraction occurs, rapid blood loss will ensue.

■ **TABLE 3-1.** Hemorrhage Classification and Physiologic Response

Hemorrhage class	Acute blood loss	% Lost	Physiologic response
1	1000 cc	15	Dizziness, palpitations, minimal blood pressure change
2	1500 cc	20-25	Tachycardia, tachypnea, sweating, weakness, narrowed pulse pressure, orthostatic hypotension
3	2000 cc	30-35	Significant tachycardia, restlessness, pallor, cool extremities, hypotension
4	≥2500 cc	40	Shock, air hunger, oliguria or anuria

Risk factors for uterine atony include uterine overdistention (multiple gestation, polyhydramnios, fetal macrosomia), prolonged oxytocin use, rapid or prolonged labor, grand multiparity, chorioamnionitis, retained placental tissue, placenta previa, and use of uterine-relaxing agents (tocolytic therapy, halogenated anesthetics, nitroglycerin).[11]

Genitourinary Tract Lacerations

The second most common cause of postpartum hemorrhage is genitourinary tract lacerations. While operative vaginal delivery remains the most significant risk factor for a genitourinary tract laceration, other sources of obstetrical trauma can contribute to this cause of hemorrhage. These sources include fetal malpresentation, fetal macrosomia, episiotomy, precipitous delivery, prior cerclage placement, Dührssen incisions, and shoulder dystocia.

A genitourinary tract laceration should be suspected if bleeding persists after a delivery despite good uterine tone. Occasionally, the bleeding may be masked due to its location, that is, broad ligament. In these circumstances, large amounts of blood loss may occur in an unrecognized hematoma. The astute obstetrician must be aware of the risk factors for this type of laceration as well as the patient's initial presenting symptoms of pain and physiological signs of shock.

Retained Products of Conception

Retained products of conception, namely, placental tissue and amniotic membranes, can inhibit the uterus from

■ **TABLE 3-2.** Causes of Postpartum Hemorrhage

Primary	Uterine atony
	Lower genital tract lacerations (perineal, vaginal, cervical, periclitoral, labial, periurethral, rectum)
	Upper genital tract lacerations (broad ligament)
	Lower urinary tract lacerations (bladder, urethra)
	Retained products of conception (placenta, membranes)
	Invasive placentation (placenta accreta, placenta increta, placenta percreta)
	Uterine rupture
	Uterine inversion
	Coagulopathy (hereditary, acquired)
Secondary	Infection
	Retained products of conception
	Placental site subinvolution
	Coagulopathy

adequate contraction and result in hemorrhage. Risk factors for retained products of conception include mid trimester delivery, chorioamnionitis, and accessory placental lobes.

Invasive Placentation

Although uncommon, invasive placentation can result in massive postpartum hemorrhage. Placenta accreta represents the abnormal attachment of the placenta to the uterine lining due to an absence of the deciduas basalis and an incomplete development of the fibrinoid layer. Placenta increta and percreta represent attachments to and through the uterine myometrium, respectively. Attempts to remove a highly invasive placenta from its attachment site will result in rapid blood loss, often necessitating emergent surgical intervention.

Major risk factors for invasive placentation include prior curettage or hysterotomy, advanced maternal age, multiparity, placenta previa, and previous cesarean delivery. As exemplified in Table 3-3, the combination of placenta previa and previous cesarean delivery should alert the physician to a substantial risk of invasive placentation and subsequent hemorrhage.[12] In these circumstances, an attempt for antepartum detection should be undertaken, and scheduled cesarean hysterectomy performed at the time of delivery if no future fertility is desired.

Uterine Rupture

Despite an uncommon incidence of 1 in 2000 deliveries, uterine rupture represents a potential catastrophic event for both mother and fetus, resulting in a significant hemorrhage if the placental implantation site is involved.[13] While prior cesarean delivery remains the most common risk factor for uterine rupture, other risk factors include multiparity, fetal malpresentation, obstructed labor, multiple gestation, prior hysterotomy or myomectomy, uterine manipulation (eg, internal podalic version), and mid- to high-operative vaginal delivery.

Uterine Inversion

Uterine inversion is a rare event, complicating approximately 1 in 2500 deliveries.[14] Uterine inversion may be complete or incomplete. In complete uterine inversion, the internal lining of the fundus crosses through the cervical os, forming a rounded mass in the vagina with no palpable fundus abdominally. Incomplete uterine inversion represents a partial extrusion of the fundus to the cervix; however, no passage through the os occurs. Both types of uterine inversion signify a need for rapid diagnosis and correction since large volume blood loss with associated shock may ensue.

The most commonly reported cause of uterine inversion is fundal placentation with excessive cord traction in the third stage of labor. Other associations include any clinical scenario with the potential for impaired uterine contraction after placental delivery, that is, uterine overdistention secondary to fetal macrosomia and prolonged oxytocin use. Other risk factors include uterine malformations and invasive placentation.

Coagulopathy

Coagulopathy represents the final major etiology of postpartum hemorrhage. Coagulopathies may be hereditary or acquired in origin. Although rare, hereditary coagulopathies may present challenging clinical courses if appropriate therapy is unavailable. In general, most of these coagulopathies are effectively treated with replacement of coagulation factors and/or additional pharmaceutical agents, that is, desmopressin (DDAVP), in the third stage of labor or at the time of cesarean delivery.

Acquired coagulopathies have numerous causes, including anticoagulant administration, sepsis, severe preeclampsia, amniotic fluid embolus, tissue necrosis (eg, retained intrauterine fetal demise and trauma), placental abruption, and consumption of clotting factors due to massive hemorrhage. Figure 3-1 reviews the pathophysiology of consumptive coagulopathy due to uterine atony.

■ TABLE 3-3. Invasive Placentation Risk with Placenta Previa and Cesarean Delivery	
Number of cesarean deliveries	**Invasive placentation risk (%)**
0	3
1	11
2	40
3	61
≥4	67

Source: Silver RM, Landon MB, Rouse DJ, et al. Maternal morbidity associated with multiple repeat cesarean deliveries. *Obstet Gynecol.* 2006;107(6):1226-1232.

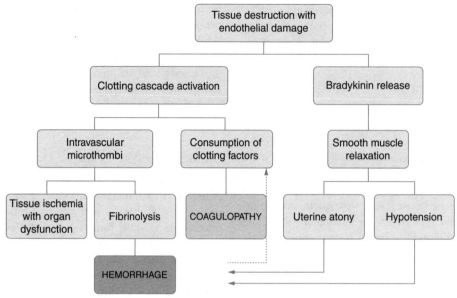

FIGURE 3-1. Pathophysiology of consumptive coagulopathy.

■ THERAPEUTIC INTERVENTIONS FOR POSTPARTUM HEMORRHAGE

When the obstetrician is faced with a postpartum hemorrhage, an organized care plan needs to be set in motion to minimize further bleeding and associated morbidity and mortality. Table 3-4 lists the components of such a care plan.

Blood Loss Needs

When faced with a postpartum hemorrhage, the first priority that a clinician should assess is his or her blood loss needs. Appropriate intravenous (IV) access is critical. This includes two large-bore IV catheters. In addition, the patient's blood type should be confirmed and held for possible cross matching needs. Finally, need for ancillary support should be assessed. This support may include additional nursing assistance, operating room staff, physician assistance, and an anesthesiology team.

Loss Estimation

Many instances of hemorrhage result in compounded morbidity secondary to an inadequate blood loss estimation on the part of the obstetrician. At the onset of a postpartum hemorrhage, it is important for the clinician to realistically estimate the amount of blood loss that has occurred. At this time, baseline laboratory evaluations of hemoglobin, hematocrit, platelet count, fibrinogen, prothrombin time, and partial thromboplastin time should be taken. If rapid laboratory assessment cannot be obtained, drawing 5 cc of blood into an empty tube and evaluating its clotting capability within 6 minutes will provide the clinician with a rough estimate of the degree of coagulopathy that exists. If the blood does not clot, the patient's fibrinogen is typically less than 200 mg/dL.

Etiology

After assessing blood loss needs and estimation, a rapid yet thorough exploration for the hemorrhage etiology

■ TABLE 3-4. Postpartum Hemorrhage Care Plan	
B	Blood loss needs
L	Loss estimation
E	Etiology
E	EBL replacement
D	Drug therapy
I	Intraoperative management
N	Nonobstetrical services
G	General complication assessment

must be undertaken. A poorly contractile uterus suggests uterine atony. If atony is not the source of bleeding, further exploration should occur. This exploration should begin with the most superior aspect of the genital tract and progress inferiorly since heavy downward blood flow may make visualization of the more inferior landmarks difficult.

Initial assessment should focus on the uterus. The most common uterine source of bleeding other than atony is retained products of conception. Figure 3-2 demonstrates proper manual exploration of the uterine cavity in order to remove retained products of conception.[15] Wrapping the examination hand with moist gauze can facilitate removal of retained amniotic membranes. If manual access to the uterine cavity is difficult or limited due to maternal body habitus or inadequate pain relief, transabdominal ultrasound may be used to assess for retained placental fragments. Once fragments are identified, appropriate removal may be undertaken via manual extraction and/or uterine curettage. Besides assessing for retained products of conception, a proper uterine examination can assess for evidence of invasive placentation, uterine rupture, and uterine inversion.

Once a uterine source has been excluded, attention should be focused on identifying a lower genitourinary tract laceration. Cervical and/or vaginal fornix lacerations are often difficult to repair due to their location. In these situations, it is best to have early assistance for retraction in order to visualize the laceration and provide adequate repair. In some instances, moving to an operating room to provide more adequate pain relief, pelvic relaxation, and visualization will save time and subsequent bleeding since a proper repair can be instituted more efficiently. In addition, lacerations that involve sites near the urethra and/or bowel may be challenging from the technical as well as visual perspectives. In these circumstances, employing additional instrumentation (eg, transurethral catheter) may protect uninjured entities and allow for a better repair.

After the most common etiologies of postpartum hemorrhage are excluded, other sources of bleeding should be assessed. Being aware of the risk factors for these etiologies will decrease diagnostic time and allow for more timely intervention.

Estimated blood loss Replacement

Understanding the patient's requirements for fluid and blood component therapy is critical to providing adequate care to the bleeding patient. Estimated blood loss (EBL) replacement begins with appropriate fluid resuscitation. Warmed crystalloid solution in a 3:1 ratio to EBL will provide the initial volume necessary to stabilize a bleeding patient. Once appropriate volume resuscitation has occurred, additional blood component therapy may be tailored to the individual patient's needs and blood loss. It is important for the clinician to understand the expected clinical response to the blood product therapy that is given (see Chap 2).

Traditionally, there has been no consensus regarding optimal blood product replacement. However, newer data from military experience suggest improved outcomes when the ratio of packed red blood cells (PRBC) to fresh frozen plasma (FFP) to platelets is 1:1:1.[16-18] In addition, hospital-based massive transfusion protocols have been successful in consumptive coagulopathy management due to postpartum hemorrhage. Stanford University Medical Center has incorporated a fixed protocol of 6:4:1 for PRBC to FFP to apheresed platelets.[19]

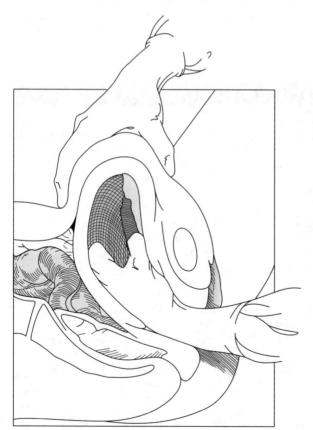

FIGURE 3-2. Manual uterine exploration.

Drug Therapy

Uterotonic medications represent the mainstay of drug therapy for postpartum hemorrhage due to uterine atony. Table 3-5 lists available uterotonic agents, their dosage, side effects, and contraindications.[20] While some reviews have questioned the efficacy of misoprostol in postpartum hemorrhage, its mild side effect profile, ease of administration, low cost, and lack of contraindications make it an attractive agent when other medications are unavailable or contraindicated.

When atony is due to tocolytic therapy, that is, those medications that impair calcium entry into the cell (magnesium sulfate, nifedipine), an additional agent to employ is calcium gluconate. Given as an intravenous push, one ampule of calcium gluconate can effectively improve uterine tone and improve bleeding due to atony.

Intraoperative Management

Intraoperative management encompasses simple conservative techniques to hysterectomy. The main objective that a clinician must keep in mind when embarking upon an operative course is to proceed efficiently with those techniques that he or she finds easy and avoid those that are either technically difficult or excessively time consuming.

Along with concurrent drug therapy, uterine atony should initially be managed with gentle bimanual massage. Figure 3-3 demonstrates the proper technique for bimanual massage.[15] Care must be taken to avoid aggressive massage that can injure the large vessels of the broad ligament.

If retained products of conception result in postpartum hemorrhage and manual extraction is unsuccessful, uterine curettage should be undertaken. While this may be performed in a delivery room, excessive bleeding mandates that an operating room be used for the procedure. Not only does moving the patient to the operating room remove potential distractions for efficient therapy, but it also allows for improved visualization, patient relaxation, ancillary support, and further operative management if the curettage is unsuccessful. A large Banjo curette should be employed with gentle traction in order to avoid uterine perforation. Transabdominal ultrasound guidance may be helpful in assisting the clinician with removal of retained placental fragments.

If uterine inversion is the source of bleeding, rapid replacement of the uterus to its proper orientation will resolve the hemorrhage. This is best accomplished in an operating room with the assistance of an anesthesiologist. The uterus and cervix should be initially relaxed with a tocolytic agent

■ TABLE 3-5. Uterotonic Medications

Agent	Dose	Route	Dosing frequency	Side effects	Contraindications
Oxytocin (Pitocin)	10-80 units in 1000 cc of crystalloid solution	First line: IV Second line: IM or IU	Continuous	Nausea, emesis, water intoxication	None
Misoprostol (Cytotec)	600-1000 µg	First line: PR Second line: PO	Single dose	Nausea, emesis, diarrhea, fever, chills	None
Methylergonovine (Methergine)	0.2 mg	First line: IM Second line: IU	Every 2-4 h	Hypertension, hypotension, nausea, emesis,	Hypertension, preeclampsia
Prostaglandin $F_{2\alpha}$ (Hemabate)	0.25 mg	First line: IM Second line: IU	Every 15-90 min (8 doses maximum)	Nausea, emesis, diarrhea, flushing, chills	Active cardiac, pulmonary, renal, or hepatic disease
Prostaglandin E_2 (Dinoprostone)	20 mg	PR	Every 2 h	Nausea, emesis, diarrhea, fever, chills, headache	Hypotension

IV, intravenous; IM, intramuscular; IU, intrauterine; PR, per rectum; PO, per oral.

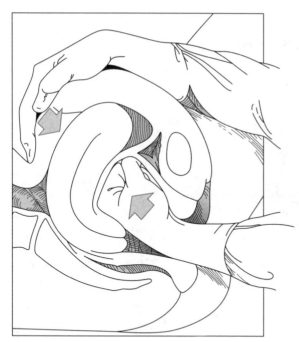

FIGURE 3-3. Bimanual massage.

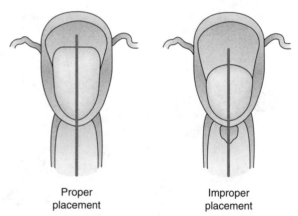

Proper placement   Improper placement

FIGURE 3-4. Placement of SOS Bakri tamponade balloon.

(eg, magnesium sulfate, terbutaline), nitroglycerin, or a halogenated anesthetic. Once adequate relaxation is accomplished, gentle pressure should be applied to the uterine fundus in order to reinvert it back into its proper abdominal location. Once reinversion has occurred, uterotonic therapy should be given to assist with uterine contraction and prevent future inversion. On rare occasions, this conservative approach for uterine reinversion is unsuccessful and therefore surgical repair by laparotomy must be performed.

Tamponade techniques are conservative approaches that may avoid further surgery or treat surface bleeding while EBL replacement is underway. A variety of techniques are available, including packing and balloon devices. Packing typically entails the use of continuous gauze (eg, Kerlex) within a sterile plastic bag or glove. The pack is left in place for approximately 12 to 24 hours while close attention is paid to the patient's vital signs, laboratory parameters, and urine output. Transurethral Foley catheter placement and prophylactic antibiotic use should be considered to prevent urinary retention and infection, respectively.

Several balloon devices are available for uterine tamponade. The most common balloon device is the SOS Bakri Tamponade Balloon (Cook Urological, Bloomington Indiana-USA). Figure 3-4 demonstrates proper placement of the

SOS Bakri Tamponade Balloon. This silicon balloon is placed within the uterus either manually or under ultrasound guidance. Once properly located, the balloon is filled with saline until bleeding stops. The balloon can hold 500 cc of saline and withstand a pressure of 300 mm Hg. Surveillance of persistent bleeding is possible as the balloon catheter drains into a collection bag. After bleeding has slowed, the balloon can be gradually deflated and subsequently removed. Tamponade balloons can be used in isolation for postpartum hemorrhage control or in conjunction with other procedures (ie, surgery or selective arterial embolization).

When bleeding continues despite conservative therapy, surgical management via laparotomy must be considered. Interventions include arterial ligation, uterine compression sutures, and hysterectomy.

The goal of arterial ligation is to decrease uterine perfusion and subsequent bleeding. Success rates have varied from 40% to 95% in published literature depending upon which arteries are ligated.[20] Arterial ligation may be performed on the uterine, utero-ovarian (Fig 3-5), and hypogastric arteries. Hypogastric artery ligation can be technically challenging and is not recommended unless the obstetrician is extremely skilled in performing the procedure. Bakri has described a bilateral looped uterine suture technique that compresses the uterine vessels against the entire thickness of the lateral uterine wall (Fig 3-6). It is recommended that a tamponade balloon be placed with the suture placement to ensure adequate hemorrhage control.[22]

Uterine compression sutures are simple, effective techniques to reduce bleeding and avoid hysterectomy. Several techniques have evolved over the past decade, including the B-Lynch suture, Hayman vertical sutures, Pereira

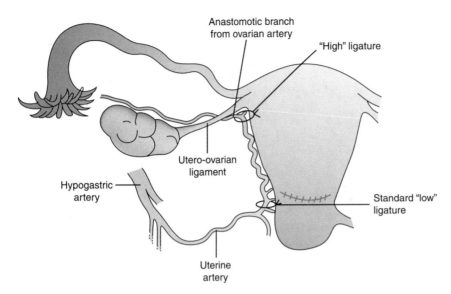

FIGURE 3-5. Uterine artery ligation.

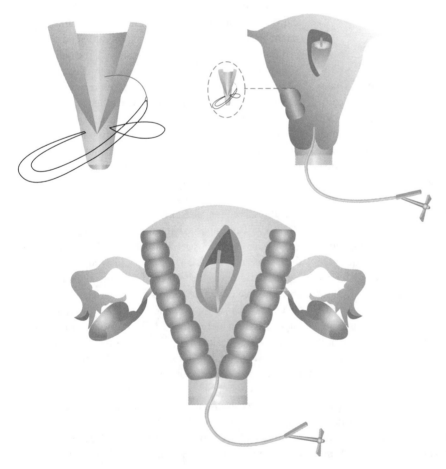

FIGURE 3-6. Bakri balloon-looped uterine vessels (BB-LUVs).

transverse and vertical sutures, and multiple square sutures.[23-28] Figures 3-7, 3-8, and 3-9 demonstrate some of these techniques. Compression sutures are best used for cases of uterine atony controlled by bimanual massage and focal invasive placentation with desire for future fertility.

Hysterectomy provides definitive therapy in cases of refractory bleeding. Since blood flow may be torrential, it is prudent for the clinician to consider performing a supracervical hysterectomy in some situations. This is especially important when the patient is unstable. Also, assistance from other surgical specialties may be necessary and a delay in consultation should be avoided.

Nonobstetrical Services

Nonobstetrical services that are particularly useful in postpartum hemorrhage management include interventional radiology, the pharmacy, and an intensive care team. Selective arterial embolization has gained success and popularity for postpartum hemorrhage management. The technique involves pelvic angiography to visualize the bleeding vessels and placement of Gelfoam (gelatin) pledgets into the vessels for occlusion. Reported success rates approximate 95%.[29] Advantages to embolization include selectivity, uterine/fertility preservation, minimal morbidity, and ability to forego or delay surgical intervention. Reported disadvantages include postembolization fever, infection, ischemic pain, and tissue necrosis. Unfortunately, a lack of rapid availability may limit its usefulness in some facilities.

In addition to interventional radiology, another nonobstetrical service that may be critical in successful postpartum hemorrhage management is the pharmacy. Recombinant

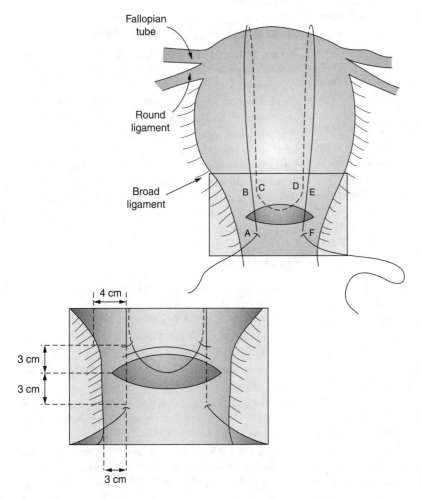

FIGURE 3-7. B-Lynch suture.

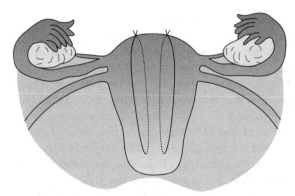

FIGURE 3-8. Hayman vertical sutures.

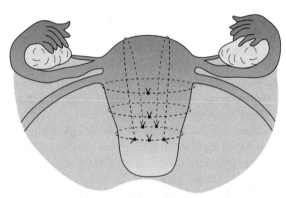

FIGURE 3-9. Pereira transverse and vertical sutures.

activated factor VIIa, RiaSTAP, and hemostatic agents can be extremely effective pharmaceutical agents in postpartum hemorrhage management. Recombinant activated factor VIIa is given as an intravenous bolus over a few minutes in doses of 60-100 μg/kg. In conjunction with other blood component therapy, recombinant activated factor VIIa can achieve rapid hemostasis within 10 to 40 minutes. Unfortunately, the half-life of the agent is relatively short (2 hours) so repeated dosing may be necessary in some cases.[30-32]

Besides recombinant activated factor VIIa, another promising pharmaceutical agent for coagulopathy management is RiaSTAP, or fibrinogen concentrate. RiaSTAP is an intravenous therapy of fibrinogen made from human plasma. Recently approved by the Food and Drug Administration (FDA), RiaSTAP has been successfully used in Europe for the treatment of massive hemorrhage due to consumptive coagulopathy (trauma, surgery, gastrointestinal hemorrhage) and congenital fibrinogen deficiency.

Hemostatic agents include fibrin sealants (eg, Tisseal), hemostatic matrices (eg, Floseal), and Gelfoam. While each of these agents has different clotting factors and mechanisms of action, they are all effective either singly or in combination for control of bleeding surfaces. These agents are particularly helpful in situations of consumptive coagulopathy associated with diffuse low-volume bleeding.

A final nonobstetrical service line to consider is an intensive care team. The patient who endures a severe postpartum hemorrhage is at risk of multiple comorbidities as noted in the following section. These comorbidities can often be avoided or dealt with more efficiently with the assistance of an intensive care team that is accustomed to the hemodynamic challenges of massive hemorrhage and transfusion.

General Complication Assessment

Once a postpartum hemorrhage has successfully been treated, the patient is still at risk for complications related to the blood loss, the therapy, or both. It is important for the obstetrician to critically assess the patient for general organ system complications. These complications include hypoperfusion injuries to the brain, heart, and kidneys, infection, persistent coagulopathy, acute lung injury due to massive transfusion requirements, and pituitary necrosis. By being aware of these potential complications, the physician can ensure that proper posthemorrhage care and consultation are available in a timely fashion so that further morbidity can be avoided.

REFERENCES

1. AbouZahr C, Royston E, eds. The global picture: the causes of maternal death. In: *Maternal Mortality: A Global Factbook.* Geneva: World Health Organization; 1991:7-11.

2. Mousa HA, Walkinshaw S. Major postpartum haemorrhage. *Curr Opin Obstet Gynecol.* 2001;13:595-603.

3. Baker R. Hemorrhage in obstetrics. *Obstet Gynecol Annu.* 1977;6:295.

4. Andolina K, Daly S, Roberts N, et al. Objective measurement of blood loss at delivery: is it more than a guess? *Am J Obstet Gynecol.* 1999;180:69S.

5. Stafford I, Dildy GA, Clark SL, et al. Visually estimated and calculated blood loss in vaginal and cesarean delivery. *Am J Obstet Gynecol.* 2008;199(5):519.

6. Pritchard JA, Baldwin RM, Dickey JC, et al. Blood volume changes in pregnancy and the puerperium. II. Red blood cell loss and changes in apparent blood volume during and following vaginal delivery, cesarean section, and cesarean section plus total hysterectomy. *Am J Obstet Gynecol.* 1962;84: 1271-1282.

7. Lu MC, Fridman M, Korst LM, et al. Variations in the incidence of postpartum hemorrhage across hospitals in California. *Matern Child Health J.* 2005;9(3):297-306.

8. Bonnar J. Massive obstetric haemorrhage. *Baillieres Best Pract Res Clin Obstet Gynaecol.* 2000;14(1):1-18.

9. Combs CA, Murphy EL, Laros RK, Jr. Factors associated with postpartum hemorrhage with vaginal birth. *Obstet Gynecol.* 1991;77:69-76.

10. Bowes WA, Jr. Clinical aspects of normal and abnormal labor. In: Creasy RK, Resnik R, eds. *Maternal-Fetal Medicine.* 4th ed. Philadelphia, PA: W B Saunders; 1999:541.

11. Fuchs K, Peretz BA, Marcovici R, et al. The "grand multipara"—is it a problem? A review of 5785 cases. *Int J Gynaecol Obstet.* 1985;23:321-325.

12. Silver RM, Landon MB, Rouse DJ, et al. Maternal morbidity associated with multiple repeat cesarean deliveries. *Obstet Gynecol.* 2006;107(6):1226-1232.

13. Combs CA, Murphy EL, Laros RK Jr. Factors associated with hemorrhage in cesarean deliveries. *Obstet Gynecol.* 1991;77:77-82.

14. Brar HS, Greenspoon JS, Platt LD, et al. Acute puerperal uterine inversion: new approaches to management. *J Reprod Med.* 1989;34:173-177.

15. Francois K, Foley MR. Antepartum and postpartum hemorrhage. In: Gabbe SG, Niebyl JR, Simpson JL, eds. *Obstetrics: Normal and Problem Pregnancies.* 5th ed. Nashville, TN: Churchill Livingston; 2007.

16. Borgman MA, Spinella PC, Perkins JG, et al. The ratio of blood products transfused affects mortality in patients receiving massive transfusions at a combat support hospital. *J Trauma.* 2007;63(4):805-813.

17. Holcomb JB, Wade CE, Michalek JE, et al. Increased plasma and platelet to red blood cell ratios improves outcome in 466 massively transfused civilian trauma patients. *Ann Surg.* 2008;248(3):447-458.

18. Cotton BA, Au BK, Nunez TC, et al. Predefined massive transfusion protocols are associated with a reduction in organ failure and postinjury complications. *J Trauma.* 2009;66(1):41-48; discussion 48-49.

19. Burtelow M, Riley E, Druzin M. How we treat: management of life-threatening primary postpartum hemorrhage with a standardized massive transfusion protocol. *Transfusion.* 2007;47(9):1564-1572.

20. Dildy GA, Clark SL. Postpartum hemorrhage. *Contemp Obstet Gynecol.* 1993;38:21-29.

21. Clark SL, Phelan JP. Surgical control of obstetric hemorrhage. *Contemp Obstet Gynecol.* 1984;24:70.

22. Bakri YN. Looped uterine sutures and tamponade balloon test (looped us-tb test) for surgical management of massive obstetric hemorrhage (Correspondence, 2009).

23. B-Lynch C, Coker A, Lawal AH, et al. The B-Lynch surgical technique for control of massive postpartum haemorrhage: an alternative to hysterectomy? Five cases reported. *Br J Obstet Gynaecol.* 1997;104:275-277.

24. Allam MS, B-Lynch C. The B-Lynch and other uterine compression suture techniques. *Int J Gynaecol Obstet.* 2005;89(3):236-241.

25. Ferguson JE, Bourgeois FJ, Underwood PB. B-Lynch suture for postpartum hemorrhage. *Obstet Gynecol.* 2000;95(6, pt 2): 1020-1022.

26. Hayman RG, Arulkumaran S, Steer PJ. Uterine compression sutures: surgical management of postpartum hemorrhage. *Obstet Gynecol.* 2002;99:502.

27. Pereira, A, Nunes, F, Pedroso, S, et al. Compressive uterine sutures to treat postpartum bleeding secondary to uterine atony. *Obstet Gynecol.* 2005;106:569.

28. Cho JH, Jun HS, Lee CN. Hemostatic suturing technique for uterine bleeding during cesarean delivery. *Obstet Gynecol.* 2000;96:129-131.

29. Ornan D, White R, Pollak J, et al. Pelvic embolization for intractable postpartum hemorrhage: long-term follow-up and implications for fertility. *Obstet Gynecol.* 2003;102(5, pt 1): 904-910.

30. Alfirevic Z, Elbourne D, Pavord S, et al. Use of recombinant activated factor VII in primary postpartum hemorrhage: the Northern European registry 2000-2004. *Obstet Gynecol.* 2007;110(6):1270-1278.

31. Franchini M, Lippi G, Franchini M. The use of recombinant activated factor VII in obstetric and gynaecological haemorrhage. *BJOG.* 2007;114(1):8-15.

32. Welsh A, McLintock C, Gatt S, et al. Guidelines for the use of recombinant activated factor VII in massive obstetric haemorrhage. *Aust N Z J Obstet Gynaecol.* 2008;48(1): 12-16.

Disseminated Intravascular Coagulopathy and Thrombocytopenia Complicating Pregnancy

CHAPTER 4

• *Philip Samuels*

Although uncommon, significant hemorrhage, coagulopathy, and need for transfusion are encountered by every practicing obstetrician. Prevention is obviously superior to treatment. By understanding the pathophysiology and events that lead to these potentially catastrophic clinical situations, we can respond more rapidly and often prevent them from becoming critical situations. Even with meticulous care, we cannot prevent all such cases. Rapid, decisive, and knowledgeable action on the part of the obstetrician can usually avert an adverse outcome. In this chapter, I cover the areas of clinical disseminated intravascular coagulopathy (DIC) and clinically significant thrombocytopenia. The best form of therapy is aimed at correcting the underlying pathophysiologic problem, as well as treating the acquired or inherent clotting problem. There are many ways to treat these clinical entities. This chapter outlines a practical approach to these patients with these complications.

■ DISSEMINATED INTRAVASCULAR COAGULOPATHY

Disseminated intravascular coagulopathy (DIC) describes a clinical scenario, but not a specific entity. It is characterized by accelerated formation of fibrin clots with simultaneous breakdown of these same clots. It is, indeed, a *consumptive* coagulopathy. The body consumes clotting factors faster than they can be produced. Normally, our body is in a constant balance between fibrin generation and fibrinolysis. When this delicate balance is disturbed and the coagulation cascade and fibrinolytic systems go unchecked, DIC can result. DIC may arise from massive activation of the coagulation system that overwhelms endogenous control mechanisms. Also, DIC may be initiated by exposure of blood to tissue factor, which triggers activation of the extrinsic clotting system. This may be the result of trauma or endotoxins damaging tissue. Also proteolytic enzyme release may trigger DIC and can occur in events such as placental abruption. This critical clinical picture, in other words, can have many etiologies. One must rapidly determine the etiology while initiating therapy.

Etiology

The most common obstetric causes of DIC are listed in Table 4-1. The most common underlying cause of mild DIC encountered by the obstetrician is probably underestimation of blood loss at the time of delivery with inadequate replacement by crystalloid or colloid. In these cases, vasospasm occurs with resultant endothelial damage and initiation of DIC. Also, in these instances, hypotension occurs which results in decreased tissue perfusion leading to local hypoxia and tissue acidosis, which can further exacerbate DIC by causing tissue release of cytokines. By keeping the patient's volume replete, DIC can often be avoided, even in the presence of profound anemia.

Following placental separation after a vaginal delivery, fibrinogen is activated to become a fibrin mesh, which covers the old placental site. This, along with uterine contraction, prevents excessive blood loss in the immediate postpartum period. The genesis of this fibrin mesh results in a 10% reduction in the concentration of clotable fibrinogen following a normal vaginal delivery. Placental abruption is a similar situation gone awry. In severe cases, the placenta partially detaches from the wall of the uterus and a retroplacental clot forms. As the clot expands, it consumes coagulation factors, which continually breakdown

■ TABLE 4-1. Causes of DIC

Common causes
- Massive hemorrhage, especially with inadequate fluid replacement with crystalloid or colloid
- Placental abruption
- Severe preeclampsia/HELLP, *not* isolated thrombocytopenia

Rare causes
- Sepsis
- Acute fatty liver of pregnancy
- Amniotic fluid embolus
- Adult respiratory distress syndrome
- Acute hemolytic transfusion reaction
- Autoimmune disease
- Malignancies
- Retained dead fetus

and this results in a consumptive coagulopathy. In these cases, the earliest laboratory sign of DIC is a significant fall in fibrinogen, which is being consumed as it is converted to fibrin. It is important to note that the concentration of clotable fibrinogen is usually greatly increased during a normal pregnancy. A concentration that may be "labeled" as normal by your laboratory may, indeed, be abnormally low for a pregnant patient. Therefore, the clinician should not be lulled into a false sense of security when the fibrinogen concentration is normal. A low-normal fibrinogen concentration may actually be a huge drop for the individual patient, representing early DIC. The clinician must rely on the overall clinical picture, because a "baseline" fibrinogen concentration is usually not available.

Severe preeclampsia and HELLP (hemolysis, elevated liver transaminases, low platelets) syndrome can result in DIC if delivery is not effected promptly. Often these patients show isolated thrombocytopenia, which should not be confused with DIC in the absence of clinical bleeding or other coagulation abnormalities. This isolated thrombocytopenia is due to increased platelet destruction by the reticuloendothelial system or decreased platelet synthesis in the bone marrow, and is not a consumptive coagulopathy. Clinical DIC in these cases is uncommon, unless the preeclampsia/HELLP is prolonged. Laboratory evidence of subclinical DIC, nevertheless, is common in preeclamptics.

There is a common misconception that a retained dead fetus commonly results in DIC. This rarely occurs and usually takes several weeks to develop. With effective cervical ripening agents, there is no reason to expectantly manage the intrauterine demise for extended periods. If, however, an unsuspected demise is discovered and it appears that the fetus expired some time previously, a coagulation profile is indicated.

Sepsis, regardless of cause, can be associated with DIC. Obviously, any infection should be treated aggressively with antibiotics. New medications such as drotrecogin alfa can greatly reduce mortality and DIC in sepsis. It, however, is associated with increased bleeding diathesis and should only be administered under the supervision of someone experienced with its use. There is no experience, however, with the use of this medication in pregnancy.

Diagnosis of DIC

The presumptive diagnosis of DIC is usually made clinically, with confirmation made through laboratory studies. Table 4-2 shows readily available diagnostic tests. Other research-based tests are available, but are not readily accessible

■ **TABLE 4-2.** Diagnosis of DIC

Clinical
- Bleeding from venipuncture and IV sites, incision sites, mucous membranes
- Profuse vaginal bleeding (postpartum and firm uterus)
- Associated shock (may be out of proportion to observed blood loss)

Laboratory studies
- Decreased fibrinogen
- Increased fibrin degradation products
- Increased D-dimer
- Prolonged prothrombin time/INR
- Prolonged aPTT (occasionally)
- Decreased antithrombin III
- Falling hemoglobin/hematocrit
- Rising LDH
- Rising bilirubin
- Examination of peripheral smear for schistocystes
- Nonclotting tube of blood

INR, international normalized ratio; LDH, lactate dehydrogenase.

■ **TABLE 4-3.** Treatment of DIC in Pregnancy

Treat inciting event
- Massive hemorrhage
  - Treat cause (uterotonic agents, repair lacerations)
- Placental abruption
  - Delivery
    - Attempt vaginal delivery if fetus and mother stable
- Preeclampsia/HELLP
  - Delivery
- Acute fatty liver
  - Delivery
- Amniotic fluid embolus
  - Cardiovascular support
  - Steroids
- Sepsis
  - Broad spectrum intravenous antibiotics
- Adult respiratory distress syndrome
  - Ventilatory support
  - Cardiovascular support
- Retained dead fetus
  - Delivery
  - (Consider) antibiotics

Blood component therapy
- See Table 4-4

to the clinician at the bedside. In obstetrics, a falling fibrinogen concentration is usually the hallmark of DIC. It is important to remember that the prothrombin time (PT) is affected by disorders of the vitamin K dependent, extrinsic clotting system (Factors II, VII, IX, X). The PT will often become prolonged before there is prolongation of the activated partial thromboplastin time (aPTT) in DIC. This is because the aPTT depends upon the intrinsic clotting system, which includes Factor VIII. Not only does Factor VIII normally increase during pregnancy, but it also increases early in the course of DIC, secondary to a release of Factor VIII/vonWillebrand's factor, from damaged endothelial cells. However, as the DIC becomes overwhelming, the aPTT will also become prolonged. Tests of fibrin degradation such as fibrin degradation products and D-dimer will also be elevated. However, in normal pregnancy, one can often find mildly elevated levels of these tests. No single test should be used in assigning a diagnosis of DIC.

Treatment

The basic treatment for DIC is to reverse the inciting event. Simultaneously while correcting the inciting event, blood component therapy should also be initiated *if needed*. Blood products should not be used frivolously, but too often we wait too long to initiate blood component therapy. DIC is more easily reversed when treated immediately. Therapies are outlined in Tables 4-3 and 4-4. It is crucial to realize that treatment should not be sequential, but that several forms of therapy should be occurring simultaneously. Therefore, if possible, two intravenous lines should be established and a Foley catheter should be in place. Aggressive fluid resuscitation can be accomplished while blood component therapy is given. In addition to the modalities listed in Table 4-4, recombinant activated factor VII can be used in life-threatening hemorrhage. This is an "off-label" use, but there is growing evidence that it is effective. A side effect is thrombotic phenomena. Therefore, it should be used only in the most refractory cases, and under the supervision of someone who is familiar with this agent. It is important to note that vitamin K and folate should be administered, as patients with DIC often develop deficiencies in these vitamins. There is some evidence that antithrombin III concentrate may promote endothelial healing and decrease fibrinolytic activity. Also, the fluid status (intake and output) must be monitored closely. It is very easy to underestimate

■ **TABLE 4-4. Blood Component Therapy for DIC in Pregnancy**

Fresh frozen plasma (FFP) (volume = 250 cc)
- Used to correct PT, aPTT, and fibrinogen. Usually use as 4 units initially and then use more as needed.
- Use for clinical hemorrhage, if INR ≥2 with bleeding, if aPTT prolonged with bleeding.
- Each unit of FFP increases the circulatory fibrinogen 5-10 mg/dL.

Cryprecipitate (volume = 35-40 cc)
- Rich in fibrinogen and used to raise fibrinogen utilizing less volume than fresh frozen plasma.
- Administer when fibrinogen <100 mg/dL or if clinical hemorrhage and fibrinogen <150 mg/dL.
- Each unit of cryoprecipitate increases the circulatory fibrinogen 5-10 mg/dL.

Platelets
- Transfuse if maternal platelets <20,000/mm³ whether or not clinical bleeding.
- Transfuse if maternal platelets <50,000/mm³ in the presence of hemorrhage.
- Each pack of pooled platelets increases the platelet count by 7,000-10,000/mm³. In DIC, transfused platelets are consumed rapidly.

PRBCs
- Increase oxygen carrying capacity (a primary priority).
- Transfuse rapidly to keep up with clinical bleeding, and try to keep hematocrit ≥25%.
- Follow electrolytes as hemolysis and RBC transfusion can lead to elevated serum potassium.
- Give one ampule of calcium after each 5 units of PRBCs since the anticoagulant in the packed units will chelate circulatory calcium.

blood loss or underestimate the volume of crystalloid/blood components administered. It is crucial to keep meticulous track of this. If the patient is not given enough volume, she could develop acute renal failure. Conversely, if an overabundance of fluid is administered, the patient can develop fluid overload and pulmonary edema.

■ THROMBOCYTOPENIA

Etiology

Thrombocytopenia (a platelet count <150,000/mm³) coincides with approximately 4% of pregnancies and is the most common reason for hematology consultation during gestation. Before diagnosing thrombocytopenia, the obstetrician must make certain that the patient does not have a platelet clumping disorder, which can give a spurious impression of thrombocytopenia. In 3 per 1000 individuals, platelets will clump in EDTA, the diluent in lavender-topped tubes used to analyze complete blood counts (CBC). In this process, platelets clump together so that many platelets are counted as a single platelet in the automatic analyzers. Examination of a peripheral smear as well as checking a platelet count in a blue-topped tube containing citrate can distinguish this from true thrombocytopenia. Those with a clumping disorder are not truly thrombocytopenic and are not at risk for bleeding. This evaluation is shown in Fig 4-1. The causes for thrombocytopenia encountered during pregnancy are listed in Table 4-5.

The most common cause for true thrombocytopenia accompanying pregnancy is gestational thrombocytopenia. This disorder occurs in about 3% of pregnancies and is more frequent than all other causes of thrombocytopenia combined. It is generally characterized by mild, progressive thrombocytopenia detected incidentally on a routine CBC. Any invasive evaluation or treatment for gestational thrombocytopenia may lead to more misadventure for the patient than the disease itself. To make this diagnosis, the patient must have no history of a bleeding diathesis outside of pregnancy. In general the platelet count should be >50,000/mm³ and there should be no evidence of platelet clumping. Fewer than 1% of uncomplicated pregnant women have a platelet count less than 100,000/mm³. Therefore, the lower the

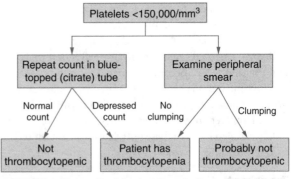

FIGURE 4-1. The method for deciding whether a patient has true thrombocytopenia or a platelet clumping disorder which affects approximately 3 per 1000 individuals. Platelet clumping is an *in vitro* process and causes a spuriously low platelet count which may result in unnecessary anxiety, work-up, and treatment.

■ **TABLE 4-5.** Causes of Thrombocytopenia During Pregnancy

Major causes
- Gestational thrombocytopenia
- Severe preeclampsia
- HELLP syndrome
- Disseminated intravascular coagulopathy
- Platelet clumping (spurious)

Uncommon causes
- Immune thrombocytopenic purpura
- Human immunodeficiency virus
- Lupus inhibitor and antiphospholipid antibody syndrome
- Systemic lupus erythematosus

Rare causes
- Thrombotic thrombycytopenic purpura
- Hemolytic uremic syndrome
- Type IIB von Willebrand's disease
- Hematologic malignancies
- Folic acid deficiency
- May-Heglin syndrome (congenital thrombocytopenia)

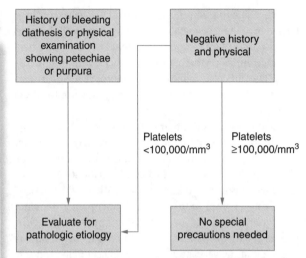

FIGURE 4-2. Evaluation of the patient after a diagnosis of thrombocytopenia has been established (Initial Evaluation of Thrombocytopenia* during Pregnancy).

maternal platelet count, the more likely the woman has an ongoing pathologic process. Pregnant women with a platelet count between 50,000/mm³ and 100,000/mm³ probably do not have a significant pathologic process. Platelet count <100,000/mm³ are infrequent, however, I feel these patients deserve a thorough evaluation. This point is illustrated in Fig 4-2. Clearly, those with platelet counts <50,000/mm³ must be evaluated by a hematologist or internist with a special interest in benign hematology.

Immune thrombocytopenic purpura (ITP) is an autoimmune disorder that results in increased platelet destruction by the reticuloendothelial system. This disorder complicates approximately 3 per 1000 pregnancies. There are two types of ITP, although they are rarely distinguished by obstetricians/gynecologists. Childhood ITP and adult-onset ITP have very different natural histories, and no observations have been made to ascertain whether or not they behave the same during pregnancy with regard to maternal and fetal/neonatal course. Childhood ITP, which also affects adolescents, usually follows an acute infection. It is characterized by an acute onset and has a rapid remission and rare relapses. Adult-onset ITP, conversely, is a chronic disorder that usually requires long-term steroid or immune globulin therapy and has frequent exacerbations and remissions.

Because it is an autoimmune disease, ITP is diagnosed in the laboratory by platelet antibody testing. The methodology of this testing is not uniform, so sensitivity and specificity vary with the laboratory used. Furthermore, traditional antibody testing cannot distinguish ITP from gestational thrombocytopenia. During pregnancy, history and physical examination are more important than laboratory testing to distinguish the two disorders. Platelet antibodies can be platelet-associated (direct, platelet-bound) or circulating (free, indirect, serum). Unfortunately, neither of these antibody classes can be used to distinguish ITP from gestational thrombocytopenia. Circulating (indirect) antiplatelet antibodies have been associated with neonatal thrombocytopenia in women with ITP. In fact, 13% to 24% of women with true ITP will give birth to infants with platelet counts <50,000/mm³. The presence of circulating antiplatelet IgG in the maternal serum can serve as a rough indicator that the pregnant woman is at risk of giving birth to a child with profound thrombocytopenia. The presence of these antibodies is only a rough indicator because their negative predictive value is excellent, but their positive predictive value is poor. This means that if these antibodies are absent, it is highly unlikely that the neonate will have a profoundly depressed platelet count at birth. The presence of these antibodies, however, indicates a risk, but not a high likelihood. Again, it is important to stress that the methodology of this testing varies between laboratories, and it is therefore safe to assume that the predictive values of these tests in predicting neonatal thrombocytopenia will also vary. It is also important to understand that ITP can be the harbinger of lupus erythematosus or other autoimmune diseases. The physician should take an appropriate history and look for physical signs that may cause suspicion for these disorders.

Most physicians feel that vaginal delivery is acceptable even in the case of an infant with an extremely low platelet count. Therefore, cordocentesis and scalp sampling for platelet count are not indicated in these patients. Nonetheless, I feel it is useful to know which patients are at risk of delivering a profoundly thrombocytopenic neonate. Therefore, I do look for circulating antiplatelet IgG in pregnant patients with true ITP. If present, I avoid operative vaginal delivery, and try to avoid scalp electrodes if possible. Furthermore, I am reticent about allowing these patients to have a prolonged second stage of labor. In any case of ITP, I notify the pediatric team so a neonatal platelet count can be obtained.

Thrombotic thrombocytopenic purpura (TTP) is a rare disorder, but one that must be considered when a pregnant patient's platelet count is severely depressed. Clinical ramifications are severe, and the disease is life-threatening. Pathologically, platelets aggregate, producing platelet thrombi that occlude arterioles and capillaries. This can produce ischemia and infarction in any organ system. It frequently affects those systems most dependent on microcirculation such as the brain and kidneys. The cause of TTP remains elusive, but probably includes the arachadonic acid/prostaglandin pathway as well as plasminogen and its activators.

TTP is a clinical diagnosis, and the disorder is characterized by a pentad of findings (Table 4-6). The classic pentad of signs/symptoms occurs in only about 40% of patients, whereas approximately 75% of patients experience the triad of microangiopathic hemolytic anemia, thrombocytopenia, and neurologic changes. TTP (non-familial) may be caused by autoantibodies against ADAMTS-13, a metalloprotease that is responsible for cleaving ultra-large von Willebrand multimers. When TTP occurs during pregnancy, it usually occurs antepartum, and possibly during the second trimester. It may be confused with HELLP (hemolysis, elevated liver transaminases, low platelets) syndrome. The degree of microangiopathic anemia is more severe in TTP and is usually readily evident on the peripheral smear. Occasionally a depressed antithrombin III level will be seen in HELLP syndrome and aid in the distinction between the two disorders. TTP is usually nonrecurring, but intermittent and chronic relapsing forms do exist, though rarely. See Chap 15 for a more detailed discussion on this disorder and differential diagnosis.

■ **TABLE 4-6. Classic Findings in Thrombotic Thrombocytopenic Purpura[a]**

- Microangiopathic, hemolytic anemia[b]
- Thrombocytopenia[b]
- Neurologic abnormalities[b]
  - Confusion
  - Headache
  - Paresis
  - Visual hallucinations
  - Seizures
- Fever
- Renal dysfunction

[a]The classic pentad is found in 40% of patients.
[b]This triad is present in 75% of patients.

Treatment

When does ITP require therapy? Spontaneous bleeding usually does not occur until the platelet count falls to around 20,000/mm^3, and surgical bleeding does not occur until the platelet count falls to about 50,000/mm^3. Many hematologists, therefore, do not empirically treat a patient until the platelet count approaches 20,000/mm^3 unless there is clinical bleeding. There is a relatively new test that may help determine which patients are at high risk. The platelet function analyzer can rapidly determine if platelets are functional by seeing how long it takes for them to aggregate when exposed to different stimuli.

The commonly used modalities for treating ITP when it exacerbates during pregnancy are listed in Table 4-7. Glucocorticoid administration remains the initial line of therapy. If rapid response is needed, intravenous methylprenisolone is used. It has an advantage over hydrocortisone as it has much less mineralocortoicoid effect. Usually 1.0 to 1.5 mg/kg *total body weight* of methylprednisolone is administered daily in two or three divided doses. An initial response is usually seen within 2 days, but in refractory cases, it may take as long as 10 days to see a maximum response. After the anticipated response is obtained, the patient should be switched to oral prednisone and the dose should be tapered to keep the platelet count arbitrarily around 100,000/mm^3. If it is not emergent, therapy can be initiated with oral prednisone on an outpatient basis. The usual starting dose

■ **TABLE 4-7.** Treatment Modalities for ITP During Pregnancy

Glucocorticoids
- Intravenous
  - Methylprednisolone 1.0-1.5 mg/kg daily in two or three divided doses
  - Prednisone 1.0 mg/kg/d>
    - Then taper

Intravenous immunoglobulin
- 0.4-1.0 g/kg/d for 3-5 days
- May be repeated

Splenectomy
- Best carried out in second trimester

Platelet transfusion
- Reserved for severe active bleeding
- May cause more rapid platelet destruction
- Each unit of platelets raising count about 7000-10,000/mm^3

■ **TABLE 4-8.** Tips for Tapering Steroids

Tapering must be individualized and patients must be observed for symptoms
- Parameters that must be taken into account when tapering glucocorticoids in order to prevent adrenal crisis
- Age
  - Patients older than 40 must be weaned very slowly
- Duration of therapy
  - No tapering needed for <1 wk of therapy
  - Rapid tapering if 1-2 wk of therapy
  - Slow taper if >2 wk of therapy
- Dosage of prednisone used
  - Taper rapidly to 40 mg/d
- Taper from 40-20 mg/d over several days
- Taper from 20 mg/d to none over an extended period of 2-4 wk, especially if duration of therapy has been >2 wk

is 1 mg/kg *total body weight* per day in a single dose. One must watch for gasttric ulcer formation when large doses are administered over extended periods. After an appropriate response, tapering should be accomplished as previously mentioned. Approximately 70% of patients respond to glucocorticoid therapy. In order to avoid adrenal crisis, it is important not to wean off prednisone too quickly if the patient has been on glucocorticoids for over 2 weeks. Tips for tapering steroids are given in Table 4-8.

For pregnant patients who fail to respond to glucocorticoids, intravenous immunoglobulin (IVIG) should be administered. The usual dose is 0.4 to 1.0 g/kg/d for 3 to 5 days. Occasionally, a dose of up to 2.0 g/kg/d will be required. The response usually begins in 2 to 3 days and usually peaks at about 5 days. This, however, is variable. The duration of response is variable, so if IVIG is being administered to raise the maternal platelet count before delivery, proper timing is essential. In general, if an adequate platelet count is needed for delivery, the course of therapy should be started 5 to 8 days before the planned induction or cesarean delivery.

If there is inadequate response to IVIG, splenectomy can be performed safely during gestation. The best time for any type of surgery during pregnancy is during the second trimester. This is before the uterus enlarges enough to interfere with surgical exposure and the risk of preterm contractions

is less. There is usually an immediate increase in platelet count after splenectomy. Splenectomy can be accomplished at the time of cesarean delivery if necessary, by extending a midline skin incision cephalad after uterine closure.

Platelet transfusion is indicated only for the profoundly thrombocytopenic patient who is experiencing clinically significant bleeding. The transfusions are given while awaiting the effect of other therapies or while preparing the patient for immediate surgery. Some advocate giving platelets at the time of surgery if the platelet count is <50,000/mm^3. At the very least, platelets should be available in the operating room for these patients. The same tenet holds for vaginal delivery in the patient with a platelet count approaching 20,000/mm^3. In the profoundly thrombocytopenic patient, the physician should thoroughly examine the vagina and perineum in the immediate postpartum period, as the risk of hematoma is high. The viability of transfused platelets is extremely short because the same antibodies and reticuloendothelial cell clearance that affect the mother's endogenous platelets also destroy and sequester the transfused platelets. Therefore, if a platelet transfusion is needed for surgery it should be started at the time of the skin incision and not earlier. Each unit of platelets will increase the maternal platelet count by about 10,000/mm^3. A scheme for treating maternal ITP is outlined in Fig 4-3. Certain technical surgical precautions should be taken when performing a cesarean delivery on a patient with severe thrombocytopenia or any other bleeding diathesis. These precautions are listed in Table 4-9.

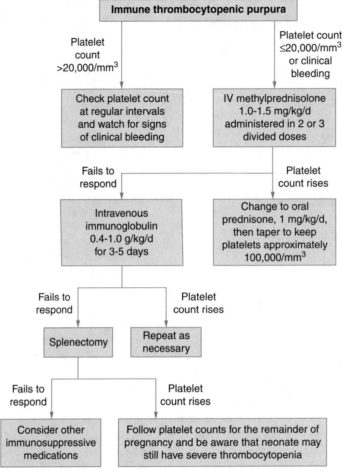

FIGURE 4-3. Management of the pregnant woman with immune thrombocytopenic purpura.

■ **TABLE 4-9. Surgical Tips for Performing a Cesarean Delivery on a Patient with a Bleeding Diathesis**

- Use a midline incision if there is clinically significant bleeding. Otherwise a Pfannenstiel incision is acceptable.
- Use electrocautery liberally, especially in opening the subcutaneous tissue.
- Close the uterus meticulously from the start. The more needle holes you put in the uterus, the more it will bleed.
- Leave the bladder flap open to prevent hematoma formation that could later lead to abscess. Cauterize the edge of the bladder flap if necessary.
- Close the peritoneum in order to prevent bleeding from the edges. This also prevents subfascial bleeding from filling the peritoneal cavity and allows placement of subfascial drains.
- If there is oozing, place subfascial drains and leave them in place until they stop draining.
- Use skin staples, even in Pfannenstiel incisions. This allows partial opening of the incision if a subcutaneous hematoma or seroma forms.
- Place a pressure dressing over the incision and leave it in place until the danger of bleeding subsides.

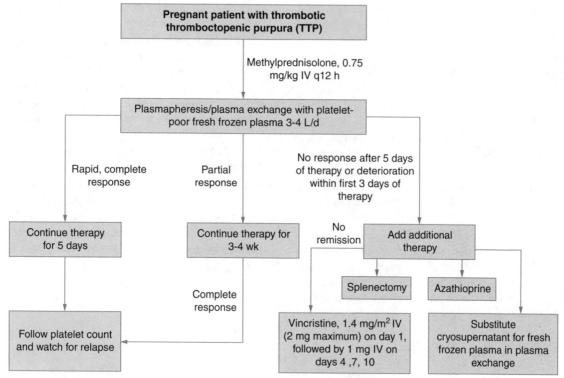

FIGURE 4-4. Management of the gravida with TTP. Before adopting this approach, the treating physician must be certain of the diagnosis. TTP is a clinical diagnosis and can mimic severe preeclampsia. The criteria for diagnosing TTP are listed in Table 4-6.

Intensive plasma manipulation is the key for treating TTP. Therapy usually entails a combination of plasmapheresis and plasma exchange with platelet-poor fresh frozen plasma (FFP, 3-4 L/d). Plasmapheresis removes platelet-aggregating substances, and plasma infusion provides some antiaggregating products, such as ADAMTS-13, which are deficient in the patient's plasma. If exchange plasmapheresis is not readily available, infusion of FFP (30 mL/kg/d) can be used as a temporizing measure. If this is done, the treating physician must be careful to watch for signs of volume overload and administer diuretics if necessary. If a patient responds to plasmapheresis, this procedure should be continued for at least 5 days. In patients who exhibit a partial response without clinical deterioration, plasmapheresis and plasma exchange should be continued for 3 to 4 wk to achieve complete remission. Also, packed red blood cells (PRBCs) should be administered to keep the hemoglobin at an acceptable concentration. The physician should also carefully monitor renal function.

Glucocorticoids should be administered to all patients with TTP immediately after diagnosis. The usual dose is 0.75 mg/kg of intravenous methylprednisolone every 12 hours until the patient recovers. Then slow tapering should be performed.

If a patient does not begin to respond within 5 days of therapy, or if her condition deteriorates within the first 3 days, other therapies should be considered including vincristine, azathioprine, and splenectomy. In refractory cases, cryosupernatant may be substituted for FFP in the plasma exchange protocol. Treatment of the pregnant patient with TTP is outlined in Fig 4-4.

SUGGESTED READING

Aster RH. Gestational thrombocytopenia. A plea for conservative management. *N Engl J Med.* 1990;323:264.

Burrows RF, Kelton JG. Low fetal risks in pregnancies associated with idiopathic thrombocytopenic purpura. *Am J Obstet Gynecol.* 1990;164:1147.

Burrows RF, Kelton JG. Fetal thrombocytopenia and its relation to maternal thrombocytopenia. *N Engl J Med.* 1993; 329:1463.

Cines DB, Dusak B, Tomaski A, et al. Immune thrombocytopenic purpura and pregnancy. *N Engl J Med.* 1982;306: 826.

Gabbe SG, Neibyl JR, Simpson JL, eds. *Obstetrics: Normal and Problem Pregnancies.* 4th ed. New York: Churchill Livingstone; 2002:1169-1176.

Hoffman R, Benz EJ, Jr, Shattil SJ, et al, eds. *Hematology: Basic Principles and Practice.* New York: Churchill Livingstone; 1991:1394-1405.

Hoffman R, Benz EJ, Jr. Shattil SJ, et al, eds. *Hematology: Basic Principles and Practice.* New York: Churchill Livingstone; 1991:1495-1500.

Jilma B. Platelet function analyzer (PFA 100): a tool to quantify congenital or acquired platelet dysfunction. *J Lab Clin Med.* 2001;138(3):152-163.

McCrae KR, Samuels P, Schreiber AD. Pregnancy-associated thrombocytopenia: pathogenesis and management. *Blood.* 1992;80:2697.

Repke JT, ed. *Intrapartum Obstetrics.* New York: Churchill Livingstone; 1996:431-446.

Rousell RH, Good RA, Pirofsky B, et al. Non-A non-B hepatitis and the safety of intravenous immunoglobulin pH 4.25. *A retrospective survey.* Vox sang 1988;54:6.

Samuels P, Bussel JB, Braitman LE, et al. Estimation of the risk of thrombocytopenia in the offspring of pregnant women with presumed immune thrombocytopenic purpura. *N Engl J Med.* 1990;323:229.

Tsai HM: Pathophysiology of thrombotic thrombocytopenic purpura. *Int J Hematol.* 2010 Jan.

Weiner CP: Thrombotic microangiopathy in pregnancy and the postpartum period. *Semin Hematol.* 1987;24:119.

Wissa I, Ebeid E, El-Shawarby S, et al. The role of recombinant activated Factor VII in major obstetric haemorrhage: the Farnborough experience. *J Obstet Gynaecol.* 2009; 29(1): 21-24.

CHAPTER 5

Hypertensive Emergencies

• *Baha M. Sibai*

Hypertensive disorders are the most common medical complications of pregnancy, affecting 5% to 10% of all pregnancies. Approximately 30% of hypertensive disorders in pregnancy are due to chronic hypertension and 70% are due to gestational hypertension–preeclampsia. The spectrum of the disease ranges from mildly elevated blood pressures with minimal clinical significance to severe hypertension and multiorgan dysfunction. Understanding the disease process and its impact on pregnancy is of utmost importance, as hypertensive disorders remain a major cause of maternal and perinatal morbidity and mortality worldwide (Table 5-1).

■ DEFINITIONS AND CLASSIFICATIONS

Hypertension is defined as a systolic blood pressure ≥140 mm Hg or a diastolic blood pressure ≥90 mm Hg. These measurements must be made on at least two occasions, no less than 6 hours and no more than a week apart. It is important to note that choosing the appropriate cuff size will help to eliminate inaccurate blood pressure measurements. Abnormal proteinuria in pregnancy is defined as the excretion of ≥300 mg of protein in 24 hours. The most accurate measurement of total urinary excretion of protein is with the use of a 24-hour urine collection. However, in certain instances the use of semiquantitative dipstick analysis may be the only measurement available to assess urinary protein. Table 5-2 lists the classification of hypertension.

Gestational Hypertension

Gestational hypertension is the elevation of blood pressure during the second half of pregnancy or in the first 24 hours postpartum, without proteinuria and without symptoms. Normalization of blood pressure occurs in the postpartum period, usually within 10 days. Treatment is generally not warranted since most patients will have mild hypertension. Gestational hypertension in and of itself has little effect on maternal or perinatal morbidity or mortality. However, approximately 46% of patients diagnosed with preterm gestational hypertension will develop preeclampsia. Those with severe gestational hypertension are at risk for adverse maternal and perinatal outcomes and should be managed like those with severe preeclampsia. If a woman with gestational hypertension receives antihypertensive therapy, she should be considered to have severe disease. Therefore, antihypertensive drugs should not be used during ambulatory management of these women.

Preeclampsia and Eclampsia

The classic triad of hypertension, proteinuria, and symptoms defines the syndrome of preeclampsia. Symptoms of preeclampsia include headache, visual changes, epigastric or right upper quadrant pain, and shortness of breath. Preeclampsia may be subdivided into mild and severe forms. The distinction between the two is based on the severity of hypertension and proteinuria as well as the involvement of other organ systems (Table 5-2). Close surveillance of patients with preeclampsia is warranted, as either type may progress to fulminant disease. Therefore, all women with suspected or diagnosed preeclampsia should be instructed to immediately report any of the symptoms listed below:

- Nausea and vomiting
- Persistent, severe headache

■ **TABLE 5-1. Adverse Outcomes in Severe Hypertensive Disorders of Pregnancy**

Maternal complications
- Abruptio placentae
- Disseminated intravascular coagulopathy
- Eclampsia
- Renal failure
- Liver hemorrhage or failure
- Intracerebral hemorrhage
- Hypertensive encephalopathy
- Pulmonary edema
- Death

Fetal-neonatal complications
- Severe intrauterine growth retardation
- Oligohydramnios
- Preterm delivery
- Hypoxia-acidosis
- Neurologic injury
- Death

■ **TABLE 5-2. Classification of Hypertension**

I. Gestational hypertension
    Mild
    - Systolic < 160 mm Hg or
    - Diastolic < 110 mm Hg
    Severe
    - Systolic ≥ 160 mm Hg or
    - Diastolic ≥110 mm Hg
II. Gestational proteinuria
    Mild (≥1 + on dipstick and <5 g/24 h)
    Severe (≥5 g/24 h)
III. Preeclampsia (hypertension + proteinuria)
    Onset >20 weeks' gestation
    Mild
    - Mild hypertension and mild proteinuria
    Severe
    - Severe hypertension and proteinuria
    - Mild hypertension and severe proteinuria
    - Persistently severe cerebral symptoms
    - Thrombocytopenia
    - Pulmonary edema
    - Oliguria (<500 mL/24 h)
IV. Chronic hypertension
    Hypertension before pregnancy
    Hypertension before 20 weeks' gestation
V. Superimposed preeclampsia
    Exacerbation of hypertension and/or
    new-onset proteinuria

- Right upper quadrant or epigastric pain
- Scotomata
- Blurred vision
- Shortness of breath
- Decreased fetal movement
- Rupture of membranes
- Vaginal bleeding
- Regular uterine contractions

A particularly severe form of preeclampsia is HELLP syndrome, which is an acronym for hemolysis (H), elevated liver enzymes (EL), and low platelet count (LP). The diagnosis may be deceptive because blood pressure measurements may be only marginally elevated. A patient diagnosed with HELLP syndrome is automatically classified as having severe preeclampsia. Another severe form of preeclampsia is eclampsia, which is the occurrence of seizures not attributable to other causes.

Chronic Hypertension

Hypertension complicating pregnancy is considered chronic if a patient is diagnosed with hypertension before pregnancy, if hypertension is present prior to 20 weeks' gestation, or if it persists longer than 6 weeks after delivery. Women with chronic hypertension are at risk of developing superimposed preeclampsia. Superimposed preeclampsia is defined as an exacerbation of hypertension and new onset of proteinuria.

■ PREECLAMPSIA

The risk to the fetus in patients with preeclampsia relates largely to the gestational age at delivery. Risk to the mother can be significant and includes the possible development of disseminated intravascular coagulation (DIC), intracranial hemorrhage, renal failure, retinal detachment, pulmonary edema, liver rupture, abruptio placentae, and death. Therefore, astute and experienced clinicians should be in charge of the care of women with preeclampsia.

Etiology

The etiologic agent responsible for the development of preeclampsia remains unknown. The syndrome is characterized by vasoconstriction, hemoconcentration, and possible ischemic changes in the placenta, kidney, liver, and brain. These abnormalities are usually seen in women with severe preeclampsia.

Pathophysiology
Cardiovascular
The hypertensive changes seen in preeclampsia are attributable to intense vasoconstriction thought to be due to increased vascular reactivity. The underlying mechanism responsible for increased vascular reactivity is presumed to be dysfunction in the normal interactions of vasodilatory (prostacyclin, nitric oxide) and vasoconstrictive (thromboxane A2, endothelins) substances. Another hallmark of severe preeclampsia is hemoconcentration. Accordingly, patients with severe preeclampsia have lower intravascular volumes and less tolerance for the blood loss associated with delivery.

Hematologic
The most common hematologic abnormality in preeclampsia is thrombocytopenia (platelet count <100,000/mm^3). The exact mechanism for thrombocytopenia is unknown. Another occasional hematologic abnormality is microangiopathic hemolysis, as seen in association with HELLP syndrome. It can be diagnosed by the presence of schistocytes on peripheral smear and by increased lactate dehydrogenase (LDH) or bilirubin levels or reduced haptoglobin levels. Interpretation of the baseline hematocrit level in a preeclamptic patient may be difficult. A low hematocrit may signify hemolysis and a high hematocrit may be due to hemoconcentration.

Renal
Vasoconstriction in preeclampsia leads to decreased renal perfusion and subsequent reductions in the glomerular filtration rate (GFR). In normal pregnancy, the GFR increases by as much as 50% above prepregnancy levels. Because of this, serum creatinine levels in nonpreeclamptic patients rarely rise above normal pregnancy levels (0.9 mg/dL). Close monitoring of urine output is necessary in patients with preeclampsia, as oliguria (defined as <500 mL/24 h) may occur due to renal insufficiency. In rare cases profound renal insufficiency may lead to acute tubular necrosis. This is usually seen in the presence of abruptio placentae, HELLP syndrome, and unrecognized severe blood loss that is not corrected.

Hepatic
Hepatic damage in association with preeclampsia can range from mildly elevated liver enzyme levels to subcapsular liver hematomas and hepatic rupture. The latter two are usually associated with HELLP syndrome. Liver lesions seen on biopsy and at autopsy include periportal hemorrhages, ischemic lesions, and fibrin deposition.

Central Nervous System
Eclamptic convulsions are perhaps the most disturbing CNS manifestation of preeclampsia and remain a major cause of maternal mortality in the third world. The exact etiology of eclampsia is unknown, but may be attributable to hypertensive encephalopathy or ischemia from vasoconstriction. Radiologic studies may show evidence of cerebral edema , particularly in the posterior hemispheres, which may explain the visual disturbances seen in preeclampsia. Other CNS abnormalities include headaches, altered mentation, scotomata, blurred vision, and, rarely, temporary blindness.

Management of Severe Preeclampsia
Any patient with severe preeclampsia should be admitted and initially observed in a labor and delivery unit (Fig 5-1). Initial work-up should include assessment for fetal well being, monitoring of maternal blood pressure and symptomatology, and laboratory evaluation. Laboratory assessment should include hematocrit, platelet count, serum creatinine, and aspartate aminotransferase (AST). An ultrasound for fetal growth and amniotic fluid index should also be obtained (Fig 5-2). Candidates for expectant management should be carefully selected. They should also be counseled regarding the risks and benefits of expectant management. Guidelines for expectant management are outlined in Table 5-3. Fetal well being should be assessed on a daily basis by nonstress testing and weekly amniotic fluid index determination. The patient should also be instructed on fetal movement assessment. An ultrasound for fetal growth should be performed every 2 to 3 weeks. Maternal laboratory evaluation should be done daily or every other day. If the patient maintains a stable maternal and fetal course, she may be expectantly managed until 34 weeks. Worsening maternal or fetal status warrants delivery, regardless of gestational age (Table 5-3). Women with a nonviable fetus should be presented with the option of pregnancy termination.

Maternal blood pressure control is essential with expectant management or during delivery. Medications can be given orally or intravenously as necessary to maintain blood pressure between 140 and 155 mm Hg systolic and 90 and 105 mm Hg diastolic. The most commonly used

```
┌─────────────────────────────────────────┐
│   Confirm diagnosis of severe preeclampsia │
└─────────────────────────────────────────┘
```

- Admit to Labor & Delivery
- Initiate magnesium sulfate seizure prophylaxis
- Antihypertensive medications, if indicated
- Continuous fetal heart rate & contractions monitoring
- Ultrasound evaluation
- Maternal assessment, including symptoms, laboratory tests

Are there contraindications to continued pregnancy?

- Eclampsia
- Pulmonary edema
- DIC
- ≥34 wk

- Acute renal failure
- Non-reassuring fetal testing
- Abruptio placentae
- <24⁰/⁷ weeks' gestation

Yes — Proceed with immediate delivery

No — Corticoid steroids

Are there additional complications?
- Persistent symptoms
- HELLP/partial HELLP syndrome
- Fetal growth restriction (<5th percentile)
- Reverse umbilical artery end-diastolic flow
- Preterm labor/preterm PROM
- 33⁰/⁷ - 33⁶/⁷

Yes — Deliver after 48 h (steroid complete)

No — 24⁰/⁷ to 32⁶/⁷ wk → Expectant management & delivery at 33⁶/⁷ wk

FIGURE 5-1. Recommended management of severe preeclampsia.

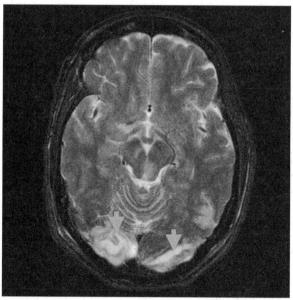

FIGURE 5-2. An ultrasound for fetal growth and amniotic fluid index.

active labor. Preeclamptic women receiving magnesium sulfate are also at risk for postpartum hemorrhage due to uterine atony. Patients should be closely monitored for at least 12 to 24 hours postpartum. Postpartum eclampsia occurs in 25% of patients; thus, MgSO₄ should be continued for 12 to 24 hours after delivery. There is usually no need for continued seizure prophylaxis beyond 24 hours postpartum. Some of these patients are at risk for pulmonary edema and exacerbation of severe hypertension at 2 to 5 days postpartum. Therefore, they should receive frequent monitoring and a short course of furosemide.

HELLP Syndrome

The specific laboratory abnormalities demonstrating hemolysis, elevated liver enzymes, and low platelets are shown in Table 5-5. The clinical presentation of patients with HELLP syndrome is highly variable. However, HELLP patients generally are multiparous, white females who present at less than 35 weeks' gestation. Sibai has noted that hypertension may be absent (20%), mild (30%), or severe (50%) in women diagnosed with HELLP syndrome. Therefore, the diagnosis of HELLP syndrome cannot necessarily be ruled out in the normotensive patient who has other signs and symptoms that are consistent with preeclampsia.

intravenous medications for this purpose are labetalol and hydralazine. The recommended dosages of medications for the acute treatment of hypertension are listed in Table 5-4. Care should be taken not to drop the blood pressure too rapidly so as to avoid reduced renal and placental perfusion. Other medications can include oral rapid-acting nifedipine.

A trial of labor is indicated in patients with severe preeclampsia if gestational age is >30 weeks and/or if cervical Bishop score is ≥6. However, an appropriate time frame should be established regarding the achievement of

■ **TABLE 5-3. Maternal/Fetal Guideline: Guidelines for Management of Severe Preeclampsia**

	Maternal	Fetal
Expeditious delivery (within 72 h)	One or more of the following: • Uncontrolled severe hypertension[a] • Eclampsia • Platelet count <100,000/mm^3 • AST or ALT >2 × upper limit of normal with RUQ or epigastric pain • Pulmonary edema • Compromised renal function[b] • Abruptio placentae • Persistent, severe headache or visual changes	One or more of the following: • Repetitive late or severe variable heart rate decelerations • Biophysical profile ≤4 on two occasions, 4 h apart • Ultrasound EFW <5th %ile • Reverse umbilical artery diastolic flow One or more of the following: • Biophysical profile >6 • Ultrasound EFW >5th %ile Reassuring fetal heart rate
Consider expectant management	One or more of the following: • Controlled hypertension • Urinary protein of any amount • Oliguria (<0.5 mL/kg/h) which resolves with hydration • AST/ALT >2 × upper limit of normal without RUQ or epigastric pain	

[a]Blood pressure persistently > 160/110 despite maximum recommended doses of two antihypertensive medications.
[b]Rise in serum creatinine of at least 1 mg/dL over baseline levels.

■ **TABLE 5-4. Acute Treatment of Hypertension**

Medication	Onset of action (min)	Dose
Hydralazine	10-20	5-10 mg IV every 20 min up to maximum dose of 30 mg
Labetalol	10-15	20 mg IV, then 40-80 mg every 10 min up to maximum dose of 300 mg or continuous infusion at 1-2 mg/min
Nifedipine	5-10	10 mg po, repeated in 30 min, (20 mg po) × 2 doses, prn; then 10-20 mg every 4-6 h up to maximum dose 240 mg/24 h
Nicardipine		As continuous infusion at 3 mg/h with increments of 0.5 mg/h (titrated according to blood pressure)
Sodium nitroprusside	0.5-5	0.25-5 µg/kg/min IV infusion Risk of fetal cyanide poisoning with prolonged treatment.

■ **TABLE 5-5.** Criteria for HELLP Syndrome

Hemolysis	• Abnormal peripheral smear
	• Total bilirubin ≥1.2 mg/dL
	• Reduced serum haptoglobin
Elevated liver enzymes	• Serum aspartate aminotransferase >70 U/L
	• Lactate dehydrogenase 2 × upper limit of normal
Low platelets	• <100,000/mm³

Differential Diagnosis

HELLP may be confused with other medical conditions, particularly in the face of normotension. A list of the differential diagnoses is found in Table 5-6. HELLP can be confused with two other specific medical conditions, acute fatty liver of pregnancy and thrombotic thrombocytopenic purpura/hemolytic uremic syndrome (TTP/HUS). The differentiation among the three entities is based on specific laboratory findings (Table 5-7).

Management

The initial evaluation in women diagnosed with HELLP syndrome should be the same as that for severe preeclampsia. The patient should be cared for at a tertiary care center. Management initially should include maternal and fetal

■ **TABLE 5-6.** Differential Diagnosis of HELLP

Acute fatty liver of pregnancy	Appendicitis with rupture
Cerebral hemorrhage	Diabetes insipidus
Gallbladder disease	Severe Gastroenteritis
Glomerulonephritis	Hemolytic uremic syndrome
Hyperemesis gravidarum	Idiopathic thrombocytopenia
Pancreatitis	Pyelonephritis
Systemic lupus erythematosis	Antiphospholipid antibody
Thrombotic thrombocytopenic purpura	Viral hepatitis, including herpes

assessment, control of severe hypertension (if present), initiation of magnesium sulfate infusion, correction of coagulopathy (if present), and maternal stabilization. Immediate delivery should be performed in patients more than 34 weeks. In patients less than 34 weeks without proven lung maturity, corticosteroids should be given and delivery planned in 48 hours, provided there is no worsening of maternal or fetal status in the meantime. The use of steroids, volume expanders, plasmapheresis, and antithrombotic agents in patients with HELLP have produced only marginal results, although some evidence suggests a benefit of steroid therapy for improvement in maternal condition. However, two recent multicenter placebo-controlled trials revealed that high-dose dexamethasone does not improve maternal outcome in patients with HELLP syndrome in the antepartum or postpartum period. Conservative management of HELLP syndrome poses a significant risk of abruptio placentae, pulmonary edema, adult respiratory distress syndrome (ARDS), ruptured liver hematoma, acute renal failure, DIC, eclampsia, intracerebral hemorrhage, and maternal death. Therefore, expectant management past 48 hours is not warranted for the potential minimal fetal benefits, when weighed against the profound maternal risk.

Patients with a favorable cervix and a diagnosis of HELLP syndrome should undergo a trial of labor, particularly if they present in labor. An operative delivery in some situations may even be harmful. However, elective cesarean section should be considered in patients, at very early gestational ages, with unfavorable cervices. O'Brien et al (2002) support the use of glucocorticoids to improve platelet counts so as to permit regional anesthesia in patients with HELLP syndrome. The anesthetist should be updated as to the trend in platelet count for patients with HELLP. Should such a patient require cesarean delivery, platelet transfusion of approximately 6 to 10 units should be initiated en route to the operating room in patients with severe thrombocytopenia. However, platelet consumption is rapid with a platelet transfusion in this setting. Intraoperative considerations should include drain placement (subfascial, subcutaneous, or both) due to generalized oozing. Postpartum management of the HELLP patient should include close hemodynamic monitoring for at least 48 hours. Serial laboratory evaluations should also be done to monitor for worsening abnormalities. Most patients should show reversal of laboratory parameters within 48 hours. Small uncontrolled studies have noted more rapid reversal of laboratory

■ TABLE 5-7. Clinical/Laboratory Findings in HELLP/TTP/HUS/AFLP

	HELLP	TTP/HUS	AFLP
Ammonia	Normal	Normal	Elevated
Anemia	±	Severe	Normal
Antithrombin III	±	Normal	Decreased
AST	Elevated	Normal	Elevated
Bilirubin	Elevated, mostly indirect	Elevated	Elevated, mostly direct
Creatinine	±	Significantly elevated	Significantly elevated
Fibrinogen	Normal	Normal	Decreased in all cases
Glucose	Normal	Normal	Decreased
Hypertension	Present	±	±
LDH	Elevated	Significantly elevated	Elevated
Proteinuria	Present	±	±
Thrombocytopenia	Present	Severe	±

HELLP, hemolysis, elevated liver enzymes, low platelet count; TTP, thrombotic thrombocytopenic purpura; HUS, hemolytic uremic syndrome; AFLP, acute fatty liver of pregnancy.

abnormalities with postpartum administration of dexamethasone. However, we do not recommend such management at our center.

Another potential life-threatening complication of HELLP syndrome is subcapsular liver hematoma. Clinical findings consistent with this complication include phrenic nerve pain. Pain in the pericardium, peritoneum, pleura, shoulder, and esophagus are consistent with referred pain from the phrenic nerve. Confirmation of the diagnosis can be obtained via the computed tomography, ultrasonography, or magnetic resonance imaging. Conservative management in a hemodynamically stable patient with an unruptured subcapsular hematoma is appropriate, provided that close hemodynamic monitoring, serial evaluations of coagulation profiles, and serial evaluation of the hematoma with radiologic studies are performed. Should the patient decompensate hemodynamically, the diagnosis of ruptured subcapsular hematoma should be entertained. If rupture of a subcapsular liver hematoma is suspected, immediate intervention is necessary. Liver hematoma rupture with hemodynamic shock is a life threatening surgical emergency. Management should involve trauma and vascular surgeons. Correction of coagulopathy and massive blood product transfusion is essential. Typically, rupture involves the right lobe of the liver. Maternal and fetal mortality is over 50%, even with immediate intervention. The current recommendation for treating rupture of subcapsular liver hematoma in pregnancy is packing and drainage, if possible.

■ ECLAMPSIA

The rate of eclampsia in the United States is 0.05% to 0.1%, and much higher in developing countries. Eclampsia continues to be a major cause of maternal and perinatal morbidity/mortality worldwide. The maternal mortality rate is approximately 4.2%. The perinatal mortality rate ranges from 13% to 30%. Eclampsia can occur antepartum (50%), intrapartum (25%), or postpartum (25%). In the postpartum period, eclampsia can develop as late as 2 weeks.

Management

During the eclamptic seizure, the main therapy is supportive care. Management of eclampsia is as follows:

1. Avoid injury: Padded bed rails, restraints
2. Maintain oxygenation: O_2, pulse oximetry, arterial blood gas assessment
3. Minimize aspiration: Lateral decubitis postion, suction
4. Initiate magnesium sulfate
5. Control blood pressure
6. Move toward delivery (corticosteroids if <30 weeks and stable condition)

Most seizures are self-limited, lasting 1 to 2 minutes. Magnesium sulfate is the drug of choice for the prevention of eclampsia and should also be used for prevention of recurrent seizures. Approximately 10% of eclamptic women receiving magnesium sulfate will have more seizures. Immediately following an eclamptic seizure, it is common to see abnormalities in the fetal heart rate pattern. These include fetal bradycardia, decreased variability, late decelerations, and reflex tachycardia. They typically resolve within 5 to 10 minutes after the convulsion. It is important not to proceed directly to cesarean delivery after a seizure, if at all possible. Vaginal delivery is the preferred birth route, even after an eclamptic seizure. Cesarean delivery should be performed for obstetric indications only. Induction of labor may be performed with oxytocin or prostaglandins, with the patient maintained on magnesium sulfate throughout her labor course. Careful attention must be given to the overall fluid status of the patient. Patients with eclampsia may have profound hemoconcentration. Because of this, close hemodynamic monitoring is required in the setting of epidural anesthesia and/or of severe blood loss. Patients who are hypovolemic will not respond well to acute blood loss, yet it is also important to limit fluids, as these patients have capillary leakage and are predisposed to developing pulmonary edema. Magnesium sulfate should be continued for 24 hours postpartum. Intracranial imaging is typically not warranted unless coma or focal neurologic signs persist, or the diagnosis is uncertain. Postpartum eclampsia is a diagnostic dilemma. Any woman seizing in the postpartum period should be considered to have eclampsia; however, other disorders must be ruled out. Patients who develop postpartum eclampsia usually will have symptoms prior to seizure activity including severe, persistent headache, blurred vision, photophobia, epigastric pain, nausea and vomiting, and transient mental status changes. Therefore, it is important to educate patients to report these symptoms to health-care providers so as to initiate preeclamptic evaluation. Eclamptics should receive $MgSO_4$ for at least 24 hours after seizure activity. If the patient has normal laboratory values and hypertension is controlled, she can be discharged in a few days with instructions to return in 1 week for outpatient evaluation.

Magnesium Sulfate

The use of magnesium sulfate in the management of preeclamptic patients is for the prevention of eclamptic seizures. The exact mode of action of $MgSO_4$ for preventing seizures is unknown, although it has been in use since the early twentieth century to prevent recurrent seizures and associated maternal/perinatal complications. The recommended regimen is presented in Table 5-8. The intravenous route is the preferred method, as intramuscular injection of magnesium sulfate is very painful and occasionally can cause gluteal abscess formation. Magnesium sulfate is not a benign medication. Patients receiving $MgSO_4$ are at increased risk for postpartum hemorrhage due to uterine atony. This should be anticipated and steps should be taken to ensure availability of crossmatched blood, if the need arises. Monitoring patients for potential

■ TABLE 5-8. Magnesium Sulfate: Dosages, Serum Levels, and Associated Findings

Magnesium doses

Loading dose:	6 g IV over 20-30 min (6 g of 50% solution diluted in 150 mL D_5W)
Maintenance dose:	2-3 g IV per hour (40 g in 1 L D_5LR at 50 mL/h)
Recurrent seizures:	Reload with 2 g over 5-10 min, 1-2 times and/or 250 mg sodium amobarbital IV

Magnesium levels and associated findings

Loss of patellar reflexes	8-12 mg/dL
Feeling of warmth, flushing, double vision	9-12 mg/dL
Somnolence	10-12 mg/dL
Slurred speech	10-12 mg/dL
Muscular paralysis	15-17 mg/dL
Respiratory difficulty	15-17 mg/dL
Cardiac arrest	20-35 mg/dL

signs of magnesium toxicity should be done throughout the course of administration; this includes eliciting deep tendon reflexes, assessing mental status, and checking respiratory rate. Table 5-8 lists the clinical findings associated with various serum magnesium levels. If a patient develops signs of magnesium toxicity, the infusion should be stopped immediately. The patient should then be evaluated for respiratory compromise by examination and pulse oximetry; oxygen should be administered and a serum magnesium level should be obtained. If magnesium toxicity is diagnosed, the patient should be treated with 10 mL of 10% calcium gluconate solution, infused over 3 minutes. Calcium competitively inhibits magnesium at the neuromuscular junction and decreases the toxic effects. The impact of calcium is transient and the patient should be closely monitored for continued magnesium toxicity. Should respiratory or cardiac arrest occur, immediate resuscitation including intubation and mechanical ventilation should be initiated.

ANTIHYPERTENSIVE AGENTS

Many agents are available for the control of hypertension. It is important to be familiar with the maternal and fetal side effects, as well as mode of action in order to choose the most effective agent for the gravida. Antihypertensive agents can exert an effect by decreasing cardiac output, peripheral vascular resistance, or central blood pressure, or by inhibiting angiotensin production. Indications for therapy are listed in Table 5-9. Commonly used drugs in pregnancy are listed in Table 5-4.

Several randomized trials compared the efficacy and side effects of intravenous bolus (IV) injections of hydralazine to either IV labetalol or oral rapid-acting nifedipine as well as oral nifedipine to IV labetalol. In general, the results of these studies suggest that either IV hydralazine or labetalol or oral nifedipine can be used to treat severe hypertension in pregnancy as long as the medical provider is familiar with the dose to be used, the expected onset of action, and potential side effects of each of these medications. Since both hydralazine and nifedipine are associated with tachycardia, it is recommended that they should not be used in patients with heart rate above 100 beats per minute (bpm). In these patients, labetalol is the appropriate drug to use. On the other hand, labetalol should be avoided in patients with bradycardia (heart reate <60 bpm), in those with asthma, and in those with congestive heart failure. In these patients, nifedipine is the drug

TABLE 5-9. Indications for Antihypertensive Therapy

I. **Antepartum and intrapartum**
   - Persistent elevations for at least 1 h
     SBP ≥160 mm Hg or
     DBP ≥110 mm Hg or
     MAP ≥130 mm Hg
   - Persistent elevations for at least 30 min
     SBP ≥200 mm Hg or
     DBP ≥120 mm Hg or
     MAP ≥140 mm Hg
   - Thrombocytopenia or congestive heart failure[a]
     SBP ≥155 mm Hg or
     DBP ≥105 mm Hg or
     MAP ≥125 mm Hg

II. **Postpartum**[b]
    SBP ≥155 mm Hg or
    DBP ≥105 mm Hg or
    MAP ≥125 mm Hg

[a]Persistent for at least 30 min.
[b]Persistent for at least 1 h.

of choice. In addition, nifedipine is associated with improved renal blood flow with resultant increase in urine output which makes it the drug of choice in those with decreased urine output, and for treatment in those with decreased urine output, and for treatment of severe hypertension in the postpartum period. There is a theoretical concern that the combined use of nifedipine and magnesium sulfate can result in excessive hypotension and neuromuscular blockage for which it was recommended that nifedipine not be used in patients receiving magnesium sulfate. However, a recent review of this subject concluded that the combined use of these drugs does not increase the risks of excessive hypotension and neuromuscular blockage in patient with severe preelampsia.

Patients with generalized swelling and/or hemoconcentration (hematocrit ≥40%) usually have marked reduction in plasma volume. The acute use of rapid-acting vasodilators (hydralazine or nifedipine) in such patients can result in excessive hypotensive response with secondary reduction in tissue perfusion and uteroplacental blood flow. Thus, such patients should receive bolus infusion of 250 to 500 mL of isotonic saline prior to the administration of vasodilators.

■ HYPERTENSIVE EMERGENCIES

On rare occasions, pregnant women may present with life-threatening clinical conditions that require immediate control of blood pressure, such as hypertensive encephalopathy, acute left ventricular failure, acute aortic dissection, or conditions characterized by increased levels of circulating catecholamines (pheochromocytoma, clonidine withdrawal, cocaine ingestion). Patients at the highest risk of these complications include those with underlying cardiac disease, chronic renal disease, hypertension requiring multiple drugs to achieve control, superimposed preeclampsia in the second trimester, and abruptio placentae in association with DIC. Although a diastolic blood pressure of 115 mm Hg, or greater, is usually considered a hypertensive emergency, this criterion is arbitrary; the rate of change of blood pressure may be more relevant than the absolute number. The combination of elevated blood pressure with evidence of new or progressive end-organ damage determines the seriousness of the clinical situation.

■ HYPERTENSIVE ENCEPHALOPATHY

Untreated essential hypertension progresses to a hypertensive crisis in up to 1% to 2% of cases. In patients with long-standing chronic hypertension, hypertensive encephalopathy is usually seen in patients with systolic blood pressure above 220 mm Hg or a diastolic above 120 mm Hg. Patients with acute onset of hypertension may develop encephalopathy at lower pressure levels than those with chronic hypertension. Normally, cerebral blood flow is approximately 50 mL/100 g tissue per minute. To maintain this level of perfusion, cerebral arterioles dilate when blood pressure falls; the converse occurs when blood pressure rises. This mechanism usually remains operative between diastolic pressures of 60 and 120 mm Hg. Hypertensive encephalopathy is considered to be a derangement of cerebral arteriolar autoregulation, which occurs when the upper limit of autoregulation is exceeded. Typically, hypertensive encephalopathy has subacute onset over 24 to 72 hours.

During a hypertensive crisis, other evidence of end-organ damage may also be present: cardiac, renal, or retinal dysfunction may arise, secondary to impaired organ perfusion, due to loss of vascular autoregulation. Ischemia of the retina (with flame-shaped retinal hemorrhages, retinal infarcts, or papilledema) may occur, causing decreased visual acuity. Impaired regulation of coronary blood flow and marked increase in ventricular wall stress may result in angina, myocardial infarction, congestive heart failure, malignant ventricular arrhythmia, pulmonary edema, or dissecting aortic aneurysm. Necrosis of the afferent arterioles of the glomerulus results in hemorrhage of the cortex and medulla, fibrinoid necrosis, and proliferative endarteritis, resulting in serum creatinine >3 mg/dL, proteinuria, oliguria, hematuria, hyaline or red blood cell casts, and progressive azotemia. Severe hypertension may result in abruptio placentae with DIC. In addition, high levels of renin, angiotensin II, aldosterone, norepinephrine, and vasopressin accompany ongoing vascular damage. These circulating hormones increase relative efferent arteriolar tone, resulting in natriurisis and hypovolemia. The impact of these endocrine changes may be important in maintaining the hypertensive crisis.

Treatment of Hypertensive Encephalopathy

The goal of hypertensive therapy is to prevent the occurrence of a hypertensive emergency. Patients at risk for hypertensive crisis should receive intensive management during labor and for 48 hours after delivery. Although pregnancy may complicate the diagnosis, once life-threatening conditions are recognized, pregnancy should not slow or alter the mode of therapy. The only reliable clinical criterion for confirming the diagnosis of hypertensive encephalopathy is prompt response to antihypertensive therapy. Headache and sensorium often clear dramatically; sometimes within 1 to 2 hours after treatment. The overall recovery may be somewhat slower in patients with uremia and in whom the symptoms have been present for a prolonged period before therapy was initiated. Sustained cerebrovascular deficits should suggest other diagnoses.

Patients with hypertensive encephalopathy or other hypertensive crises should be hospitalized. Intravenous lines should be inserted for the administration of fluids and medications. Although there is a tendency to restrict sodium intake in patients with a hypertensive emergency, volume contraction from natriuresis may be present. A marked drop in diastolic blood pressure with a concommittent rise in heart rate upon rising from the supine position is evidence of volume contraction. Infusion of normal saline solution during the first 24 to 48 hours to achieve volume expansion should be considered. Saline infusion may help decrease the activity of the renin-angiotensin-aldosterone axis and result in better blood pressure control. Simultaneous repletion of potassium losses with continuous monitoring of blood pressure, volume status, urinary output, electrocardiographic readings, and mental status is mandatory. An intra-arterial line may provide the most accurate blood pressure readings. Laboratory studies include complete blood count with differential, reticulocyte count, platelet count, and blood chemistries. A urinalysis can be obtained to survey for protein, glucose, blood, casts, and bacteria. Assessment for end-organ damage in the central nervous system, retinas, kidneys, and cardiovascular system should be done periodically. Antepartum patients should undergo continuous electronic fetal heart rate monitoring.

Lowering Blood Pressure

The drug of choice in hypertensive crisis is sodium nitroprusside. Other drugs such as nitroglycerin, nifedipine, trimetaphan, labetalol, and hydralazine can also be used. There are risks associated with too rapid or excessive lowering of blood pressure. The aim of the therapy is to reduce the mean arterial pressure by no more than 15% to 25%. Small reduction in blood pressure in the first 60 minutes of therapy, working toward a systolic level of 155 to 160 mm Hg and a diastolic level of 100 to 110 mmHg, is recommended. In chronic hypertensives, who have a rightward shift of the cerebral autoregulation secondary to medial hypertrophy of the cerebral vasculature, lowering blood pressure too rapidly may result in cerebral ischemia, stroke, or coma. Coronary blood flow, renal perfusion, and uteroplacental blood flow also may deteriorate, resulting in myocardial infarction, acute renal failure, fetal distress, or death. Hypertension that proves increasingly difficult to control is an indication for delivery. If the patient's outcome appears grave, consideration of and preparation for possible perimortem cesarean delivery should be made.

Sodium Nitroprusside

Sodium nitroprusside causes arterial and venous relaxation by interfering with both the influx and intracellular activation of calcium. It is given as an intravenous infusion at 0.25 to 5.0 µg/kg/min. The onset of action is immediate and its effect may last 3 to 5 minutes after discontinuation. Thus, hypotension caused by nitroprusside should subside within a few minutes of discontinuing the drip because of the short half-life. If it does not, other causes of low blood pressure should be considered. The effect of nitroprusside on uterine blood flow is unclear. Nitroprusside is metabolized into thiocyanate, which is excreted in the urine. Cyanide can accumulate as a result of large doses (>10 µg/kg/min) or prolonged administration (>48 hours), if there is renal insufficiency or if there is decreased hepatic metabolism. Signs of toxicity include anorexia, disorientation, headache, fatigue, restlessness, tinnitus, delirium, hallucinations, nausea, vomiting, and metabolic acidosis. When infused at less than 2 µg/kg/min, however, cyanide toxicity is unlikely. A maximum rate of 10 µg/kg/min should never be continued for more than 10 minutes. The few published reports regarding nitroprusside use in pregnancy have stated that thiocyanate toxicity rarely occurs if used in standard doses. Indeed, tachyphylaxis generally occurs before toxicity. Whenever toxicity is suspected, however, therapy should be initiated with 3% sodium nitrite at a rate not to exceed 5 mL/min, up to a maximum of 15 mL. Next, administration of 12.5 g of sodium thiosulfate in 50 mL of 5% dextrose in water infused over a 10-minute period should be started.

Nitroglycerin

Nitroglycerin is an arterial, but mostly venous dilator. It is given as an intravenous infusion at an initial rate of 5 µg/min that is gradually increased every 3 to 5 minutes, titrated to blood pressure, to a maximum dose of 100 µg/min. It is the drug of choice in preeclampsia associated with pulmonary edema and for control of hypertension associated with tracheal manipulation. Side effects include a headache, tachycardia, and methemoglobinemia. It is contraindicated in hypertensive encephalopathy because it increases cerebral blood flow and intracranial pressure.

■ SUMMARY

Patients with severe preeclampsia, HELLP syndrome, and hypertensive emergencies are at risk of maternal and perinatal morbidity and mortality. Every effort should be made to optimize outcomes for both. The risk to the fetus relates largely to the gestational age at delivery. Risks to the mother can be significant and include development of DIC, intracranial hemorrhage, renal failure, retinal detachment, pulmonary edema, liver rupture, abruptio placentae, and death. Therefore, astute and experienced clinicians should provide care for these women.

SUGGESTED READINGS

Aali BS, Nejad SS. Nifedipine or hydralazine as a first-line agent to control hypertension in severe preeclampsia. *Acta Obstet Gynecol Scand.* 2002;81:25-30.

Barton JR, Hiett AK, Conover WB. The use of nifedipine during the postpartum period in patients with severe preeclampsia. *Am J Obstet Gynecol.* 1990;162:788-792.

Belfort MA, Anthony J, Kirshon B. Respiratory function in severe gestational proteinuric hypertension: the effects of rapid volume expansion and subsequent vasodilation with verapamil. *Br J Obstet Gynaecol.* 1991;98:964-972.

Bolte AC, Van Geijn HP, Dekker GA. Management and monitoring of severe preeclampsia (Review). *Eur J Obstet Gynecol Reprod Biol.* 2001;96:8-20.

Chames MC, Livingston JC, Ivester T, et al. Late postpartum eclampsia: a preventable disease? *AM J Obstet Gynecol.* 2002;186:1174-1177.

Diagnosis and management of preeclampsia and eclampsia. *ACOG Practice Bulletin, No 33.* 2002;99:159-167.

Katz VL, Farmer R, Kuller JA. Preeclampsia into eclampsia: toward a new paradigm. *Am J Obstet Gynecol.* 2000;182: 1389-1396.

MacKay AP, Berg CJ, Atrash HI. Pregnancy related mortality from preeclampsia and eclampsia. *Obstet Gynecol.* 2001;97: 533-538.

Magee L, Sadeghi S. Prevention and treatment of postpartum hypertension. *Cochrane Database Syst Rev.* 2005;1: CD004351.

Magee LA, Cham C, Waterman EJ, Ohlsson A, Von Dadelszen P. Hydralazine for treatment of severe hypertension in pregnancy: meta analysis. *BMJ.* 2003;327:955-960.

Magee LA, Miremadi S, Li J, Cheng C, et al. Therapy with both magnesium sulfate and nifedipine does not increase the risk of serious magnesium-related maternal side effects in women with preeclampsia. *Am J Obstet Gynecol.* 2005;193: 153-163.

Magee LA, von Dadelszen P. The management of severe hypertension. *Semin Perinatol.* 2009;33:138-142.

O'Brien JM, Shumate SA, Satchwell SL, et al. Maternal benefit of corticosteroids therapy in patients with HELLP (hemolysis, elevated liver enzymes, and low platelet count) syndrome: impact on the rate of regional anesthesia. *Am J Obstet Gynecol.* 2002;186:475-479.

Report of the National High Blood Pressure Education Program Working Group on High Blood Pressure in Pregnancy. *Am J Obstet Gynecol.* 2000;183: 1S-22S.

Scardo JA, Vermillion ST, Newman RB, et al. A randomized, double-blind, hemodynamic evaluation of nifedipine and labetalol in preeclamptic hypertensive emergencies. *Am J Obstet Gynecol.* 1999;181(4):862-866.

Sibai BM, Barton JR. Expectant management of severe preeclampsia remote from term: patient selection, treatment, and delivery indications. *Am J Obstet Gynecol.* 2007;196: 514.e1-514.e9.

Sibai BM, Mabie WC, Harvey CJ, Gonzalez AR. Pulmonary edema in severe preeclampsia: analysis of thirty-seven consecutive cases. *Am J Obstet Gynecol.* 1987;156:1174-1178.

The Magpie Trial Collaborative Group. Do women with preeclampsia and their babies benefit from magnesium sulfate? The Magpie Trial. *Lancet.* 2002;359:1877-1890.

Vadhera RB, Pacheco LD, Hankins GDV. Acute antihypertensive therapy in pregnancy-induced hypertension. Is Nicardipine the answer? *Am J Perinatol.* 2009;26(7):495-499.

Vigil-De Gracia P, Lasso M, Ruiz E, et al. Severe hypertension in pregnancy: hydralazine or labetalol. A randomized clinical trial. *Eur J Obstet Gynecol Reprod Biol.* 2006;128: 157-62.

Witlin AG, Mattar F, Sibai BM. Postpartum stroke: a twenty-year experience. *Am J Obstet Gynecol.* 2000;183:83-88.

Obesity in the Obstetric Intensive Care Patient

CHAPTER 6

• *Jordan H. Perlow*

The clear but unfortunate trend toward a sedentary lifestyle and unhealthful eating habits has contributed to the so-called "obesogenic" state of American society. Ironically, and despite the decades long availability of dietetic, fat-free, low-fat, sugar-free, and low-calorie foods and beverages, not to mention the ubiquitous presence of health clubs in most communities, there are more obese Americans today than at any previous time in our history. While the number of obese Americans stood at just 13% in 1962, presently, nearly two-thirds of US women are overweight or obese, with the highest prevalence in the non–Hispanic-Black population. Since 1980, obesity rates have doubled for adults and tripled for those aged 12 to 19 years. Only one state (Colorado) has a current prevalence of obesity less than 20%. This unfortunate "state of the weight" in the United States may ultimately undo the steady gains in overall health we have enjoyed as Americans since the dawn of the twentieth century, and now contributes to the deaths of 300,000 Americans annually.

The remarkably high prevalence of this condition and its significant negative impact on overall health makes its prevention and treatment a top priority for all health-care disciplines. Obese women are at significantly increased risk for myriad medical complications, cancers, and premature sudden death (Table 6-1). Coexisting diabetes is a particularly significant co-morbidity and affects nearly 10 million US obese women, with its prevalence having increased 61% since 1991. Nearly 4% of the overall adult female population is both obese and diabetic. Obesity in pregnancy has also been recognized as a significant contributor to an increased use of health-care resources, contributing to the ever-increasing costs of care.

Obesity should be of particular interest and importance to those providing health care to women because age-adjusted rates of obesity for women of all races significantly exceeds those for males. As with many other adverse health measures, disparity in obesity exists. African Americans are now noted to have a 51% higher prevalence of obesity, when compared to Caucasians, while the increased prevalence for Hispanics is noted at 21%. Additionally, disparity in obesity rates amongst children is noted with the startling finding that 1 in 7 low-income preschool-aged children are now obese. The percentage of overweight children (ages 6-11) has doubled since the early 1980s, while the percentage of overweight adolescents has nearly tripled! African American women incur the greatest number of years of life lost to obesity-related premature mortality.

Obesity has long been perceived as a risk factor in pregnancy. Research over several decades has consistently demonstrated that the obese gravida is at risk for adverse perinatal outcome. While statistically significant risks for complications affecting fetal, neonatal, and maternal well-being have been demonstrated uniformly in the literature, the busy practitioner of contemporary obstetrics needs no "p value" or "relative risk" statistic to be keenly aware of the prevalence of obesity within the gravid population, and the complications and challenges posed by obesity in the care of these patients. Even the most dreadful of obstetric complications, maternal death, appears to be on the rise in the twenty-first century, with obesity considered a primary contributor. Thus, these patients are indeed at risk and deserving our intense efforts to minimize morbidity and mortality when possible, and thus improve

61

■ **TABLE 6-1.** Medical Complications of Obesity

Sudden death	Gout
Stroke	Osteoarthritis
Coronary artery	Digestive diseases
disease	Cholelithiasis
Hypertension/	Hiatus hernia
Cardiomyopathy	Pulmonary function impairment,
Thromboembolic	obstructive sleep apnea/
disease	pulmonary hypertension,
Diabetes mellitus	asthma
Dyslipidemias	Hepatic steatosis
Carcinoma	Endocrine abnormalities
Colon	Menstrual disorders
Gallbladder	Infertility
Ovary	Polycystic ovary disease
Endometrium	Psychosocial disorders
Breast	Depression, mood, and
Cervix	anxiety disorders
Compromised	
obstetric outcome	
Anesthetic	
complications	
Dermatologic	
diseases	
Acanthosis	
nigricans	
Gragilitas cutis	
inguinalis	

■ **TABLE 6-2.** Body Mass Index and Obesity

Definition	BMI (kg/m²)	Obesity class
Underweight	<18.5	
Normal	18.5-24.9	
Overweight	25.0-29.9	
Obese	30.0-34.9	I
	35.0-39.9	II
Extreme obesity	≥40	III

an individual's weight status, and as such to determine if one is obese.

$$Body\ mass\ index = \frac{Patient\ Weight\ (kg)}{Patient\ Height\ (m^2)}$$

Categories of obesity have also been defined (Table 6-2). The term "overweight" refers to an excess of body weight compared to set standards, with the excess weight coming from muscle, bone, fat, and/or body water. Obesity, however, is defined as "an excess of body fat frequently resulting in impairment of health." Therefore, rarely, an individual (bodybuilder) could be overweight but not obese. Obesity is usually caused by an excess of caloric intake versus expenditure; however, its cause is primarily multifactorial accounting for 99% of all patients with obesity. A small percent may be caused by a diverse group of neurologic and endocrine disorders (Table 6-3). An adult with a BMI >30 kg/m² is considered to be obese, while an individual with a BMI calculation between 25 and 29.9 kg/m² is considered overweight. Recently, the terms "very obese" and "extremely obese" were utilized to indicate Class II and Class III obesity in an evaluation of obesity during pregnancy and health-care utilization. Other methods of estimating body fat and body fat distribution include measurements of skinfold thickness and waist circumference, calculation of waist-to-hip circumference ratios, and techniques such as ultrasound, computed tomography, and magnetic resonance imaging.

Unfortunately, the most severe degree of obesity, Class 3 obesity (BMI ≥40) is increasing rapidly, and is associated with the most morbid health complications. Nearly 6% of the adult population and more than 14% of non–Hispanic-Black women can now be classified as such. During

perinatal outcome. As such, the complications of obesity and its relation to the obstetric intensive care patient cannot be overemphasized. This chapter will serve to inform the reader of the various aspects of critical obstetric care for the obese gravida, reviewing antepartum, intrapartum, and postpartum considerations.

■ DEFINITIONS AND PREVALENCE

Obesity has been defined and described in a variety of descriptive ways. Terms such as severe, extreme, super, massive, morbid, and even "grotesque" appear in the literature to describe different degrees of obesity. Historically, standardized descriptive definitions were lacking; however, currently the body mass index (BMI) is used to categorize

TABLE 6-3. Obesity: Differential Diagnosis (<1% of Etiology)	
Hypothyroidism	Insulinoma
Prader Willi syndrome	Adiposogenital dystrophy
Laurence-Moon syndrome	Partial lipodystrophy
Hypothalamic pathology	Polycystic ovaries
Craniopharyngioma	Cushing syndrome
Hypogonadism	

TABLE 6-4. Obesity and Perinatal Outcome: Fetal/Neonatal Risk

Preterm birth
Increased perinatal mortality
Low Apgar scores
Intrauterine growth restriction
Low birth weight
Macrosomia/large for gestational age
Post dates
Shoulder dystocia/birth trauma
Intensive care nursery admission
Neonatal/childhood obesity
Congenital malformations
  Spina bifida, omphalocele, heart defects, multiple
  anomalies

pregnancy, 25% of women have been noted to be >200 lb at their first prenatal visit, and more than 10% are >250 lb. Approximately 1 in 20 women will be ≥300 lb when initiating prenatal care. The ubiquity and increasing prevalence of obesity only serves to magnify the consequences of associated adverse perinatal outcomes.

Given the health implications of obesity and the desire to minimize risks, pharmacologic and surgical approaches to the treatment of obesity have been developed, when lifestyle modification is unsuccessful. Bariatric surgery has become quite common and is seen not uncommonly among patients of reproductive age. A BMI of 40 (or 35 in the presence of other medical co-morbidities) is a general indication for consideration of bariatric surgery. While patients undergoing these procedures have shown overall improvements in health measures and reduced mortality, reports have shown an increased risk for gastric band complications during pregnancy and nutritional deficiencies have been reported. Gastrointestinal hemorrhage and other procedure-related complications, including fetal and maternal death, have been reported during pregnancy. Pregnant patients with a history of gastric surgery for obesity should be counseled appropriately and surveillance during prenatal care heightened. Patients with this surgical history with abdominal complaints should be evaluated thoroughly and without delay, and physical findings consistent with an acute abdomen should be evaluated with a low threshold for surgical consultation and exploration.

Perinatal Outcomes

Perinatal outcome is compromised among pregnancies complicated by obesity (Tables 6-4 and 6-5). The obese pregnant woman and her fetus are at risk for a variety of complications during pregnancy, with even a significant percentage of maternal deaths now determined to be associated with obesity. Some risks are inherent to chronic medical

conditions commonly seen in this patient population, such as pregestational diabetes and chronic hypertension. Other risks are independent of preexisting disease, and include greater risks for hypertensive disorders of pregnancy,

TABLE 6-5. Obesity and Perinatal Outcome: Maternal Risks

Infection
Maternal mortality
  Aspiration/failed intubation
  Hemorrhage
  Thromboembolism
  Stroke
Dysfunctional labor
Cesarean section: Primary/repeat/emergent
Failed vaginal birth after cesarean (VBAC)
Cesarean section
  Operative and anesthetic morbidities
  Increased blood loss
  Increased endometritis
  Prolonged operative time
  Failed epidural placement/failed intubation
  Respiratory complications (atelectasis, pneumonia)
  Wound infection/dehiscence
  Thromboembolism
Medical Complications (see Table 6-1)
  Chronic hypertension
  Diabetes: Pregestational and gestation DM
  Preeclampsia
Prolonged hospitalization
Urinary tract infection

gestational diabetes, labor abnormalities, postpartum hemorrhage, and cesarean delivery. Those women requiring cesarean section run further perioperative risks of blood loss, infection, and thrombotic complications. The neonate born to the obese mother has also been noted to be at significantly increased risk for adverse outcome including congenital malformations, low Apgar scores, intrauterine growth restriction, preterm delivery, low birth weight, macrosomia/large for gestational age, birth trauma, and intensive care requirement.

■ PATHOPHYSIOLOGY

Physiologic Changes in the Obese Pregnant Patient

In pregnancy, blood volume and cardiac output increase approximately 40% with further increases of cardiac output during labor and delivery, reaching values 80% greater than prepregnancy values. Obesity accentuates these changes as blood volume and cardiac output expand in proportion to the increase in fat and tissue mass.

Obese patients have marked abnormal changes in respiratory physiology (Table 6-6). In fact, obese gravidae have markedly diminished functional residual capacity, and except for residual volume, all lung volumes, vital capacity and total lung capacity are reduced. Obese parturients have also been shown to have diminished Po_2 and chest wall/lung compliance. Total compliance in obesity diminishes by an average of 50%, which is equivalent to placing a 50-lb weight on the chest and abdomen of a non-obese patient! These respiratory changes in the obese parturients cause the work of breathing to be increased three times the normal. Morbid obesity may

---

■ TABLE 6-6. Physiology: Obesity and Cardiopulmonary Function

Diminished lung volumes and capacities
Decreased lung/chest wall compliance
Decreased breathing efficiency/gas exchange
Relative hypoxia
    Pulmonary shunt→Cardiac compensation
    Blood/plasma volume≠cardiac work
    Ischemia/infarction→↓cardiac efficiency
(cardio)-Failure-(respiratory)
    cor pulmonale
Pulmonary hypertension←Obesity/Hypoventilation
    Syndrome (Pickwickian syndrome)

---

also be associated with obstructive sleep apnea, which can predispose to right-sided heart failure and secondary pulmonary hypertension. Given the increased mortality rate associated with pulmonary hypertension of any cause, appropriate evaluation of obese patients with a history of obstructive sleep apnea or sleep disorders is recommended. Treatment with nasal continuous positive airway pressure (CPAP) may be helpful and improve outcome. The increase in cardiac work in these patients should also be considered in the evaluation of underlying cardiac dysfunction. Consideration for performing maternal echocardiography is reasonable, especially for Class III obese patients and those with coexisting hypertension to rule out cardiomyopathy.

■ INTRAPARTUM MANAGEMENT

The intrapartum management of the obese patient in labor is truly a multidisciplinary team effort (Table 6-7). The obstetrical physician, labor and delivery nurse, obstetric anesthesiologist, and nurse anesthetist form the primary components of the team. Medical consultants who have evaluated the patient for coexisting medical complications should be notified of the patient's admission to labor and delivery, or called upon for consultation if previously unrecognized medical complications are diagnosed. A thorough history and physical examination should be undertaken upon the patients admission to labor and delivery.

Given the marked physiologic changes occurring in the obese gravid patient and the high probability of coexisting medical complications, it is suggested that obese patients at highest risk (eg, Class II, III) have an anesthesia consultation; preferably during the antepartum period, or at the time of admission to labor and delivery. In addition to careful evaluation of the patient's cardiovascular and pulmonary status, meticulous assessment of the patient's airway is critical. This cannot be overemphasized, as it has been reported that 80% of all anesthesia-related maternal mortality occurred among obese patients and the inability to accomplish endotracheal intubation was the principal cause. Securing intravenous access and accurate blood pressure monitoring may also prove challenging due to the obese body habitus. The use of central venous access and an arterial line may be helpful in individual cases.

Particular attention should be given to the obese gravida's laboring position with the left lateral position preferred to increase maternal oxygenation and uteroplacental blood flow and prevent aorto-caval compression. Obese patients may also benefit from elevation of the head

■ **TABLE 6-7. Obesity and Pregnancy: Intrapartum and Postpartum Management of Challenges**

Obesity-related problem/risk solutions/adjuncts	Potential
Increased respiratory work/lateral laboring	Epidural anesthesia, oxygen, left myocardial O^2 requirement position
Difficult peripheral IV access	Central IV line
Inaccurate or difficult BP monitoring	Arterial line
Preexisting cardiopulmonary disease	Continuous ECG, ABG, CXR, pulse oximetry, prenatal echocardiography/cardiology, pulmonary consultations
Increased risks of general anesthesia, epidural catheter	Anesthesia consultation/prophylactic
Difficult emergent regional placement	Prophylactic epidural catheter/regional anesthesia
Difficult intubation probable	Capability for awake intubation/fiberoptics
Aspiration risks	Prophylactic epidural
	H2 antagonist (Ranitidine HCl 50 mg IV q 6-8 h, 45 min prior to surgery) or PPI omeprazole 40 mg IV qd.
	Sodium citrate with citric acid (Bictra) (30 mL of 0.3 M prior to anesthesia)
	Metoclopramide (10 mg IV over 1-2 min, 45 min prior to surgery)
	NPO status in labor
Thromboembolic risks	Low-dose heparin (5000-10,000 units SQ every 8-12 h) TED hose (thigh high)
	Sequential pneumatic compression device (thigh high)
	Early post operative ambulation
	Minimize operative/immobilization times
Endometritis/wound infection	Prophylactic antibiotic (broad spectrum, prior to incision)
	Thorough skin preparation
	Pelvic/wound irrigation (consider placing antibiotics in the irrigant)
	Surgical drains
	Subcutaneous sutures

and chest to prevent airway closure and improve oxygenation as well as overall comfort. Continuous pulse oximetry will provide the clinician with important information with respect to maternal oxygen saturation and allow for ongoing evaluation of hypoxemia and guide the administration of supplemental oxygen as needed. Another important aspect of labor management includes maximizing pulmonary function and decreasing myocardial oxygen requirements. Recall that the obese gravida's respiratory work requirement is approximately three times that for the gravida of ideal body weight. Epidural anesthesia is beneficial, as it decreases respiratory work, improves oxygenation, and by decreasing the perception of pain, can decrease the release of catecholamines, which cause increased cardiac work (output).

Operative Management

Perhaps the most important aspect of epidural anesthesia lies in the fact that in an emergent situation, should cesarean section be required, a regional anesthetic can be administered through the existing catheter. It has been shown that neonatal outcome is not compromised by this approach. This is critically important as at least 90% of maternal deaths from anesthetic causes are attributed to general anesthesia, primarily due to complications of aspiration of gastric contents and failed endotracheal intubation.

The risks of general anesthesia for the obese parturient are intensified due to greater difficulty in intubation secondary to anatomic barriers, a greater gastric volume with lower pH and diminished barrier pressure (difference between lower esophageal sphincter tone minus intragastric pressure). Therefore, regional anesthesia should be considered the anesthetic of choice unless contraindications exist. Such contraindications may include coagulopathy, thrombocytopenia, maternal therapeutic anticoagulation, recent use of low-molecular-weight heparin, hemodynamic instability, acute hemorrhage, and infection over the site of planned needle insertion. With increased utilization of regional anesthesia, one would anticipate a significant impact on the reduction of anesthetic-related maternal mortality. Also, as it has been shown that the placement of regional anesthesia is often difficult in the obese gravida, as evidenced by the increased number of attempts needed, the "prophylactic" placement of an epidural catheter nonemergently in the obese laboring patient should be strongly considered in the intrapartum management of these patients.

Other benefits of regional anesthesia include reduction in postoperative pulmonary complications in obese patients. Long-acting spinal or epidural narcotics may be administered for postoperative analgesia, and their use reduces risks of respiratory depression from parenteral narcotics. Additionally, patients treated in this manner will ambulate earlier, which is likely to decrease risk of thromboembolic complications.

As acidic aspirate from the patient's stomach can cause severe pulmonary injury, patients should receive prophylactic administration of a non-particulate antacid (30 mL of 0.3 M sodium citrate; Bicitra) just prior to anesthesia induction (general or regional) and have the dose repeated each hour if surgery continues beyond 1 hour for the patient with regional anesthesia. In patients at high risk for aspiration, the use of an H2 receptor blocker (eg, ranitidine, 150 mg po or 50 mg IV), proton-pump inhibitors [PPIs] (eg, omeprazole, 40 mg IV), and/or dopamine antagonists (eg, metoclopramide, 10 mg slowly IV) administered during labor may be helpful in reducing the sequelae of aspiration should this potentially lethal complication occur. At least 60 minutes are required for H2 antagonists to decrease gastric acidity to a "safe pH" if given parenterally. Therefore, their use is preferred on admission and during labor rather than in the acute situation. For scheduled cases or inductions of obese gravidae, ranitidine may be administered the night prior to surgery and then repeated on admission to the hospital and at appropriate intervals thereafter. Bicitra should also be administered in addition to an H2 receptor blocker if cesarean section is required. These prophylactic measures will raise the gastric pH >3.0 in nearly 99% of patients. The importance of these measures cannot be overemphasized as pneumonitis and respiratory failure resulting from aspiration of gastric contents has been the most common single cause of maternal mortality related to anesthetic causes accounting for 25% of 2700 maternal deaths from 1979 to 1986, and given the inherent respiratory compromise which exists for these patients.

In situations where evaluation of the patient's airway indicates the probability of difficult intubation, awake intubation and fiberoptic laryngoscopy should be considered. The environment of care should be capable of attending to these specialized needs or consideration for maternal transport to a fully equipped facility with specialists capable of managing these anesthetic challenges should be undertaken. Therefore, to decrease the risk of maternal morbidity and mortality associated with general anesthesia in the obese gravida, regional anesthesia should be considered the anesthesia of choice for cesarean delivery when not contraindicated.

Recent data indicate that obesity doubles the likelihood for cesarean section even among a "low-risk" obese population receiving midwifery care and that over the past 20 years, obesity-related cesarean deliveries have tripled. Furthermore, the risk for emergent cesarean section is also increased. The obese gravida has been uniformly found to be at increased risk for perioperative morbidity associated with cesarean section. These morbidities include the unsuccessful initial placement of the epidural catheter and the need for extended time periods to surgically deliver the fetus when compared to controls. These findings again emphasize the potential benefit of the "prophylactic epidural," as discussed above. Other risks noted for the obese gravida undergoing cesarean section include prolonged operative and delivery times, increased blood loss, prolonged hospitalization, and a nearly 10-fold increase in postoperative endomyometritis and wound infection. Furthermore, the success rate for VBAC (failed vaginal birth after cesarean) in the massively obese woman has been found to be just 15% with more than 50% of these VBAC attempts complicated by infectious morbidity. Given the potential need for urgent cesarean section in the course of VBAC and the potential for significant surgical and anesthetic morbidity for these women, counseling for

VBAC in this population should be tailored to include these important unique issues.

Various adjuncts to perioperative care have been utilized to prevent morbidities associated with cesarean section in the obese population. Infectious complications of cesarean section are particularly common among the obese population undergoing cesarean section. Prophylactic antibiotics have been found to be the most significant protective factor in the reduction of postoperative wound infection and endometritis. H2 receptor blockers, PPIs, and metoclopramide to prevent the risk of aspiration (discussed above), thromboembolic preventative stockings, intermittent sequential compression devices for the lower extremities, and low-dose prophylactic unfractionated or fractionated heparin to decrease thromboembolic complications have not been studied in the setting of randomized clinical trials. Therefore, there is little definitive data regarding the utility of these adjuncts, specifically in the obese obstetric population.

Cesarean Section "Pearls" for the Obese Gravida

1. **O:** OXYGEN: Decrease maternal myocardial oxygen requirement with adequate analgesia; preferably the "prophylactic epidural." Increase fetal oxygenation by laboring/positioning the patient at a "left-tilt." Monitor maternal oxygen saturation and supplement oxygen as needed.
2. **B:** BLOOD: Blood loss is greater and postpartum hemorrhage risk is increased. Be sure to supplement patients during prenatal care with iron if anemic. Have the patient typed and crossed as necessary, as the potential need for blood transfusion is foreseeable.
3. **E:** EQUIPMENT: Be certain to have appropriate equipment that can withstand the weight of the obese gravida; surgical table, commode, wheelchair. Be sure that surgical instruments are appropriately sized. The Alexis Retractor can help provide excellent exposure.
4. **S:** STAFF: Having sufficient and appropriately trained staff is critical. Surgical assistance is required; not optional. Anesthesiology staff trained in fiberoptic intubation may be critical to a good outcome. Compassion, in addition to skill is mandatory from all staff members.
5. **I:** INTUBATION RISK: Failed intubation is a cause of maternal death, especially in the obese gravida. A "prophylactic epidural" can minimize this risk and should be strongly considered. Preoperative measures to reduce gastric acidity should be taken.
6. **T:** THROMBOPROPHYLAXIS: Pregnancy is a risk factor for life-threatening deep venous thrombosis. Additive risks are cesarean section and obesity. Take measures to prevent this complication. Sequential compression devices should be uniformly placed preoperatively, and individual consideration given to the use of heparin.
7. **Y:** YES, WE CAN!: While the challenges of caring for the obese gravida can be numerous, especially the seemingly insurmountable operative difficulties of cesarean section in the extremely obese, a positive attitude, combined with good physician-patient communication, meticulous preparation, and ongoing provider education will contribute to positive outcomes in these high-risk scenarios.

Nevertheless, while further study is encouraged, it is suggested that the potential benefit of reducing significant life-threatening morbidities among the obese gravid population would outweigh the potential risks of these prophylactic interventions. Given that maternal obesity is a high-risk factor for maternal mortality and a large proportion of that mortality is related to thromboembolic complications, it would seem that a risk/benefit evaluation would favor the use of low-dose pharmacologic thromboprophylaxis in the obese population, particularly those women with a BMI $\geq$40 (Class III obesity). It is suggested that sequential compression devices be placed on the lower extremities preoperatively. The patient can then be administered 5000 to 10,000 units of unfractionated heparin subcutaneously every 8 to 12 hours postoperatively until the patient is fully ambulatory. Alternatively, an adjusted dose protocol to achieve subtherapeutic peak anti-factor Xa heparin activity levels of 0.11 to 0.25 U/mL may be considered. This regimen has been used among obese patients undergoing gastric bypass surgery and found to be effective and with minimal complications. Patients who may receive or who have received regional anesthesia *are not* candidates for low-molecular-weight heparin due to an increased risk of spinal and epidural hematoma formation.

Incision Choice

Given a lack of randomized clinical trials, the incision of choice for cesarean section in obese patients is not entirely clear. Nevertheless, it has been shown that vertical skin incisions are associated with an approximate 12-fold greater risk of wound complications (defined as the necessity to reopen the wound) compared to a transverse incision. While a vertical incision may offer the most rapid entry into the obese abdominal cavity, stated benefits of the transverse incision include a more secure closure, less fat transaction, and less postoperative pain. Perhaps the most compelling reason to utilize a transverse incision in the obese gravida is its association with a diminished risk for atelectasis and hypoxemia postoperatively and decreased pain leading to earlier ambulation and deep breathing, all critically important given the increased risk for pulmonary and thromboembolic complications. Criticisms of the Pfannenstiel incision include the placement of a surgical wound in the warm, moist intertriginous area beneath the panniculus, potentially increasing the risk of infection, more difficult surgical exposure, and the inability to explore the upper abdomen.

A suggested approach would include the cephalad retraction of the pannus utilizing Montgomery straps. This permits exposure of the lower abdomen, allowing the low transverse abdominal incision to be made through a minimum of adipose tissue (Fig 6-1). At times, however, the pannus may be too large to accomplish retraction and doing so may lead to marked cardiorespiratory compromise in the patient with a massive panniculus or the retraction results in the pannus becoming a vertical "wall" of tissue prohibiting access to the lower abdomen. In this situation, or alternatively, a transverse or vertical periumbilical incision may be utilized. This allows for excellent exposure without pannus retraction and the potential for cardiorespiratory compromise (Fig 6-2). The incision circumvents the intertriginous area beneath the pannus and avoids the thick and edematous portion of the panniculus transected in "high Pfannenstiel" or low vertical incisions. The supraumbilical vertical skin incision with a fundal uterine incision with breech extraction of the vertex fetus (in conjunction with bilateral tubal ligation) has been shown to have similar postoperative morbidity in morbidly obese patients when compared to a low transverse abdominal incision. Some have advocated the superiority of surgical technique using less sharp dissection and greater use of manual manipulation of the tissues as in the Joel-Cohen incision and Misgav Ladach method for cesarean section. These techniques have yet to be studied specifically in the obese population, but in principle

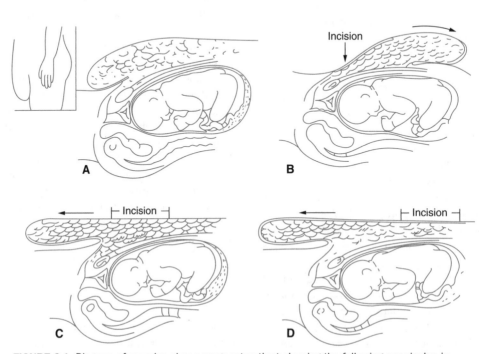

FIGURE 6-1. Diagram of massive obese pregnant patient showing the following panniculus in place: (A). placement of a Pfannensteil incision following retraction of the panniculus, (B). location of a low midline vertical incision above the panniculus, and (C). placement of a midline vertical incision higher in the abdomen and (D) periumbilically.

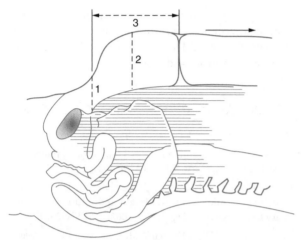

FIGURE 6-2. Possible sites of abdominal incisions. The panniculus retracted in the direction of the solid arrow.
1 = low suprasymphyseal transverse abdominal incision;
2 = high suprasymphyseal transverse abdominal incision;
3 = low vertical midline abdominal.
A supraumbilical vertical or transverse incision may be considered after careful individual assessment of body habitus.

they are worthy of consideration for this high-risk group. At times it may be helpful to use vacuum extraction assistance at the time of cesarean section on markedly obese patients. The forces generated with fundal pressure as the vertex is typically delivered at cesarean section will be dissipated throughout the large abdominal body mass of the patient and is therefore often times not helpful in assisting with delivery. One cannot overstate the importance of preparedness. Having sufficient surgical assistance, appropriate-sized instruments and ideally a preoperative assessment of body habitus and its relation to the surgical approach are critical to achieve the best outcome possible given challenging clinical circumstances.

Uterine closure can be undertaken in the usual manner with close attention to hemostasis. Operative times are longer and blood loss greater in this population. Often, visualization of the operative field can be compromised and obviously, care must be taken with sharp instruments in a "visually challenged" surgical field. As needle-stick injuries occur commonly and given the risks for infectious disease transmission through these accidents, consideration for blunt-tip needle use should be given. These needles work well with cesarean section. The use of a specific retractor for the obese patient (Alexis-O; Applied Medical, Rancho Santa Margarita, CA) may assist in providing exposure to the surgical site. Fascial closure requires special attention. If a vertical incision is utilized, a Smead-Jones- or modified Smead-Jones closure is preferred (Fig 6-3). Skillful transverse fascial closure, which provides the majority of wound strength during the healing process, is critical. A simple running suture is appropriate utilizing #1 or #2 delayed absorbable or permanent suture. Wide "bites"

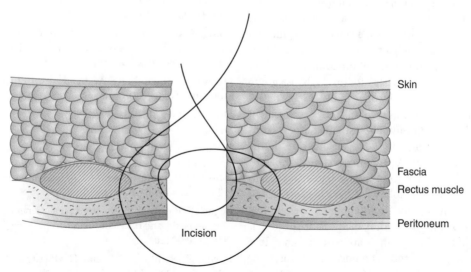

Skin

Fascia
Rectus muscle

Peritoneum

Incision

FIGURE 6-3. Diagram showing placement of a Smead-Jones suture.

incorporating more than 1 cm of fascial tissue from the cut edge should be utilized, stitch intervals should be no greater than 1 cm apart and excessive tension should be avoided to prevent fascial necrosis, the primary cause of dehiscence. The placement of closed surgical drains within the subcutaneous tissue has been studied in randomized fashion and while results have been conflicting, the preponderance of literature would suggest a decreased likelihood of wound complications with obliteration of the subcutaneous space with either sutures or closed suction drainage when the subcutaneous tissue is at least 2 cm in depth. An individualized surgical approach to the clinical situation is always appropriate.

Sterile skin staples may be used for skin closure; however, one should be careful not to remove them prematurely in the obese patient. Good clinical judgement and close wound inspection prior to hospital discharge will determine which patients may need to return as outpatients for staple removal several days post discharge.

At least daily postoperative patient evaluation should focus on early detection of complications, including pneumonia, atelectasis, urinary tract infection, endometritis, wound infection, and deep venous thrombosis (DVT). Early ambulation and incentive spirometry is encouraged to minimize pulmonary and thrombotic risks, respectively. Finally, these patients should be given thorough discharge instructions including the signs and symptoms of wound infection and dehiscence, endomyometritis, thromboembolic complications (DVT and pulmonary embolism), and diligent follow-up with respect to the continued management of any existing medical complications.

In conclusion, the management and care of the obese gravida is extremely challenging and laden with significant risks. Our interventions and attention to detail may allow us to markedly improve perinatal outcome and reduce maternal morbidity and mortality for this high-risk group of pregnant women. Hopefully one's efforts in this regard will also allow for the development of a physician-patient relationship built upon mutual trust and rapport, contributing to a "long-term" influence of our care on the patient's obese condition. As prevention should always be the hallmark of the best medical approach to disease management, it should be emphasized here in closing that appropriate follow-up for counseling on weight loss opportunities, be they behavioral, medical, or surgical, is critical. Weight loss through these approaches can reduce risk in future pregnancy, and in no uncertain terms, these patients should be counseled to achieve a normal BMI prior to subsequent pregnancy. Preconception counseling should be strongly recommended. Truly, any impact made in this regard has the potential for tremendous health benefit over the patient's entire life and in subsequent pregnancy.

BIBLIOGRAPHY: RECOMMENDED READINGS

Epidemiology

Adams TD, Gress RE, Smith SC, et al. Long-term mortality after gastric bypass surgery. *N Engl J Med.* 2007;357:753-761.

Bibbins-Domingo K, Coxson P, Pletcher MJ, Lightwood J, Goldman L. Adolescent overweight and future adult coronary heart disease. *N Engl J Med.* 2007;357:2371-2379.

Chu SY, Bachman DJ, Callaghan WM, et al. Association between obesity during pregnancy and increased use of health care. *N Engl J Med.* 2008;358:1444-1453.

Dietz WH, Robinson TN. Clinical practice. Overweight children and adolescents. *N Engl J Med.* 2005;352:2100-2109.

Flegal KM, Carroll MD, Ogden CL, Curtin LR. Prevalence and trends in obesity among US Adults, 1999-2008. *JAMA.* 2010 Jan 13. [Epub ahead of print]

Fontaine KR, Redden DT, Wang C, Westfall AO, Allison DB. Years of life lost due to obesity. *JAMA.* 2003 Jan 8;289(2):187-193.

Frank B Hu, *Obesity Epidemiology.* New York, NY: Oxford University Press; 2008. ISBN 978-0-19-531291-1.

Huda SS, Brodie LE, Sattar N. Obesity in pregnancy: prevalence and metabolic consequences. *Semin Fetal Neonatal Med.* 2009 Nov 5. [Epub ahead of print]

Mokdad AH, Ford ES, Bowman BA, et al. Prevalence of obesity, diabetes, and obesity-related health risk factors, 2001. *JAMA.* 2003;289:76-79.

Must A, Spadano J, Coakley EH, Field AE, Colditz G, Dietz WH. The disease burden associated with overweight and obesity. *JAMA.* 1999 Oct 27;282(16):1523-1529.

Overweight and Obesity. Available at http://www.cdc.gov/obesity/. Accessed December 20, 2009.

Owan T, Litwin SE. Is there a cardiomyopathy of obesity? *Curr Heart Fail Rep.* 2007;4:221-228.

Pereira MA, Kottke TE, Jordan C, O'Connor PJ, Pronk NP, Carreón R. Preventing and managing cardiometabolic risk: the logic for intervention. *Int J Environ Res Public Health.* 2009;6:2568-2584. Epub Sep 30, 2009.

Pischon T, Boeing H, Hoffmann K, et al. General and abdominal adiposity and risk of death in Europe. *N Engl J Med.* 2008; 359:2105-2120.

Pischon T, Nothlings U, Boeing H. Obesity and cancer. *Proc Nutr Soc.* 2008;67:128-145.

Power ML, Schulkin J. *The Evolution of Obesity.* Baltimore, MD: Johns Hopkins University Press; 2009. ISBN 978-0-8018-9262-2.

Stewart ST, Cutler DM, Rosen AB. Forecasting the effects of obesity and smoking on U.S. life expectancy. *N Engl J Med.* 2009;361:2252-2260.

Yanovski SZ, Yanovski JA. Obesity. *N Engl J Med.* 2002;346:591-602.

Yurcisin BM, Gaddor MM, DeMaria EJ. Obesity and bariatric surgery. *Clin Chest Med.* 2009;30:539-553.

Obesity and Perinatal Outcome

Arendas K, Qiu Q, Gruslin AJ. Obesity in pregnancy: preconceptional to postpartum consequences. *Obstet Gynaecol Can.* 2008;30:477-488.

Callaway LK, O'Callaghan M, McIntyre HD. Obesity and the hypertensive disorders of pregnancy. *Hypertens Pregnancy.* 2009;4:1-21.

Catalano PM. Management of obesity in pregnancy. *Obstet Gynecol.* 2007;109:419-433.

Freedman MA, Preston LW, George WM. Grotesque obesity: a serious complication of labor and delivery. *S Med J.* 1972;65:732-736.

Gross T, Sokol RJ, King K. Obesity in pregnancy: risks and outcome. *Obstet Gynecol.* 1980;56:446-450.

Lewis DF, Chesson AL, Edwards MS, Weeks JW, Adair CD. Obstructive sleep apnea during pregnancy resulting in pulmonary hypertension. *S Med J.* 1998;91:761-762.

Lu GC, Rouse DJ, DuBard M, Cliver S, Kimberlin D, Hauth JC. The effect of the increasing prevalence of maternal obesity on perinatal morbidity. *Am J Obstet Gynecol.* 2001;185:845-849.

Maasilta P, Bachour A, Teramo K, Polo O, Laitinen LA. Sleep-related disordered breathing during pregnancy in obese women. *Chest.* 2001;120:1448-1454.

Nelson SM, Matthews P, Poston L. Maternal metabolism and obesity: modifiable determinants of pregnancy outcome. *Human Reprod Update.* 2009 Dec 4. [Epub ahead of print].

Perlow JH, Morgan MA, Montgomery DM, Towers CV, Porto M. Perinatal outcome in pregnancy complicated by massive obesity. *Am J Obstet Gynecol.* 1992;167:958-962.

Wax JR. Risks and management of obesity in pregnancy: current controversies. *Curr Opin Obstet Gynecol.* 2009;21:117-123.

Bariatric Surgery and Pregnancy

Alexander CI, Liston WA. Operating on the obese woman-a review. *BJOG.* 2006;113:1167-1172.

American College of Obstetricians and Gynecologists. ACOG Practice Bulletin. Bariatric Surgery and Pregnancy. Number 105. June 2009.

Beard JH, Bell RL, Duffy AJ. Reproductive considerations and pregnancy after bariatric surgery: current evidence and recommendations. *Obes Surg.* 2008;18:1023-1027.

Guelinckx I, Devlieger R, Vansant G. Reproductive outcome after bariatric surgery: a critical review. *Human Reprod Update.* 2009;15:189-201.

Maggard MA, Yermilov I, Li Z, et al. Pregnancy and fertility following bariatric surgery: a systematic review. *JAMA.* 2008;300:2286-2296.

Sheiner E, Balaban E, Dreiher J, Levi I, Levy A. Pregnancy outcome in patients following different types of bariatric surgeries. *Obes Surg.* 2009;19:1286-1292.

Wax JR, Cartin A, Wolff R, Lepich S, Pinette MG, Blackstone J. Pregnancy following gastric bypass surgery for morbid obesity: maternal and neonatal outcomes. *Obes Surg.* 2008;18:540-544.

Wax JR, Cartin A, Wolff R, Lepich S, Pinette MG, Blackstone J. Pregnancy following gastric bypass surgery for morbid obesity: effect of surgery-to-conception interval on maternal and neonatal outcomes. *Obes Surg.* 2008;18:1517-1521.

Weintraub AY, Levy A, Levi I, Mazor M, Wiznitzer A, Sheiner E. Effect of bariatric surgery on pregnancy outcome. *Int J Gynaecol Obstet.* 2008;103:246-251.

Obesity and Surgical Risks, Cesarean Section

Beattie PG, Rings TR, Hunter MF, Lake Y. Risk factors for wound infection following caesarean section. *Aust N Z J Obstet Gynaecol.* 1994;34:398-402.

Berghella V, Baxter JK, Chauhan SP. Evidence-based surgery for cesarean delivery. *Am J Obstet Gynecol.* 2005;193:1607-1617.

Chauhan SP, Magann EF, Carroll CS, et al. Mode of delivery for the morbidly obese with prior cesarean delivery: vaginal versus repeat cesarean section. *Am J Obstet Gynecol.* 2001;185:349-354.

Dodd JM, Anderson ER, Gates S. Surgical techniques for uterine incision and uterine closure at the time of caesarean section. *Cochrane Database Syst Rev.* 2008 Jul 16;CD004732.

Gallup DG. Modifications of celiotomy techniques to decrease morbidity in obese gynecologic patients. *Am J Obstet Gynecol.* 1984;150:171-178.

Gross TL. Operative considerations in the obese pregnant patient. *Clin Perinatol.* 1983;10:411-421.

Greer JA. Prevention of venous thromboembolism in pregnancy. *Best Pract Res Clin Haematol.* 2003;16:261-278.

Hema KR, Hohanson R. Techniques for performing caesarean section. *Best Pract Res Clin Obstet Gynaecol.* 2001; 15: 17-47.

Houston MC, Raynor BD. Postoperative morbidity in the morbidly obese parturient woman: supraumbilical and low transverse abdominal approaches. *Om J Obstet Gynecol.* 2000;182:1033-1035.

Kamran SI, Downey D, Ruff RL. Pneumatic sequential compression reduces the risk of deep vein thrombosis in stroke patients. *Neurology.* 1998 Jun;50(6):1683-1688.

Krebs HB, Helmkamp FB. Transverse periumbilical incision in the massively obese patient. *Obstet Gynecol.* 1984;63: 241-245.

Magann EF, Chauhan SP, Rodts-Palenik S, et al. Subcutaneous stitch closure versus subcutaneous drain to prevent wound disruption after cesarean delivery: a randomized clinical trial. *Am J Obstet Gynecol.* 2002;186: 1119-1123.

Nielsen TF, Hokegard KH. Postoperative cesarean section morbidity: a prospective study. *Am J Obstet Gynecol.* 1983;146: 911-916.

Owens SM, Brozanski BS, Meyn LA, Wiesenfeld HC. Antimicrobial prophylaxis for cesarean delivery before skin incision. *Am J Obstet Gynecol.* 2009;114:573-579.

Perlow JH. Preventing needlestick injuries in obstetrics and gynecology: how can we improve the use of blunt tip needles in practice? *Obstet Gynecol.* 2008;111:1443-1444.

Perlow JH, Morgan MA. Massive obesity and perioperative cesarean morbidity. *Am J Obstet Gynecol.* 1994;170: 560-565.

Pisegna JR. Switching between intravenous and oral pantoprazole. *J Clin Gastroenterol.* 2001;32:27-32.

Ramsey PS, White AM, Guinn DA, et al. Subcutaneous tissue reapporximation alone or in combination with drain, in obese women undergoing cesarean delivery. *Obstet Gynecol.* 2005;105:967-973.

Shepherd MF, Rosborough TK, Schwartz ML. Heparin thromboprophylaxis in gastric bypass surgery. *Obes Surg.* 2003 Apr;13(2):249-253.

Sicuranza BJ, Tisdall LH. Cesarean section in the massively obese. *J Reprod Med.* 1975;14:10-11.

Smaill F, Hofmeyr GJ. Antibiotic prophylaxis for cesarean section. *Cochrane Database Syst Rev.* 2002;(3):CD000933.

Sullivan S, Williamson B, Wilson LK, Korte JE, Soper D. Blunt needles for the reduction of needlestick injuries during cesarean delivery: a randomized controlled trial. *Obstet Gynecol.* 2009;114:211-216.

Wolfe HM, Gross TL, Sokol RJ, Bottoms SF, Thompson KL. Determinants of morbidity in obese women delivered by cesarean. *Obstet Gynecol.* 1988;71:691-696.

Obesity, Pregnancy, and Anesthetic Morbidity and Mortality

Conklin KA. Can anesthetic-related maternal mortality be reduced? *Letter: Am J Obstet Gynecol.* 1990;163:253-254.

Endler GC. The risk of anesthesia in obese parturients. *J Perinatol.* 1990;10:175-179.

Endler GC, Mariona FG, Sokol RJ, Stevenson LB. Anesthesia-related maternal mortality in Michigan, 1972 to 1984. *Am J Obstet Gynecol.* 1988;159:187-193.

Hood DD, Dewan DM. Anesthetic and obstetric outcome in morbidly obese parturients. *Anesthesiology.* 1993;79: 1210-1218.

Jones T. Morbid obesity: a risk factor for maternal mortality. *Int J Obstet Anesth.* 2007;16:384-385. Epub 2007 Jul 20.

Maeder EC, Barno A, Mecklenburg F. Obesity: a maternal high-risk factor. *Obstet Gynecol.* 1975;45:669-672.

May JW, Greiss Jr FC. Maternal mortality in North Carolina: a forty-year experience. *Am J Obstet Gynecol.* 1989;161: 555-561.

Soens MA, Birnbach DJ, Ranasinghe JS, van Zundert A. Obstetric anesthesia for the obese and morbidly obese patient: an ounce of prevention is worth more than a pound of treatment. *Acta Anaesthesiol Scand.* 2008; 52:6-19.

CHAPTER 7

Thromboembolic Disease Complicating Pregnancy

• *Christina S. Han and Michael J. Paidas*

Thromboembolic disease is a major contributor to both perinatal and maternal morbidity and mortality worldwide, accounting for 14.9% of maternal deaths in 2006, according to the World Health Organization.[1] In developed countries, thromboembolism has risen above hemorrhage and hypertension as the leading cause of maternal mortality.[2] Venous thromboembolic diseases (VTE)—such as deep venous thrombosis (DVT), pulmonary embolism (PE), septic pelvic thrombophlebitis (SPT), and ovarian vein thrombosis (OVT)—complicate 0.76 to 1.72 per 1000 pregnancies.[3] The cornerstones of VTE management lie in prevention, accurate diagnosis, and prompt treatment. This chapter will review the etiology, diagnosis, treatment, and prevention of VTE.

■ REGULATION OF HEMOSTASIS

A detailed discussion of the clotting system, the anticoagulant system, and the fibrinolytic system is beyond the scope of this manual and can be found elsewhere in more comprehensive textbooks. A practical and user-friendly version of the complex regulatory pathways of hemostasis and fibrinolysis is presented in Fig 7-1.

Pregnancy

As a result of physiologic changes in pregnancy, VTE occurs at a rate that is fourfold higher compared to the nonpregnant state.[4] The postpartum period is even more thrombogenic, with VTE twice as likely as a given 6-week period during pregnancy. That VTE does not occur more often is remarkable, given the paradoxical challenges presented to the hemostatic system during pregnancy.

During early placentation, syncytiotrophoblasts penetrate maternal uterine vessels to establish the primordial uteroplacental circulation. Subsequently, endovascular extravillous cytotrophoblasts invade decidual and superficial myometrial spiral arteries, orchestrating a morphological conversion of these vessels to achieve high-volume, low-resistance blood flow into the intervillous space. Fetal survival requires that these processes occur in the absence of either significant decidual hemorrhage (ie, abruption) or intervillous thrombosis. To ensure maternal survival, decidual hemorrhage must be avoided throughout pregnancy.

The most profound hemostatic challenge is faced by mothers during the third stage of labor. Following separation of the placenta from the uterine wall after delivery of the infant, hemostasis must be rapidly achieved in 140 remodeled spiral arteries to avoid potentially catastrophic hemorrhage. While local factors such as high decidual tissue factor (aka thromboplastin) expression contribute to this placental site hemostasis, dramatic changes in the mother's expression of clotting and anticlotting factors are also required to meet this hemostatic challenge.

In addition to an innate hypercoagulability, venous stasis and vascular trauma complete Virchow's classic triad.[5] (See Fig 7-2.) Venous stasis is present as a result of mechanical impedance of the lower extremity vasculature by the gravid uterus, and estrogen-mediated vascular dilation.[6] Endothelial damage is often present during the puerperium, especially with operative delivery, hypertensive disease, tobacco use, and infections.

Risk Factors

In a review of International Classification of Disease-9 (ICD-9) codes from over nine million pregnancy

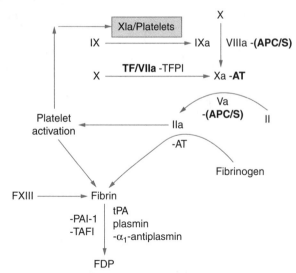

FIGURE 7-1. Hemostatic and fibrinolytic pathways. The primary initiator of coagulation is tissue factor (TF) which is not normally expressed by cells in contact with the circulation (ie, endothelial cells). Following vascular disruption, perivascular, cell membrane–bound TF complexes with plasma-derived factor VII or its more active form (VIIa) to directly convert factor X to Xa. TF/VIIa can also indirectly generate Xa by converting factor IX to IXa, which, in turn, complexes with factor VIIIa to convert X to Xa. Factor Xa, once generated, complexes with its cofactor, Va, to convert prothrombin (factor II) to thrombin (IIa). Thrombin activates platelets and cleaves fibrinogen to generate fibrin monomers, which spontaneously polymerize and are cross-linked by thrombin-activated factor XIIIa to form a stable clot. Clotting is restrained by a series of anticoagulant proteins. The initial anticoagulant response is by TF pathway inhibitor (TFPI) that binds to the TF/VIIa/Xa complex to rapidly stop TF-mediated clotting. However, thrombin-activated factor XIa maintains clotting by serving as an alternative activator of factor IX on the surface of platelets. Thus, effective inhibition of the clotting cascade requires prevention of factor IXa- and Xa-mediated clotting. Activated protein C and protein S (APC/S) complex serve this function by inactivating factors VIIIa and Va, respectively. However, the most crucial endogenous anticoagulant system involves antithrombin (AT) inactivation of thrombin and Xa directly. Finally, fibrinolysis breaks down the fibrin clot. Fibrinolysis is mediated by tissue-type plasminogen activator (tPA) that binds to fibrin where it activates plasmin. Plasmin, in turn, degrades fibrin but can be inactivated by α2-antiplasmin embedded in the fibrin clot. Fibrinolysis is primarily inhibited by type-1 plasminogen activator inhibitor (PAI-1), the fast inactivator of tPA. Thrombin activatable fibrinolytic inhibitor (TAFI) is an alternative antifibrinolytic protein.

admissions and over 73,000 postpartum admissions in the United States National Inpatient Sample (NIS), a list of medical and obstetrical risk factors for VTE was identified. See Tables 7-1 and 7-2 for a listing of common risk factors in the development of VTE.

Thrombophilia

Patients with underlying hypercoagulable states are at even higher risk for VTE and other obstetric adverse outcomes. These thrombophilic states can be divided into inheritable mutations and acquired disorders.

Inheritable Thrombophilia

The most common significant inherited thrombophilias include heterozygosity for the Factor V Leiden (FVL) mutation heterozygosity, and prothrombin G20210A (PGM) gene mutations. Rarer causes of inherited thrombophilias include: antithrombin (AT) deficiency, protein S deficiency, and protein C deficiency. See Table 7-3 for a summary of these thrombophilias, their respective inheritance patterns, and risks of thromboses.

Acquired Thrombophilia

The most common acquired thrombophilia is antiphospholipid antibody syndrome (APAS). Approximately 2% of APAS patients will experience a VTE in pregnancy, accounting for approximately 14% of VTE events in pregnancy. Diagnosis of APAS requires one clinical criterion and one laboratory criterion, as defined at the international consensus conference in 2006.[8] (See Table 7-4)

APAS is a thrombogenic disorder that arises from autoimmune targeting of proteins binding to exteriorized anionic phospholipids on endothelial cell membranes, such as cardiolipin and phosphatidylserine. In more than half of APAS patients, the responsible antibodies arise as a result of underlying disorders such as systemic lupus erythematosus (SLE). Diseases such as SLE induce endothelial compromise, which expose the anionic phospholipids that bind to specialized proteins, creating neoantigens recognized by the immune system. The antiphospholipid antibodies increase the thrombogenic potential by inhibiting anionic phospholipid-binding endogenous anticoagulants (such as β2-glycoprotein-I, annexin V, antithrombin, thrombomodulin, proteins C and S) and inducing procoagulants (such as tissue factor, plasminogen activator inhibitor-1, von Willebrand factor, and activation of complement).

The type and concentration of antiphospholipid antibody predict its pathogenicity. Low-positive anticardiolipin IgG and IgM are seldom associated with medical

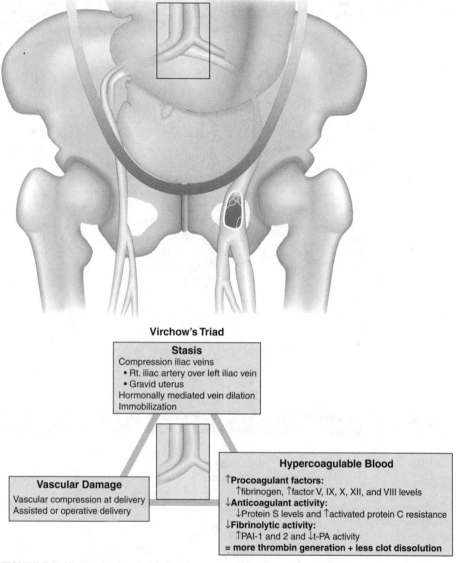

Virchow's Triad

Stasis
Compression iliac veins
• Rt. iliac artery over left iliac vein
• Gravid uterus
Hormonally mediated vein dilation
Immobilization

Vascular Damage
Vascular compression at delivery
Assisted or operative delivery

Hypercoagulable Blood
↑**Procoagulant factors:**
  ↑fibrinogen, ↑factor V, IX, X, XII, and VIII levels
↓**Anticoagulant activity:**
  ↓Protein S levels and ↑activated protein C resistance
↓**Fibrinolytic activity:**
  ↑PAI-1 and 2 and ↓t-PA activity
= **more thrombin generation + less clot dissolution**

FIGURE 7-2. Virchow's classic triad of hypercoagulability.

complications. Medium or high titers of anticardiolipin and presence of lupus anticoagulant are associated with fourfold higher rates of thrombosis.

■ DEEP VENOUS THROMBOSIS

Diagnosis

Most cases of VTE in pregnancy occur in the lower extremities, with predisposition (~90%) for the left lower extremity, secondary to the anatomical compression of the left iliac vein by the right iliac and ovarian arteries.[9,10] The clinical diagnosis of DVT is complicated by nonspecific symptoms that overlap with physiologic changes in pregnancy, such as lower extremity edema. In one report, clinical suspicion for DVT was confirmed in only 10% of pregnant patients, compared to approximately 25% in the nonpregnant population.[11] Accurate prompt diagnosis is essential to decreasing maternal and fetal morbidity, and may require a combination of various modalities.

■ **TABLE 7-1. Medical Conditions and the Risk of VTE[4]**

Complication	Odds Ratio (OR)	95% CI
Thrombophilia	51.8	38.7-69.2
History of thrombosis	24.8	17.1-36.0
Antiphospholipid antibody syndrome	15.8	10.9-22.8
Lupus	8.7	5.8-13.0
Heart disease	7.1	6.2-8.3
Sickle cell disease	6.7	4.4-10.1
Obesity	4.4	3.4-5.7
Diabetes	2.0	1.4-2.7
Hypertension	1.8	1.4-2.3
Smoking	1.7	1.4-2.1
Substance abuse	1.1	0.7-1.9

CI, confidence interval.

■ **TABLE 7-2. Obstetric Conditions and the Risk of VTE[4]**

Complication	OR	95% CI
Transfusion	7.6	6.2-9.4
Disorders of fluid, electrolyte, and acid-base balance	4.9	4.1-5.9
Postpartum infection	4.1	2.9-5.7
Anemia	2.6	2.2-2.9
Hyperemesis	2.5	2.0-3.2
Antepartum hemorrhage	2.3	1.8-2.8
Cesarean versus vaginal delivery	2.1	1.8-2.4
Multiple gestation	1.6	1.2-2.1
Postpartum hemorrhage	1.3	1.1-1.6
Preeclampsia and gestational hypertension	0.9	0.7-1.0
Preterm labor	0.9	0.7-9.5
Thrombocytopenia	0.6	0.8-4.1

■ **TABLE 7-3. The Risk of VTE in Pregnant Patients With a Thrombophilia[7]**

Condition	Inheritance	Prevalence in European populations	Risk of thrombosis without prior history	Risk of thrombosis with prior history
Antithrombin deficiency	AD	0.02%-1.1%	3.0%-7.2%	11%-40%
Prothrombin mutation (PGM)	AD			
Homozygous		0.02%	2.8%	>10%
Heterozygous		2.9%	0.37%-0.5%	>10%
Factor V Leiden (FVL)	AD			
Homozygous		0.07%	1.5%	>10%
Heterozygous		5.3%	0.26%	>10%
Compound Heterozygous FVL/PGM		0.17%	4.7%	
Protein C deficiency	AD	0.2%-0.3%		0.8%-1.7%
Protein S deficiency	AD	0.03%-0.13%		<1%-6.6%
Hyperhomocysteinemia	AR	<5%		OR 6.1
Elevated factor VII	AD			~0.1%
Elevated factor VIII	AD			~0.1%
Elevated factor XI	AD			~0.1%

AD, autosomal dominant.

■ TABLE 7-4. Diagnosis of Antiphospholipid Antibody Syndrome		

Clinical criteria	Obstetrical	• History of three unexplained consecutive spontaneous abortions ≤10 wk gestational age (GA), or
		• History of one unexplained fetal death ≥10 wk GA (morphologically and karyotypically-normal), or
		• History of preterm delivery <34 wk GA, as a sequelae of preeclampsia or uteroplacental insufficiency, including the following:
		  • Non-reassuring fetal testing indicative of fetal hypoxemia (eg, abnormal Doppler flow velocimetry waveform)
		  • Oligohydramnios (amniotic fluid index ≤5 cm)
		  • Intrauterine growth restriction (IUGR) <10th percentile
		  • Placental abruption

	Non-obstetrical	• Arterial thrombosis, including: cerebrovascular accidents, transient ischemic attacks, myocardial infarction, amaurosis fugax • Venous thromboembolism (VTE), including: deep venous thrombosis (DVT), pulmonary emboli (PE), or small vessel thrombosis

Laboratory criteria		Should be present on two occasions, >12 wks apart, and no more than 5 years prior to clinical manifestation:
		• **Anticardiolipin antibody**
		  • IgG or IgM isotype, present in medium or high titers (ie, >40 GPL or MPL, or >99th percentile), or
		• **Anti-β2GPI antibody**
		  • IgG or IgM isotype (>99th percentile), or
		• **Lupus anticoagulant** in plasma, utilizing one of the following tests:
		  • Dilute Russell viper venom time (dRVVT)
		  • Lupus anticoagulant

Clinical Signs and Symptoms

- Acute onset of symptoms
- Unilateral extremity erythema, pain, warmth, edema
- May have reflex arterial spasm, with cool, pale extremity and decreased pulses ("phlegmasia alba dolens")
- Lower abdominal pain
- Homan sign
- A risk assessment model combining physical findings with risk factors has been developed by Wells and associates for use in nonpregnant populations, allowing a determination of pretest probabilities.[12] (see Table 7-5)

Laboratory Studies

- D-dimer: D-dimer is the breakdown product of cross-linked fibrin and elevations may be detected by enzyme-linked immunosorbent assay (ELISA) in acute thrombotic events outside of pregnancy. In normal pregnancy, however, physiologic elevations of D-dimer are found in a gestational-age dependent fashion, with 84% of women in the first trimester with a normal D-dimer, 33% in the second trimester, and 1% in the third trimester.[13] D-dimer levels further peak at the time of delivery and early puerperium. Obstetrical complications such as placental abruption, preeclampsia, and sepsis can also elevate D-dimer levels. Therefore, although D-dimer plays an important role in the exclusion of VTE in nonpregnant populations, its use in pregnancy is still highly debated.

Imaging

- Compression Doppler ultrasonography: The primary diagnostic tool for DVT is compression ultrasonography.

■ **TABLE 7-5. DVT Clinical Characteristic Scoring System (High ≥3, Moderate = 1-2; Low ≤0)**

Characteristic	Score
Active cancer	+1
Immobilization (cast, paralysis, or paresis)	+1
Bed rest >3 d or surgery within 12 wk	+1
Local tenderness along deep venous system	+1
Entire leg swollen	+1
Asymmetric calf swelling >3 cm measured 10 cm below tibial tuberosity	+1
Pitting edema only in symptomatic leg	+1
Collateral non-varicose superficial veins	+1
Prior DVT	+1
Alternative diagnosis at least as likely as DVT	−2

Compression color Doppler ultrasound is both highly sensitive (92%) and specific (98%) for popliteal and femoral vein thrombosis, but slightly less effective for evaluating calf vein thrombosis with a sensitivity of only 50%-70% and specificity of 60%.[14] Isolated iliac vein thrombosis can sometimes be diagnosed by placing patients in the left lateral decubitus position and assessing Doppler flow variations with respirations. If these sonographic findings are abnormal, venous thrombosis can be diagnosed and treatment started. Conversely, if the sonographic findings are normal and the patient has no other risk factors (eg, history of VTE, thrombophilia, or clinical progression), the study can be repeated in a week and if negative, no treatment is required. However, contrast venography or venous MRI should be performed if the sonographic findings are normal but there is a high index of suspicion.

- Ascending contrast venography: Contrast venography was previously considered the gold standard for diagnosing DVT in pregnancy, with a negative predictive value of 98%. However, given its invasive nature and high rate of complication, contrast venography has fallen out of favor. Contrast agents are injected into lower extremity veins and the venous system of the leg and pelvis are evaluated radiographically. When used with an abdominal lead shield it exposes the fetus to very low levels of radiation (0.0005 Gy), well below that associated with childhood cancers and teratogenicity. Chemical phlebitis and thrombosis occurs in 3% of cases.

- Impedance plethysmography: Impedance plethysmography is a noninvasive measurement of differentials in electrical resistance in the extremity, a reflection of blood volume changes induced by inflation and deflation of a pneumatic thigh cuff. Although sensitivity is high for obstructions at proximal veins, sensitivity is only 50% in smaller calf vessels.[15] False positives are also high secondary to the mechanical obstruction from the gravid uterus.

- Magnetic resonance imaging (MRI): Magnetic resonance imaging (MRI) is useful for detecting thigh and pelvic vein thrombosis. Although the safety of MRI in pregnant women is yet to be proven, no adverse effects have been noted. The use of IV gadolinium in pregnancy remains under debate. At high and repeated doses of intravenous gadolinium, teratogenicity in animals has been observed.[16] Gadolinium-induced nephrogenic systemic fibrosis has been observed in adult populations. This concern carries over the placenta to the fetal circulation, where persistent concentration of gadolinium in the amniotic fluid may be present. Currently, gadolinium is classified as a category C drug by the US Food and Drug Administration and can be used if benefits of diagnosis of PE outweigh the risks.[17]

In summary, compression Doppler ultrasound is recommended as the initial test in pregnant women with suspected DVT. If this study proves positive for a DVT, treatment should be initiated. With equivocal test results, venous MRI (for pelvic thromboses) are performed as detailed in Fig 7-3.

General DVT Management Principles

- Heparin anticoagulation (see separate section for details)
  - Therapeutic anticoagulation should be for 12 to 20 weeks.
  - Prophylactic anticoagulation should be initiated after initial treatment, for 6 to 12 weeks and until the patient reaches 6 weeks postpartum.
  - For complicated DVTs, including those involving the iliofemoral vessels, prophylaxis is recommended for 4 to 6 months.
  - Conversion to oral warfarin may be considered in the postpartum period, if the patient is compliant with drug level monitoring.

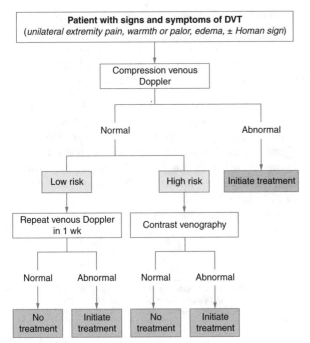

FIGURE 7-3. Ruling out DVT in pregnancy.

- Leg elevation
- Warm moist heat packs to decrease swelling and provide symptomatic relief
- Avoidance of sequential compression stocking devices in the presence of a DVT

■ PULMONARY EMBOLISM

Pulmonary embolism (PE) complicates approximately 1 in 2500 pregnancies. A thrombotic obstruction in the pulmonary vascular tree results in obstruction to pulmonary arterial blood flow, vasoconstriction of small arterial vessels, and progressive loss of alveolar surfactant. In pregnancy, thromboemboli most commonly originate in the iliac vessels.

Diagnosis

Clinical Signs and Symptoms
- Acute onset of symptoms
- Dyspnea, tachypnea, pleuritic chest pain, hemoptysis
- Tachycardia
- Cyanosis
- Syncope
- Pleural friction rub
- Fixed S2

Laboratory Studies
- D-dimer (see DVT).
- Arterial blood gases (ABG): In nonpregnant patients with PE, ABG may reveal hypoxemia, hypocapnia, and respiratory alkalosis. Although patients with PE may display hypoxia, 17% of patients will have a normal PaO_2. A decreased PaO_2 is also not overly specific, since the supine position may lower Pao_2 by as much as 15 mm Hg in the third trimester. In addition, respiratory alkalosis is a very common feature that is present in both normal pregnancy and PE.

Imaging
- Compression Doppler ultrasonography: Normal venous ultrasound does not necessarily rule out pulmonary emboli. Fewer than 30% of unselected patients with PE have sonographic/radiographic signs of a DVT at the time of presentation. Conversely, since the treatment of DVT and PE both involve anticoagulation, therapy can be initiated for positive Doppler ultrasound of the extremity alone.
- Electrocardiogram: An ECG may reveal right bundle branch block, right axis shift, Q wave in leads III and aVF, S wave in leads I and aVL >1.5 mm, T wave inversions in leads III and aVF or new onset of atrial fibrillation. However, these cardiac findings are insensitive predictors since they require large pulmonary artery occlusions.
- Echocardiogram: Echocardiographic findings include right ventricular dilation and hypokinesis, tricuspid regurgitation, and pulmonary artery dilation. Only 30% to 40% of patients with PE have echocardiogram findings on transthoracic echocardiogram (TTE).[18] Transesophageal echocardiogram (TEE) allows for direct imaging of the main pulmonary artery, significant portion of the right pulmonary artery, and proximal portion of the left pulmonary artery, allowing for an improved sensitivity of 58% to 97% and specificity of 88% to 100%.[19]
- Chest x-ray (CXR): Findings of PE on CXR include pulmonary parenchymal abnormality, atelectasis, pleural effusion, cardiomegaly, ipsilateral hemidiaphragm, pulmonary artery enlargement, and wedge-shaped perfusion defects. However, these findings are neither sensitive nor specific, and are seen in both healthy patients and those with PE. A quarter of patients with

PE exhibit normal CXR.[20] CXR exposes the fetus to less than 0.001 rad of radiation, well below the 5-rad cut-off for adverse effects of spontaneous abortion, teratogenicitiy, and perinatal morbidity.

- Ventilation/perfusion scan (V/Q scan): The initial evaluation of a suspected PE should be a V/Q scan. However, the scan must be interpreted in the context of clinical probability. Only negative and low probability scans in the setting of a low clinical risk, and high probability scans in the setting of high clinical risks are considered diagnostic. Non-diagnostic scans (ie, intermediate probability) or low probability scans in high-risk patients (eg, thrombophilia, suggestive ECG, or echocardiogram) should be followed up with a color Doppler compression ultrasound study of the lower extremities. Fetal radiation exposure from a V/Q scan is less than 0.012 rad from the [99]technetium perfusion scan and 0.019 rad from the [133]Xenon ventilation scan. Although the amount of total exposure is less than 0.031 rad, radiation exposure can be further limited by triaging with the perfusion study first. Since a normal perfusion study requires no further testing, radiation exposure may be reduced by more than half.
- Pulmonary angiography (PA): PA once was considered the gold-standard for diagnosis of PE outside of pregnancy, and is often obtained in high-risk patients with negative compression ultrasound. A negative PA excludes clinically relevant PE. However, radiation exposure is greater than that from spiral computed tomographic pulmonary angiography, and its sensitivity may actually be lower for subsegmental emboli.[21] Fetal radiation exposure from PA is 0.05 rad from the brachial route, and 0.22 to 0.33 rad from the femoral route.
- Spiral computed tomographic pulmonary angiography (CT-PA): The reported sensitivities of CT-PA compared with PA vary widely (64%-93%). While CT-PA is relatively sensitive and specific for diagnosing central pulmonary artery thrombi, it is insensitive for diagnosing subsegmental clots. Therefore, CT-PA appears to have a role as a rule-in test for large central emboli, but cannot exclude smaller peripheral lesions. Like compression ultrasonography, an equivocal V/Q scan in a high-risk patient with a positive CT-PA should require therapy, but a negative CT-PA in a high-risk setting should prompt pulmonary angiography or MRI angiography. Advantages of CT-PA over V/Q scanning include relative decrease in fetal radiation, easier technique, and straightforward interpretation. CT-PA, with appropriate abdominal

shielding and employing minimal fluoroscopy, exposes the fetus to 0.013 rad for the entire examination, compared to the 0.031 rad for V/Q scan. Conversely, however, CT-PA exposes maternal breast tissue to increased levels of irradiation, compared to a V/Q scan.

In summary, V/Q scan after a normal CXR should be considered the first-line test, with or without compression Doppler ultrasonography of the lower extremities. Confirmation in the non-diagnostic population should be performed with spiral CT-PA. Figures 7-4 and 7-5 summarize two recommended algorithms for diagnosis of PE.[22] Table 7-6 summarizes the radiation exposure of each recommended imaging modality.

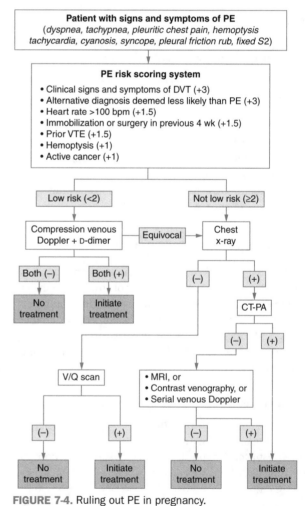

FIGURE 7-4. Ruling out PE in pregnancy.

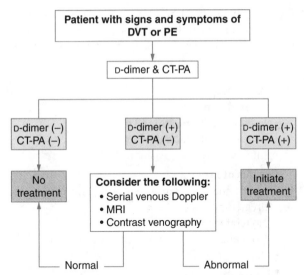

FIGURE 7-5. Alternative algorithm utilizing D-dimer and CT-PA.

■ TABLE 7-6. Fetal Radiation Exposures[23]

Imaging modality	Radiation exposure (in milliGray)	Radiation exposure (in rad)
Chest x-ray		<0.001
Contrast venography (limited), with abdominal shield	<0.5	<0.05
Contrast venography (full), without abdominal shield	3.1	0.31
V/Q scan: [99]technetium perfusion scan	<0.12	0.012
V/Q scan: [133]Xenon ventilation scan	<0.19	0.019
Spiral CT-PA	<0.13	0.013
Pulmonary angiography (brachial)	<0.5	0.05
Pulmonary angiography (femoral)	2.2-3.3	0.22-0.33

Fetal effects
5 rads = Increased risk of spontaneous abortion, teratogenicity, and perinatal morbidity.
1 rad = Marginally increased risk of childhood leukemia (from 1/3000 baseline to 1/2000)[24]

General PE Management Principles

- Heparin anticoagulation (see separate section for details)
  - Therapeutic anticoagulation should be initial treatment for 12 to 20 weeks.
  - For patients with PE, prophylactic anticoagulation is recommended for 4 to 6 months.
- Maintain maternal PaO_2 above 70 mm Hg or O_2 saturation of >94%.

■ PELVIC THROMBOSES

There are two types of pelvic thromboses: septic pelvic thrombophlebitis (SPT) and ovarian vein thrombosis (OVT). The two entities may share the same pathogenesis, clinical manifestations, and often the same patient. Incidence of pelvic thromboses is approximately 1 in 3000 deliveries (1 in 9000 vaginal deliveries and 1 in 800 cesarean deliveries). Risk factors include cesarean delivery, pelvic surgery, infection, and underlying malignancy.[25]

Septic Pelvic Thrombophlebitis

SPT is an uncommon complication of pelvic infection. It is more common after cesarean than vaginal delivery but has also been reported after gynecologic procedures. Thrombus formation in the pelvic veins appears to result from inflammatory cytokine induction of tissue factor expression in the endothelium of pelvic vessels.

Clinical Signs and Symptoms
- Nonspecific symptoms
- Spiking fevers, despite adequate antibiotic coverage
- May have multiple infected emboli
- Usually present within a few days after delivery or surgery
- Often present without abdominal tenderness

Laboratory Testing
- Complete blood count: Leukocytosis of >12,000/µL occurs in 70% to 100% of patients with SPT.[26]
- Blood culture: Blood cultures should be obtained in the evaluation of postpartum fever, particularly with persistent spiking fevers. Negative blood culture would point to the diagnosis of SPT, while positive blood cultures may enable targeted alterations in antibiotic regimen.

Imaging
MRI or CT may aid in the diagnosis of SPT. CT imaging may reveal enlargement of affected vein, with mural enhancement, and low-density vessel lumen. MRI reveals

hyperintensity in thrombosed vessels compared to those with normal flow. However, as a surgical specimen revealing thrombosis in the pelvic vasculature is the only gold standard in confirmation of SPT diagnoses, the utility of imaging modalities remains unproven.

General Management Principles

Traditional management was a course of therapeutic anticoagulation. Clinical response was considered both therapeutic and diagnostic with defervescence expected in 48 to 72 hours and the recommended duration of treatment ranging from 7 to 10 days to a full 6 weeks of anticoagulation. However, a recent study has called into question the role of anticoagulation in SPT. In a small study of 14 patients with CT documented SPT, eight received continued antibiotic therapy alone (ampicillin, gentamicin, and clindamycin) and six received a combination of heparin and antibiotic therapy. No difference was noted in the duration of fever between the two groups.[27]

Ovarian Vein Thrombosis

OVT typically presents with acute pain 2 to 3 days postpartum (with or without fever). It occasionally can be mistaken for appendicitis in a postpartum patient. Moreover, OVT can occur in the absence of infection and has been described in antepartum patients. The incidence of OVT is 1 in 4000 deliveries. Thrombosis can be diagnosed with CT or MRI and is most commonly noted in the right ovarian vein. Treatment for OVT is the same as outlined for SPT.

■ TREATMENT OF VTE

Prompt treatment with anticoagulation should be initiated upon diagnosis of DVT or PE. In some cases, particularly in setting of high suspicion of acute PE, without contraindication to anticoagulation, empiric treatment may be initiated prior to completion of diagnostic evaluation. Five categories of treatment are available to the nonpregnant population: heparins, warfarin, surgery, IVC filter, and thrombolytic therapy. However, secondary to teratogenicity and increased risks of bleeding, a unique understanding of the risks of benefits of each therapy in pregnancy is necessary in the management of obstetrical VTE.

Heparins

The current armamentarium of heparin and its derivatives includes unfractionated heparin (UFH), biologic low-molecular-weight heparin (LMWH), and synthetic pentasaccharide inhibitors of factor Xa. All forms of heparin are administered via an injectable route, either subcutaneous or intravenous.

General Concepts

Actions of heparin
- Enhances antithrombin (AT) activity
- Increases factor Xa inhibitor activity
- Inhibits platelet aggregation

Benefits of heparin
- Levels may be monitored and adjusted during pregnancy
- No teratogenicity
- Does not cross placenta or enter breast milk
- Rapidly reversible

Disadvantages of heparin
- Requires injection
- Not as effective in prophylaxis of patients with mechanical heart valves
- Required therapeutic doses display inter-patient variability due to variable levels of heparin-binding proteins such as vitronectin, fibronectin, von Willebrand factor, platelet factor 4, and histidine-rich glycoprotein during pregnancy.

Goals for drug monitoring levels
- Anti-factor Xa activity:
  - Therapeutic levels: 0.6 to 1.2 U/mL
  - Prophylactic levels: 0.1 to 0.2 U/mL
- Activated partial thromboplastin time (aPTT): Therapeutic levels between 1.5 and 2.5 times control values
- Heparin levels (Protamine assay) between 0.2 and 0.4 U/mL for therapy

Unfractionated Heparins

Route of administration: Subcutaneous or intravenous
Dosing
- Intravenous UFH for therapeutic treatment: Initial treatment is with intravenous bolus of UFH at 80 U/kg, followed by continuous infusion of 18 U/kg/h. Titration is performed every 6 hours until therapeutic aPTT, heparin, or anti-factor Xa level is achieved. A common weight-based algorithm is listed in Table 7-7.[28]
- Subcutaneous UFH for therapeutic treatment: Conversion from intravenous to subcutaneous UFH may be undertaken when any of these three criteria are met: (1) clinical improvement is noted; (2) completion of 5 days of IV treatment after uncomplicated VTE; or

■ **TABLE 7-7.** Practical Weight-Based Guidelines for Heparin Dosage[28]

1. **Bolus dose:** 80 U/kg of total body weight
2. **Maintenance dose:** 18 U/kg/h (25,000 U heparin in 250 mL D5W)
3. **Adjustments:** Assess aPTT values every 4-6 h and make adjustments made based on the aPTT values obtained. Adjustments may be rounded off to the nearest 100 U.

aPTT value	Adjustment
<35 sec (<1.2 × control)	Repeat 80 U/kg bolus, then increase infusion rate by 4 U/kg/h.
35-45 sec (1.2-1.5 × control)	Repeat 40 U/kg bolus, then increase infusion rate by 2 U/kg/h.
46-70 sec (1.6-2.3 × control)	No change in dosing.
71-90 sec (2.4-3.0 × control)	Decrease infusion by 2 U/kg/h.
>90 sec (>3.0 × control)	Stop infusion for 1 h, then decrease by 3 U/kg/h.

4. **Laboratory monitoring**
   - CBC
     - Check prior to initiation of therapy.
     - Recheck platelet count in 3-7 d after initiation of therapy.
   - aPTT
     - Check prior to initiation of therapy.
     - Recheck 6 h after initiation of therapy and after any dosage change.
     - When two consecutive aPTTs are noted in therapeutic range (50-70 sec), frequency of aPTT checks may be decreased to every 24 h.
5. For postpartum patients transitioning to oral warfarin, give first dose of warfarin as soon as aPTT in therapeutic range.

(3) completion of 7 to 10 days of IV treatment after large thrombosis or massive PE. Dosing for subcutaneous UFH is 10,000 to 15,000 units every 8 to 12 hours. Steady state is achieved in subcutaneous UFH after 4 doses (or 48 hours) in 99% of patients.[29]

- Subcutaneous UFH for prophylactic treatment: Prophylactic treatment with UFH should be dosed at 5000 units subcutaneously twice daily. Given decreases in plasma levels with advanced gestation, empiric increases may be employed, with 7500 units twice daily in the second trimester or 10,000 units twice daily in the third trimester.

Monitoring

- aPTT: Therapeutic levels of aPTT is laboratory-specific, and should be confirmed with your lab. The general goal is aPTT of 1.5 to 2 times control (or heparin level of at least 0.2 U/mL) 6 hours after injection. It is important to realize that aPTT is not reliable in patients with lupus anticoagulant.
- Anti-factor Xa: This test is used as an alternative in lupus anticoagulant patients. Goal for therapeutic treatment is 0.6 to 1.2 U/mL, while prophylactic is 0.1 to 0.2 U/mL.

Timing of anticoagulation, relative to delivery

- For prophylactic doses, optimal timing of delivery is 4 hours after dosing.
- For therapeutic doses, aPTT should be checked pre-operatively.
- Anticoagulation can be restarted safely 6 hours after vaginal delivery and 8 to 12 hours after cesarean delivery.

Reversing UFH activity

- Protamine sulfate reverses the action of heparin by binding to the heparin molecules. Dosage is protamine 1 mg intravenously for every 100 units of residual heparin. Administration should be slower than 20 mg/min, with no more than 50 mg over 10 minutes.

Low-Molecular-Weight Heparins

Route of administration: Subcutaneous only.
Dosing
- Enoxaparin (Lovenox):
  - Therapeutic: 1 mg/kg subcutaneously every 12 hours
  - Prophylactic: 40 mg subcutaneously daily, or 30 mg subcutaneously every 12 hours

- Dalteparin sodium (Fragmin):
  - Therapeutic: 100 units/kg subcutaneously every 12 hours
  - Prophylactic: 5000 units subcutaneously daily
- Tinzaparin (Innohep): 175 IU/kg subcutaneously daily

Monitoring
- Anti-factor Xa levels should be titrated to 0.6 to 1.2 U/mL for therapy. Optimal timing for checking levels is 4 hours after the fourth administration of an adjusted dose. Adjustments should be an increase or decrease of 10% to 25% of previous dose.
- Conversion from LMWH to UFH at approximately 36 weeks gestation is recommended to avoid increased risk of bleeding and complications from regional anesthesia.

Timing of medication, relative to delivery
- For prophylactic doses, optimal timing of delivery is 12 hours after dosing.
- For therapeutic doses, optimal timing of delivery is 18 to 24 hours after dosing.
- Anticoagulation can be restarted safely 6 hours after vaginal delivery and 8 to 12 hours after cesarean delivery.

Reversing LMWH activity
- Unlike UFH, protamine sulfate does not completely reverses the activity of LMWH. However, its use may be recommended to decrease amount of bleeding. Dosage is calculated at 1 mg per 100 anti-Xa units of LMWH.

Synthetic Low-Molecular-Weight Heparins
Synthetic heparin pentasaccharides, such as fondaparinux or idraparinux, bind to AT with high affinity. Its use in pregnancy has been uncommon because safety profiling has thus far been inadequate. Indications for synthetic LMWH heparin use include patients with heparin-induced thrombocytopenia (HIT), secondary to the lack of interaction with platelet factor 4 in these synthetic forms. Initial in vitro studies reveal absence of placental transfer at recommended doses; however, small amounts of fondaparinux have been detected in umbilical cord blood following multiple doses in pregnancy.[30] Fondaparinux is labeled as class B in pregnancy.

Route of administration: Subcutaneous only
Dosing
- Fondaparinux

- Therapeutic: 5 to 10 mg subcutaneously per day, based on body weight, with an average of approximately 0.1 mg/kg.
  - <50 kg: 5 mg/d
  - 50 to 100 kg: 7.5 mg/d
  - >100 kg: 10 mg/d
- Prophylactic: 2.5 mg subcutaneously per day.
- Idraparinux (weekly fondaparinux)
  - Not recommended in pregnancy secondary to its long-acting nature.

Monitoring: Monitoring can be performed with anti-factor Xa levels, as noted above.

Reversing: No antidote is known.

Heparins and Neuraxial Analgesia[31]
The following recommendations are from the American Society of Regional Anesthesia and Pain Medicine 2003 consensus guidelines on neuraxial anesthesia and anticoagulation.

UFH and neuraxial analgesia
- IV UFH should be discontinued with the onset of labor.
- Subcutaneous UFH should be stopped 24 hours prior to planned induction of labor or cesarean delivery, or with the onset of spontaneous labor.
- Timing of neuraxial analgesia placement:
  - Neuraxial anesthesia can be administered when the aPTT returns to normal.
  - If anticoagulation with IV heparin is needed in patients with recent epidural catheterization, heparin should not be given for at least 1 hour after the epidural catheter has been inserted or removed.
- Timing of neuraxial analgesia removal:
  - Remove the epidural catheter 2 to 4 hours after the last heparin dose, after confirmation of the patient's normal coagulation status.

LMWH and neuraxial analgesia
- Timing of neuraxial analgesia placement:
  - Prophylactic (low-dose) LMWH: Neuraxial block should not be performed until at least 12 hours after the last dose of prophylactic (low-dose) LMWH, secondary to concerns regarding spinal hematoma formation.
  - Therapeutic (high-dose) LMWH: Neuraxial block should not be performed until at least 24 hours after the last dose of therapeutic (high-dose) LMWH.

- Timing of neuraxial analgesia removal:
  - Once-daily LMWH regimen: An epidural catheter may be maintained, but the catheter should not be removed for at least 10 to 12 hours after the last LMWH dose.
  - Twice-daily LMWH regimen: For patients receiving a twice-daily LMWH regimen, an epidural catheter should be removed prior to initiation of LMWH thromboprophylaxis. If an epidural is to be maintained with the twice-daily regimen, the catheter may be left indwelling overnight and removed the following day, with the first dose of LMWH administered 2 hours after catheter withdrawal.
- Timing of anticoagulation after delivery and neuraxial analgesia:
  - Once-daily LMWH regimen: Administer the first dose at least 6 to 8 hours postoperatively.
  - Twice-daily LMWH regimen: Administer the first dose no earlier than 24 hours postoperatively, and only in the presence of adequate surgical hemostasis.
  - Following removal of an indwelling epidural catheter postoperatively, in setting of either single or twice daily LMWH, initiate LMWH after at least 2 hours have elapsed.

Complications/Side-Effects

- Hemorrhage: Risks increase with concomitant aspirin use, recent surgery, thrombocytopenia, and liver disease.
- Heparin-induced thrombocytopenia: HIT occurs in 3% of patients, and has two forms. The early-onset, transient form occurs secondary to heparin-induced platelet aggregation. A delayed-onset, immune-mediated form occurs approximately 2 weeks after initiation of therapy, secondary to formation of IgG. Diagnosis can be confirmed with a heparin-platelet factor 4 antibody test (ELISA) for HIT.
- Cessation is mandatory for the immune-mediated form, but is less frequently seen with LMWH compared to unfractionated forms. We recommend checking a platelet count 1 week after initiation of therapy, or sooner if there is a higher index of suspicion for HIT.
- Osteoporosis: This rare side-effect is more common when doses of UFH are greater than 15,000 U/day for more than 6 months. We recommend supplementation with 1500 mg of calcium each day. Bone densitometry can be considered postpartum for patients on long-term anticoagulation, with subsequent referral to medical or reproductive endocrinology specialist.

Direct Thrombin Inhibitor

Direct thrombin inhibitors may offer advantages over heparin because they do not bind plasma proteins, do not rely on levels of AT, resist neutralization by platelet factor 4, and inhibit both fibrin-bound- and circulating thrombin.[32] This class of hirudin-like medications can be used in patients who experience HIT or local adverse reaction from UFH or LMWH. The following are the types of commercially-available direct thrombin inhibitors in the United States:

- **Lepirudin** is a bivalent recombinant form of hirudin that is approved for treatment of acute thrombosis with HIT. This medication is pregnancy category B, however, literature is limited to case reports of successful use in pregnancy.[33]
- **Bivalirudin** is bivalent synthetic polypeptide analog of hirudin, and is also pregnancy category B.
- **Argatroban** is a univalent synthetic direct thrombin inhibitor with a very short half-life, and is also pregnancy category B.

Direct Factor Xa Inhibitor

Direct factor Xa inhibitors are a new class of anticoagulants and include the oral rivaroxaban (Xarelto), and investigational apixaban and otamixaban. This class of anticoagulants is FDA-approved for prevention of VTE in patients who have undergone orthopedic surgery. No trials or case reports have been reported to date in pregnancy.

Warfarin

Actions of warfarin
- Inhibition of the action of vitamin K, which is a cofactor in the synthesis of the final molecular forms of factors VII, IX, X, and prothrombin
- Readily crosses placenta
- Does not concentrate in breast milk

Disadvantages of warfarin
- Exposure between 7 to 12 weeks of gestation is linked to a 33% risk of embryopathy. Stigmata includes nasal hypoplasia, stippled epiphysis, and central nervous system abnormalities including: agenesis of the corpus callosum, Dandy-Walker malformation, midline cerebellar atrophy, and ventral midline dysplasia with optic atrophy.
- Risk of placental and fetal hemorrhage throughout pregnancy.

- Risk of warfarin-induced paradoxical thromboembolism, secondary to rapid inhibitory effect of warfarin on the anticoagulant protein C, compared to the other clotting factors.

Indications in obstetrics
- Mechanical heart valve: Use of UFH or LMWH in patients with older-generation prosthetic heart valves has shown an increase in thrombogenic complications, including fatal valve thrombosis. The risk of fatal maternal valve thrombosis may outweigh the risks of warfarin to the fetus between 12 and 36 weeks' gestation.
- Postpartum period.

Route of administration: Oral only

Dosing
- Initial dosing: 5 to 10 mg for 2 days, with subsequent titration.
- UFH or LMWH should always be maintained during the initial *4 days* of Warfarin therapy *and* until a therapeutic international normalized ratio (INR) is achieved.

Monitoring
- INR: This test is the ratio of the patient's prothrombin time (PT) over the mean population PT adjusted for the effects of the local lab's thromboplastin. Warfarin dose should be adjusted to the patient's INR, with goal for 2.0 to 3.0. Warfarin has a peak effect at 36 to 72 hours after initiation of therapy, with a half-life of 36 to 42 hours.

Reversal of warfarin action
- Vitamin K or fresh-frozen plasma can be used to reverse the effects of warfarin, with normalization of the PT within 6 hours of an oral or subcutaneous 5-mg dose of vitamin K.

Inferior Vena Cava Filter

Percutaneous placement of an inferior vena cava (IVC) filter provides a mechanical obstacle to the deportment of clots present in the distal inferior vena cava, thereby preventing passage of emboli that have showered from lower extremity VTE. Multiple filter compositions and shapes are available today. Retrievable IVC filters may prove ideal for pregnant patients requiring this therapy.

Indications for use
- Contraindications to anticoagulation:
  - Recent surgery
  - Hemorrhagic stroke
  - Active bleeding

- Adverse reactions to or ineffectiveness of prior anticoagulation:
  - Recurrent PE despite adequate anticoagulation
  - Prior serious hemorrhagic complication
  - Allergic reactions
- Massive PE with significant compromise of pulmonary vascular tree, with high risk of fatality if recurrent PE occurs.

Surgery and Thrombolytic Therapy

Surgical embolectomy should be reserved for life-threatening settings. Massive PE with hemodynamic instability should be the only indication for thrombolytic therapy (ie, tPA, urokinase, and streptokinase) in pregnancy, given the high risk that these agents will induce abruption. However, no controlled studies exist examining the efficacy and safety of thrombolytic therapy in pregnancy. In a review of 172 pregnant patients treated with thrombolytic therapy, the maternal mortality rate was 1.2%, the fetal loss rate was 6%, and maternal complications from hemorrhage occurred in 8%.[34]

■ PREVENTION

Recurrence Risk

Among pregnant patients who have had a previous VTE during pregnancy, recurrence risks of 2.4% to 10% have been reported.[35] In a review of hospital discharge data from 1085 women with pregnancy-associated VTE and 7625 women with unprovoked VTE, recurrence risk was 5.8% and 10.4%, respectively.[36]

Indications for Prophylaxis

- In the following patients populations, if not already receiving therapeutic anticoagulation, antepartum DVT prophylaxis should be considered:
  - Thrombophilias
    - High-risk (FVL homozygosity, PGM homozygosity, AT deficiency, compound heterozygous FVL/PGM) thrombophilia.
    - Low-risk thrombophilia (FVL heterozygosity, PGM heterozygosity, protein C deficiency, protein S deficiency) with personal or family (first-degree relative with VTE at <50 years of age) history of VTE.
  - Antiphospholipid antibody syndrome (would require prophylactic aspirin treatment, along with therapeutic anticoagulation if a history of VTE is present.)

- Prior VTE that occurred in the setting of the following:
  - Recurring condition, or
  - During pregnancy, or
  - During oral contraceptive pill use
- Postpartum DVT prophylaxis should be considered in the following:
  - All patients receiving antepartum prophylactic anticoagulation, unless the indication is only for prevention of recurrent fetal loss in the setting of a low-risk thrombophilia.
  - Low-risk thrombophilia without history of prior VTE, if patient requires a cesarean delivery or has other risk factors for VTE (eg, obesity, prolonged immobilization)
  - Prior VTE with nonrecurring condition
  - Obesity (BMI $\geq$30 kg/m^2)

Mechanical Preventative Measures

- Left-lateral decubitus positioning during the third trimester displaces the gravid uterus and allows for improved venous return from lower extremities.
- Pneumatic compression stockings: Pneumatic compression stockings improve blood flow, decrease stasis, increase blood flow in the femoral vessels by 240%, and increase fibrinolysis. In a meta-analysis of moderate-risk surgery, they were shown to decrease the incidence of DVT by 60%. Since pneumatic compression stockings have no hemorrhagic risk, and have been shown to be an effective means of DVT prophylaxis in gynecologic oncology surgery, they should be an ideal device for prophylaxis in high-risk pregnant patients (eg, thrombophilic patients at prolonged bed rest or who are undergoing a cesarean delivery).
- Graduated elastic compression stockings: Graduated elastic compression stockings have been shown to increase femoral vein flow velocity in late pregnancy but their role in decreasing VTE in pregnancy is yet to be defined.

Pharmacologic Preventative Measures

Please see the previous section on heparins for prophylactic dosing and drug monitoring.

■ Summary

- Clinical signs and symptoms of DVT and PE are frequently unreliable, and diagnostic imaging should be employed. For DVT, compression Doppler ultrasonography is standard. For PE, a combination of V/Q scanning, spiral CT, or lower extremity compression Doppler ultrasonography can be utilized, depending on clinical suspicion.
- Treatment with Heparin and LMWH is standard during the antepartum period, should be prompt, and should continue for a total of 12 to 20 weeks of therapeutic anticoagulation.
- Prophylaxis during the antepartum and postpartum periods should be considered in patients without VTE who are at risk for developing VTE.

SUGGESTED READINGS

1. Marik PE, Plante LA. Venous thromboembolic disease and pregnancy. *N Eng J Med.* 2008;359:2025.
2. James AH, Jamison MG, Brancazio LR, Myers MR. Venous thromboembolism during pregnancy and the postpartum period: incidence, risk factors, and mortality. *Am J Obstet Gynecol.* 2006;194:1311-1315.
3. Bourjeily G, Paidas M, Khalil H, et al. Pulmonary embolism in pregnancy. *Lancet.* 2009 Nov; Epub.
4. Miyakis S, Lockshin MD, Atsumi T, et al. International consensus statement on an update of the classification criteria for definite antiphospholipid syndrome (APS). *J Thromb Haemost.* 2006;4:295-306.
5. Ginsberg JS, Greer I, Hirsch J. Use of antithrombotic agents during pregnancy. *Chest.* 2001;119:122S.
6. Van Belle A, Buller HR, Huisman MV, et al. Effectiveness of managing suspected pulmonary embolism using an algorithm combining clinical probability, D-dimer testing, and computed tomography. *JAMA.* 2006 Jan; 295(2):172-179.
7. Horlocker TT, Wedel DJ, Benzon H, et al. Regional anesthesia in the anticoagulated patient: defining the risks (the second ASRA Consensus Conference on Neuraxial Anesthesia and Anticoagulation). *Reg Anesth Pain Med.* 2003;28:172.
8. Gabbe SG, Niebyl JR, Simpson JL, et al. Thromboembolic disorders. In: *Obstetrics: Normal and Problem Pregnancies.* 5th ed. Philadelphia, PA: Churchill Livingstone Elsevier; 2007:1064-1076.

REFERENCES

1. Khan KS, Wojdyla D, Say L, et al. WHO analysis of causes of maternal death: a systematic review. *Lancet.* 2006;367:1066-1074.
2. Chang J, Elam-Evans LD, Berg CJ, et al. Pregnancy-related mortality surveillance: United States, 1991-1999. *MMWR Surveill Summ.* 2003;52:1.

3. Marik PE, Plante LA. Venous thromboembolic disease and pregnancy. *N Eng J Med*. 2008;359:2025.

4. James AH, Jamison MG, Brancazio LR, Myers MR. Venous thromboembolism during pregnancy and the postpartum period: incidence, risk factors, and mortality. *Am J Obstet Gynecol*. 2006;194:1311-1315.

5. Bourjeily G, Paidas M, Khalil H, et al. Pulmonary embolism in pregnancy. *Lancet*. 2009 Nov; Epub.

6. Goodrich S, Wood JE. Peripheral venous distensibility and velocity of venous blood flow during pregnancy or during oral contraceptive therapy. *Am J Obstet Gynecol*. 1964;90:740.

7. Gabbe SG, Niebyl JR, Simpson JL, et al. Thromboembolic disorders. In: *Obstetrics: Normal and Problem Pregnancies*. 5th ed. Philadelphia, MA: Churchill Livingstone Elsevier; 2007:1064-1076.

8. Miyakis S, Lockshin MD, Atsumi T, et al. International consensus statement on an update of the classification criteria for definite antiphospholipid syndrome (APS). *J Thromb Haemost*. 2006;4:295-306.

9. Gherman RB, Goodwin TM, Leung B, et al. Incidence, clinical characteristics, and timing of objectively diagnosed venous thromboembolism during pregnancy. *Obstet Gynecol*. 1999;94:730.

10. Greer IA. Prevention and management of venous thromboembolism in pregnancy. *Clin Chest Med*. 2003;24:123.

11. Ginsberg JS, Greer I, Hirsch J. Use of antithrombotic agents during pregnancy. *Chest*. 2001;119:122S.

12. Wells PS, Hirsh J, Anderson DR, et al. A simple clinical model for the diagnosis of deep-vein thrombosis combined with impedance plethysmography: potential for an improvement in the diagnostic process. *J Intern Med*. 1998;243: 15-23.

13. Kovac M, Mikovic Z, Rakicevic L, et al. The use of D-dimer with new cutoff can be useful in diagnosis of venous thromboembolism in pregnancy. *Eur J of Ob Gyn & Rep Biol*. 2009 Oct; Epub ahead of print.

14. Gaitini D. Current approaches and controversial issues in the diagnosis of deep venous thrombosis via duplex Doppler ultrasound. *J Clin Ultrasound*. 34(6):289-297.

15. Wells P, Hirsh J, Anderson DR, et al. Comparison of the accuracy of impedance plethysmography and compression ultrasound in outpatients with clinically suspected deep venous thrombosis. A two center paired-design prospective trial. *Thromb Haemost*. 1995;74:1423-1427.

16. Okuda Y, Sagami F, Tirone P, et al. Reproductive and developmental toxicity study of gadobenate dimeglumine formulation (E7155)—Study of embryo-fetal toxicity in rabbits by intravenous administration. *J Toxicol Sci*. 1999;24(Suppl 1): 79-87.

17. Chen MM, Coakley FV, Kaimal A, et al. Guidelines for computed tomography and magnetic resonance imaging use during pregnancy and lactation. *Obstet Gynecol*. 2008 Aug;112(2, Pt 1):333-340.

18. Gibson NS, Sohne M, Buller HR. Prognostic value of echocardiography and spiral computed tomography in patients with pulmonary embolism. *Curr Opin Pulm Med*. 2005 Sep;11(5):380-384.

19. Leibowitz D. Role of echocardiography in the diagnosis and treatment of acute pulmonary thromboembolism. *J Am Soc Echocardiogr*. 2001 Sept;14(9):921-926.

20. Elliott CG, Goldhaber SZ, Visani L, et al. Chest radiographs in acute pulmonary embolism: Results from the International Cooperative Pulmonary Embolism Registry. *Chest*. 2000 Jul;118:33-38.

21. Wittram C, Waltman AC, Shepard JA, et al. Discordance between CT and angiography in the PIOPED II study. *Radiology*. 2007 Sep;244(3):883-889.

22. Van Belle A, Buller HR, Huisman MV, et al. Effectiveness of managing suspected pulmonary embolism using an algorithm combining clinical probability, D-dimer testing, and computed tomography. *JAMA*. 2006 Jan;295(2): 172-179.

23. Brent RL. The effect of embryonic and fetal exposure to x-ray, microwaves, and ultrasound: counseling the pregnant and nonpregnant patient about these risks. *Semin Oncol*. 1989;16:347-368.

24. Stewart, A, Kneale, GW. Radiation dose effects in relation to obstetric x-rays and childhood cancers. *Lancet*. 1970;1: 1185-1188.

25. Wysokinska EM, Hodge D, McBane RD II. Ovarian vein thrombosis: incidence of recurrent venous thromboembolism and survival. *Thromb Haemost*. 2006 Aug;96(2):126-131.

26. Witlin AG, Sibai BM. Postpartum ovarian vein thrombosis after vaginal delivery: a report of 11 cases. *Obstet Gynecol*. 1995 May;85(5, Pt 1):775-780.

27. Brown CE, Stettler RW, Twickler F., et al. Puerperal septic pelvic thrombophlebitis: Incidence and response to heparin theory. *Am J. Obstet Gynecol*. 1999;181:143–148.

28. Raschke RA, Reilly BM, Guidry JR, et al. The weight-based heparin dosing nomogram compared with a "standard care" nomogram. A randomized controlled trial. *Ann Intern* Med. 1993 Nov; 119:874.

29. Prandoni P, Bagatella P, Bernardi E, et al. U se of an Algorithm for Administering Subcutaneous Heparin in the Treatment of Deep Venous Thrombosis. *Ann Int Med*. 1998;129(4):299-302.

30. Lagrange F, Vergnes C, Brun JL, et al. Absence of placental transfer of pentasaccharide (Fondaparinux, Arixtra) in the

dually perfused human cotyledon in vitro. *Thromb Haemost*. 2002 May;87(5):831-835.

31. Horlocker TT, Wedel DJ, Benzon H, et al. Regional anesthesia in the anticoagulated patient: defining the risks (the second ASRA Consensus Conference on Neuraxial Anesthesia and Anticoagulation). *Reg Anesth Pain Med*. 2003;28:172.

32. Hirsh J, O'Donnell M, Weitz JI. New anticoagulants. *Blood*. 2005;105:453-463.

33. Chapman ML, Martinez-Borges AR, Mertz HL. Lepirudin for treatment of acute thrombosis during pregnancy. *Obstet Gynecol*. 2008 Aug;112(2, Pt 2):432-433.

34. Turrentine MA, Braems G, Ramirez MM. Use of thrombolytics for the treatment of thromboembolic disease in pregnancy. *Obstet Gynecol Surv*. 1995;50:534.

35. Brill-Edwards P, Ginsberg JS, Gent M, et al. Safety of withholding heparin in pregnant women with a history of venous thromboembolism. *N Eng J Med*. 343;1439-1444.

36. White RH, Chan WS, Zhou H, et al. Recurrent venous thromboembolism after pregnancy-associated versus unprovoked thromboembolism. *Thromb Hemost*. 2008;100(2): 246-252.

CHAPTER 8

Cardiac Disease in Pregnancy

• *Stephanie R. Martin*

Cardiac disease complicates approximately 4% of all pregnancies in the United States; however, these patients are at a disproportionate increase in risk for maternal deaths (10%-25%).[1,2] Congenital cardiac lesions are three times more common than acquired, adult-onset abnormalities in pregnant patients. Intensive care unit (ICU) admissions due to maternal cardiac disease comprise up to 15% of obstetric ICU admissions, yet these patients account for up to 50% of all maternal deaths in the ICU.[3-9]

Common complaints of normal pregnancy such as dyspnea, fatigue, palpitations, orthopnea, and pedal edema mimic symptoms of worsening cardiac disease and can create challenges for the clinician when evaluating a pregnant patient with cardiac disease. Nevertheless, these patients are at risk of developing cardiac decompensation and adverse pregnancy outcomes based on the type of cardiac lesion.

In this chapter, we will review valvular, congenital, and acquired cardiac lesions and their impact on pregnancy management. Each section will address the concerns specific to the relevant abnormality including key points in antepartum management, anesthetic and delivery issues.

■ PHYSIOLOGIC CHANGES OF SINGLETON PREGNANCY

Comprehensive understanding of the normal physiologic adaptations to pregnancy is essential to the successful management of patients with cardiac disease. Conditions which may be asymptomatic while nonpregnant can deteriorate in the pregnant state. Table 8-1 outlines key physiologic changes in a normal singleton gestation. Multiple gestations can be expected to have more dramatic physiologic changes. Table 8-2 provides an overview of changes in cardiovascular evaluations during pregnancy.

■ COUNSELING THE PATIENT

Establishing baseline cardiac function is essential for pregnant cardiac patients. Functional status for patients with cardiac disease is commonly classified according to the New York Heart Association (NYHA) classification system as outlined in Table 8-3. Patients with NYHA Class I or II have less risk of complications compared to those in Class III or IV.[10] Table 8-4 classifies various cardiac abnormalities according to maternal death risk estimates; however, the patient's particular history is not included in these estimates.[11]

In a recent study of over 600 pregnancies complicated by maternal cardiac disease, four predictors for maternal complications were identified:[12]

1. Prior cardiac event (heart failure, transient ischemic attack, stroke, or arrhythmia)
2. Prepregnancy New York Heart Association class > II
3. Left heart obstruction (mitral valve area <2 cm^2, aortic valve area <1.5 cm^2, peak left outflow gradient >30 mm Hg)
4. Ejection fraction <40%

■ **TABLE 8-1. Expected Physiologic Changes Occurring the Antepartum, Intrapartum, and Postpartum Periods**

Antepartum
- Blood volume increases by 20%-50%
- In nonpregnant females total blood volume is ~60-70 mL/kg
- Systemic vascular resistance decreases by 20%
  - Accounts for majority of drop in BP
  - Accommodates increase in circulating volume without increase in BP
- Blood pressure (taken in sitting position)
  - BP ≥140/90 abnormal at any time in gestation
  - BP decreases to lowest point at 28 wk
  - After 28 wk, BP increases to nonpregnant level by term
- Mean arterial pressure unchanged
- Heart rate increases by 10-15 bpm
- Stroke volume increases by 30%
- Cardiac output increases by 30%-50%
  - CO = heart rate × stroke volume. Majority of increase is from stroke volume
  - Half of the expected increase occurs by 8 wk
  - Peaks end of second trimester, sustained to term
  - 6 L/min by term
- Pulmonary capillary wedge pressure (preload to left heart) unchanged
- Central venous pressure (preload to right heart) unchanged
- Pulmonary vascular resistance decreases 30%
- Hypercoagulable state
  - Increased fibrinogen
  - Platelets unchanged
- Dilutional anemia despite 30% increase in red cell mass

Intrapartum
- During a contraction:
  - 300-500 mL of blood enters circulation
  - heart rate increases
  - cardiac output increases by 30%
  - blood pressure increases by 10-20 mm Hg
- Supine position may decrease cardiac output by 20%

Postpartum
- Postpartum diuresis between days 2-5
- Cardiac output increases by 50% in the immediate postpartum period
- Stroke volume increases 60% in the immediate postpartum period
- Reflex bradycardia occurs (−15%)
- These changes persist for 2 wk after delivery

■ **TABLE 8-2. Changes in Cardiovascular Tests during Pregnancy**

Cardiovascular exam	Findings in pregnancy
Chest x-ray	Apparent cardiomegaly Enlarged left atrium Increased vascular markings
Electrocardiography	Right axis deviation Right bundle branch block ST segment depression of 1 mm on left precordial leads Q waves in lead III T wave inversion in leads III, V2, and V3
Echocardiography	Trivial tricuspid regurgitation Pulmonary regurgitation Increased left atrial size Increased left ventricular end-diastolic dimensions by 6%-10% Mitral regurgitation Pericardial effusion

■ **TABLE 8-3. New York Heart Association Functional Classification System**

Class I	No limitations of physical activity. Ordinary physical activity does not precipitate cardiovascular symptoms such as dyspnea, angina, fatigue, or palpitations.
Class II	Slight limitation of physical activity. Ordinary physical activity will precipitate cardiovascular symptoms. Patients are comfortable at rest.
Class III	Less than ordinary physical activity precipitates symptoms that markedly limit activity. Patients are comfortable at rest.
Class IV	Patients have discomfort with any physical activity. Symptoms are present at rest.

■ TABLE 8-4. Maternal Mortality Associated with Pregnancy

Group 1—Mortality <1%
Atrial septal defect
Ventricular septal defect
Patent ductus arteriosus
Mitral stenosis—NYHA class I & II
Pulmonic/tricuspid valve disease
Corrected Tetralogy of Fallot
Bioprosthetic valve

Group 2—Mortality 5%-15%
2A
  Mitral stenosis—NYHA class III & IV
  Aortic stenosis
  Coarctation of aorta without valvular involvement
  Uncorrected Tetralogy of Fallot
  Previous myocardial infarction
  Marfan syndrome with normal aorta
2B
  Mitral stenosis with atrial fibrillation
  Artificial valve

Group 3—Mortality 25%-50%
Pulmonary hypertension
  Primary
  Eisenmenger Syndrome
Coarctation of aorta with valvular involvement
Marfan syndrome with aortic involvement
Peripartum cardiomyopathy with persistent left
  ventricular dysfunction

Source: From Clark SL, Phelan JP, Cotton DB eds. *Critical Care Obstetrics: Structural Cardiac Disease in Pregnancy.* Oradell, NJ: Medical Economics Company; 1987.

The risk of maternal complications was directly proportional to the number of risk factors identified as outlined below:

No. of predictors	Risk of cardiac event in pregnancy
0	5%
1	27%
>1	75%

The most commonly encountered cardiac events are pulmonary edema and dysrhythmias. Maternal mortality is of highest risk for patients with coronary artery disease, pulmonary hypertension, endocarditis, cardiomyopathy, and dysrhythmias.[13,14]

Neonatal complications are more likely to occur in patients with NYHA class > II, anticoagulation during pregnancy, smoking, multiple gestation, and left heart obstruction. These complications include small for gestational age infants, delivery before 34 weeks gestation and neonatal death.[15] Structural cardiac anomalies (excluding autosomal dominant disorders) occur in 2% to 18% of fetuses born to patients with a history of congenital cardiac disease. Therefore fetal echocardiogram is recommended for all pregnant patients with structural cardiac defects. Table 8-5 outlines the risks of congenital cardiac disease by maternal disorder.

General Principles of Management

Management details for each condition are addressed separately.

Preconception Care

- Baseline evaluation of cardiac function
- Counseling regarding pregnancy risk for mother and fetus
- Consultation with cardiologist and maternal fetal medicine specialist, if possible
- Review of current medications to determine appropriateness of continuing during pregnancy

■ TABLE 8-5. Risk of Fetal Cardiac Abnormality by Maternal Lesion

Risk of Fetal Congenital Cardiac Abnormality	
Lesion	Risk if mother is affected (%)
Tetralogy of Fallot	2-4.5
Aortic coarctation	4-14.1
Atrial septal defect	4.6-11
Ventricular septal defect	6-15.6
Pulmonary stenosis	5.3-6.5
Aortic stenosis	8-17.9
Persistent ductus arteriosus	4.1
Marfan syndrome	50
22q11 deletion syndromes	50

- Routine preconception care as for all patients: assessment of immunization status, screening for genetic diseases as indicated, supplemental folic acid

Antepartum Care
- A team approach to antepartum care is recommended and should include maternal fetal medicine, cardiology and anesthesia as indicated, particularly for patients with congenital cardiac disease.
- Patients should be evaluated regularly for signs and symptoms of cardiac decompensation.
- Fetal echocardiogram between 20 and 24 weeks' gestation is indicated in the presence of congenital heart disease in mother.
- Periodic ultrasound to assess fetal growth.
- Antepartum fetal surveillance starting at 30 to 34 weeks.

Labor and Delivery Care
- Attention to I and Os. Maintain all IV fluids on a pump.
- Avoid supine positioning.
- Supplemental oxygen.

- Cesarean delivery is not routinely recommended in the setting of maternal cardiac disease.
- Endocarditis prophylaxis is no longer recommended for any genitourinary procedures, even in patients with the highest risk lesions.[16]

VALVULAR CARDIAC DISEASE

Valvular abnormalities may be congenital or acquired. However, the majority is acquired secondary to rheumatic fever which accounts for 90% of cardiac disorders in pregnancy worldwide. The degree of risk for the development of complications (particularly dysrhythmias and pulmonary edema) depends on the specific valve lesion, number of valves involved, and the degree of valvular obstruction, particularly of the mitral and aortic valves. The mitral valve is most commonly affected followed in order of decreasing frequency by aortic, tricuspid, and pulmonic valves. Table 8-6 presents a summary of relative maternal and fetal risk in patients with valvular abnormalities.[17] Each valvular lesion will be addressed in the sections that follow. Table 8-7 outlines common cardiac medications and their effects on uterine blood flow and the fetus.

■ TABLE 8-6. Classification of Valvular Heart Lesions According to Maternal and Fetal Risks

Low maternal and fetal risks	High maternal and fetal risks	High maternal risks
Asymptomatic aortic stenosis with a low mean outflow gradient (<50 mm Hg); normal LV systolic function	Severe aortic stenosis with or without symptoms	Ejection fraction <40%
Aortic regurgitation, NYHA Class I or II with normal LV function	Aortic regurgitation, NYHA Class III or IV	Previous heart failure
Mitral regurgitation, NYHA Class I or II, normal LV function	Mitral stenosis, NYHA Class II, III, or IV	Previous stroke or transient ischemic attack
Mitral valve prolapse with none to moderate mitral regurgitation, normal LV function	Mitral regurgitation, NYHA Class III or IV	
Mild to moderate mitral stenosis, no pulmonary hypertension	Aortic or mitral valve disease with pulmonary hypertension	
Mild to moderate pulmonary valve stenosis	Aortic or mitral valve disease with LV dysfunction	
	Maternal cyanosis	
	NYHA Class III or IV	

■ **TABLE 8-7.** Cardiovascular Drugs Commonly Used in the Obstetric Intensive Care Setting and Their Effects on Uterine Blood Flow and the Fetus

Drug (FDA class)	Dose	Uterine blood flow (UBF)	Fetal effects
Inotropic agents			
Digoxin (C)	Loading dose 0.5 mg IV over 5 min, then 0.25 mg IV q 6 h × 2. Maintenance 0.125-0.375 mg IV/PO q.d.	No change	Placental transfer Higher maternal maintenance dose required for fetal effect Not teratogenic
Dopamine (C)	Initiate with 5 μg/kg/min and titrate by 5-10 μg/kg/min to max. 50 μg/kg/min	Directly ↓ UBF May ↑ UBF with improved maternal hemodynamics	No known adverse fetal effects
Dobutamine (B)	Initiate with 1.0 μg/kg/min and titrate up to 20 μg/kg/min		No known adverse fetal effects
Epinephrine (C)	Endotracheal, 0.5-1.0 mg q 5 min; IV 0.5 mg bolus and follow with 2-10 μg/kg/min infusion		Not teratogenic
Vasodilators			
Nitroprusside (C)	Initiate with 0.3 μg/kg/min and titrate to 10 μg/kg/min	↑ UBF unless significant ↓ in maternal BP	No known adverse fetal effects Potential for fetal cyanide toxicity Avoid prolonged use
Hydralazine (C)	5-10 mg IV q 15-30 min; total dose 30 mg		Not teratogenic
Nitroglycerin (B)	0.4-0.8 mg sublingual 1-2 in of dermal paste, IV infusion 10 μg/min, titrate up by 10-20 μg/min p.r.n.		Not teratogenic
Beta blockers			
Propranolol (C)	1 mg IV q 2 min as needed	May ↓ by ↑ uterine tone and/or ↓ maternal BP	Not teratogenic Readily crosses placenta Fetal bradycardia IUGR Category D if used in 2nd or 3rd trimester
Labetalol (C)	10-20 mg IV followed by 20-80 mg IV q 10 min to total dose of 150 mg		
Atenolol (D)	5 mg IV over 5 min, repeat in 5 min to a total dose of 15 mg		
Metoprolol (C)z	5 mg IV over 5 min; repeat in 10 min		
Esmolol (C)	500 ug/kg IV over 1 min with infusion rate of 50-200 μg/kg/min		No known adverse fetal effects Rapid metabolism (1/2 life 11 min) also occurs in the fetus

(Continued)

■ TABLE 8-7. Cardiovascular Drugs Commonly Used in the Obstetric Intensive Care Setting and Their Effects on Uterine Blood Flow and the Fetus (*Continued*)

Drug (FDA class)	Dose	Uterine blood flow (UBF)	Fetal effects
Calcium channel blockers			
Verapamil (C)	2.5-5 mg IV bolus over 2 min, repeat in 5 min and then q 30 min p.r.n. to a max dose 20 mg	Mild ↓ UBF	Not teratogenic
Nifedipine (C)	10 mg PO, repeat every 6 h		
Diltiazem (C)	20 mg IV bolus over 2 min, repeat in 15 min		
Vasoconstrictors			
Ephedrine sulphate (C)	10-25 mg slow IV bolus, repeat q 15 min p.r.n × 3	No effect	Not teratogenic 70% of maternal blood level in the fetus
Metaraminol (C)	Initiate with 0.1 mg/min and titrate to 2 mg/min	Mild ↓ UBF	No data available
Antidysrhythmic agents			
Lidocaine (B)	1 mg/kg bolus; repeat 1/2 bolus at 10 min as needed × 4; infusion at 1-4 mg/min; total dose 3 mg/kg	No effect	Not teratogenic Rapidly crosses placenta
Procainamide (C)	100 mg over 30 min, then 2-6 mg/min infusion; total dose 17 mg/kg		
Quinidine (C)	15 mg/kg over 60 min, then 0.02 mg/kg/min infusion		
Bretylium (C)	5 mg/kg IV bolus, then 1-2 mg/min infusion	↓ UBF	Unknown
Phenytoin (D)	300 mg IV, then 100 mg every 5 min to a total of 1000 mg	No effect	Teratogenic Fetal Hydantoin syndrome
Amiodarone (D)	5 mg/kg IV over 3 min, then 10 mg/kg/day		Teratogenic Transient bradycardia Prolonged QT
AV Node blocking agents			
Adenosine	6 mg IV bolus over 1-3 s, followed by 20 mL saline bolus; may repeat at 12 mg in 1-2 min × 2	↑ or ↓ UBF	No known adverse fetal effects
Verapamil	As stated above		
β-Blockers	As stated above		
Digoxin	As stated above		

Source: From McAnulty JH. Heart and other circulatory diseases. In: Bonica JJ, McDonald JS, eds. *Principles and Practice of Obstetric Analgesia and Anesthesia*, 2nd ed. Baltimore, MD: William & Wilkins, 1995;1019-1020.

Pulmonic Stenosis

Key Points

- Isolated lesions most commonly an acquired abnormality as a result of endocarditis in intravenous drug abusers
- Well tolerated in pregnancy with minimal risk of right heart failure

Recommended Workup and Clinical Findings

- Echocardiogram to evaluate severity of right outflow obstruction (>60 mm Hg consistent with severe obstruction)

Potential Complications

- Right heart failure if severe obstruction

Medical Therapy

- Generally not indicated

Anticoagulation

- Not indicated

Anesthetic Issues

- Epidural acceptable

Labor and Delivery

- Reserve cesarean for usual obstetric indications, not demonstrated to improve outcome

Tricuspid Lesions

- Isolated lesions most commonly a result of endocarditis in intravenous drug abusers
- Well tolerated in pregnancy with minimal risk of right heart failure
- Rarely clinically significant in pregnancy

Mitral Stenosis

Key Points

Figure 8-1 is a diagram of mitral stenosis.

- Most common valvular lesion in pregnancy.
- Stenosis of the mitral valve impedes flow of blood from left atrium to the left ventricle.
- Elevated left atrial pressures necessary to maintain adequate left ventricular filling through restricted opening.
- Patients with moderate or severe stenosis are most likely to develop cardiac complications.

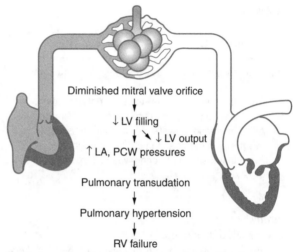

Diminished mitral valve orifice
↓
↓ LV filling
↓ ↘ ↓ LV output
↑ LA, PCW pressures
↓
Pulmonary transudation
↓
Pulmonary hypertension
↓
RV failure

FIGURE 8-1. Pathophysiology of mitral stenosis. LV, left ventricle; LA, left atrium; PCW, pulmonary capillary wedge; RV, right ventricle.

- Patients may be asymptomatic until physiologic changes of pregnancy unmask the disease.
- Symptomatic patients may undergo balloon valvulotomy during pregnancy.

Recommended Workup and Clinical Findings

- Echocardiogram to establish severity of stenosis and size of left atrium
  - Symptoms unusual until valve area <2 cm^2
  - Moderate mitral stenosis: 1 to 1.5 cm^2 valve area
  - Severe mitral stenosis: <1 cm^2 valve area
- ECG to exclude atrial fibrillation from enlarged left atrium. May show left atrial enlargement; right ventricular hypertrophy and right atrial enlargement in cases of pulmonary hypertension.
- Auscultation: loud first heart sound, an opening snap and rumbling diastolic murmur.

Potential Complications

- Pulmonary edema, atrial fibrillation, and supraventricular tachycardia are the most common maternal complications.
- Sixty percent develop the initial episode of pulmonary edema antepartum, at a mean gestational age of 30 weeks.
- Thromboembolism can develop as a result of left atrial dilation. May present as a stroke.

Key Avoids

Avoids: mitral stenosis

1. Avoid tachycardia (decreases diastolic ventricular filling time).
2. Avoid fluid overload (may cause atrial fibrillation, pulmonary edema, and right ventricular failure).
3. Avoid decrease in systemic vascular resistance/ hypotension (decrease in cardiac output).
4. Avoid increase in pulmonary vascular resistance (hypoxia).

Therapy
- Two goals of therapy:
  1. Prevent tachycardia: pain management, beta blockers. Goal HR <100 bpm.
  2. Maintain left ventricular filling (preload) to over- come obstruction. Inadequate preload may not be able to overcome obstruction and lead to inadequate left ventricular filling and drop in cardiac output.
- Diuretics to treat pulmonary edema as needed.
- Digoxin to treat atrial fibrillation as needed.

Anticoagulation
- Consider if left atrium dilated or if chronic atrial fibrillation.

Anesthetic Issues
- Epidural acceptable; may help in control of tachycar- dia in labor by managing pain.
- Avoid abrupt sympathetic blockade which can decrease preload.

Labor and Delivery
- Tocolytic agents that cause tachycardia are contraindi- cated for premature labor (ie, terbutaline).
- Hemodynamic monitoring for severe mitral stenosis.
- Consider assisted second stage of labor.
- Reserve cesarean for usual obstetric indications, not demonstrated to improve outcome.

Mitral Insufficiency

Key Points

Figure 8-2 is a diagram of mitral insufficiency

- Well tolerated in pregnancy.
- Commonly secondary to mitral valve prolapse.

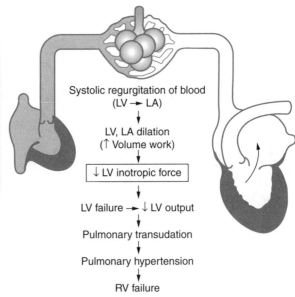

Systolic regurgitation of blood
(LV → LA)

↓

LV, LA dilation
(↑ Volume work)

↓

↓ LV inotropic force

↓

LV failure → ↓ LV output

↓

Pulmonary transudation

↓

Pulmonary hypertension

↓

RV failure

FIGURE 8-2. Pathophysiology of mitral insufficiency. LV, left ventricle; LA, left atrium; RV, right ventricle.

- Longstanding regurgitation may lead to ventricular dysfunction or atrial enlargement.

Recommended Workup and Clinical Findings
- ECG to assess severity of regurgitation and evaluate left atrial enlargement and ventricular function
- ECG to exclude atrial fibrillation from enlarged left atrium. May show left atrial enlargement

Potential Complications
- Rarely, pulmonary edema or dysrhythmias

Key Avoids

Avoids: mitral insufficiency, aortic insufficiency

1. Avoid arrhythmia (immediate treatment, if occurs).
2. Avoid bradycardia (increases regurgitation).
3. Avoid increase in systemic vascular resistance (increases regurgitation).
4. Avoid myocardial depressant drugs.

Medical Therapy
- Necessary only in presence of ventricular dysfunction or dysrhythmias

Anticoagulation
- Consider if left atrium dilated or if chronic atrial fibrillation.

Anesthetic Issues
- Epidural acceptable

Labor and Delivery
- Reserve cesarean section for usual obstetric indications, not demonstrated to improve outcomes.

Aortic Stenosis/Idiopathic Hypertrophic Subaortic Stenosis (IHSS)

Key Points
Figure 8-3 is a diagram of aortic stenosis.

- IHSS is autosomal dominant in inheritance with similar risks and management to aortic stenosis. It is characterized by hypertrophy of the ventricular septum which can obstruct left ventricular outflow.
- When isolated, stenosis is often due to bicuspid aortic valve. If multiple valves involved, usually rheumatic in origin.
- Valve diameter normally 3 to 4 cm^2.
- Mild disease (valve area >1.5 cm^2, peak gradient <50 mm Hg) tolerated well in pregnancy.

- Severe disease (valve area <1 cm^2, peak gradient >75 mm Hg or an ejection fraction <55%) are at significant risk, preconception correction recommended.
- **Stenotic valve leads to fixed cardiac output.**
- Presence of symptoms worsens outcomes. Patients with severe disease should limit activity.
- Complications may develop from underperfusion or excessive flow. Consequences of underperfusion typically more life-threatening than pulmonary edema from fluid overload. Goal pulmonary artery wedge pressures (if measured) is 15 to 17 mm Hg.
- Use diuretics cautiously to avoid underperfusion.

Recommended Workup and Clinical Findings
- Echocardiogram to evaluate size of aortic valve opening, gradient of flow across the valve and ejection fraction.
- ECG may show left ventricular hypertrophy and left atrial enlargement. Arrhythmias possible if significant left atrial enlargement.
- Harsh systolic ejection murmur.

Potential Complications
- If unable to overcome obstruction and maintain adequate cardiac output:
  - Angina: due to decreased coronary perfusion
  - Syncope: due to poor cerebral perfusion
  - Sudden death: due to arrhythmias
- Hypervolemia may lead to pulmonary edema.

Key Avoids

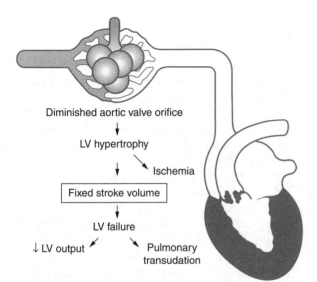

> **Avoids: aortic stenosis**
>
> 1. Avoid hypotension: necessary to maintain coronary perfusion.
> 2. Avoid decreased venous return: ie, excessive blood loss, position, Valsalva.
> 3. Avoid bradycardia: cardiac output maintained by heart rate and stroke volume. If stroke volume limited by obstruction, bradycardia can worsen cardiac output.
> 4. Avoid hypervolemia: may lead to pulmonary edema.

Diminished aortic valve orifice
↓
LV hypertrophy
↓ ↘ Ischemia
Fixed stroke volume
↓
LV failure
↓LV output ↙ ↘ Pulmonary transudation

FIGURE 8-3. Pathophysiology of aortic stenosis, LV, left venticle.

Medical Therapy
- Necessary in presence of dysrhythmias

Anticoagulation
- Not indicated

Anesthetic Issues
- Epidural should be used with great caution to avoid hypotension. Narcotic epidural may be acceptable.

Labor and Delivery
- Reserve cesarean section for usual obstetric indications, not demonstrated to improve outcomes.
- Avoid exertion. Consider shortened second stage of labor.
- Pulmonary edema may develop postpartum due to autotransfusion effect.

Aortic Insufficiency

Key Points
Figure 8-4 is a diagram of aortic insufficiency.

- Well tolerated in pregnancy.
- Significant long standing regurgitation may lead to left ventricular dysfunction.

Recommended Workup and Clinical Findings
- Echocardiogram to assess severity of regurgitation and evaluate left atrial enlargement and ventricular function

Potential Complications
- Complications unlikely. Risk related to underlying left ventricular dysfunction.

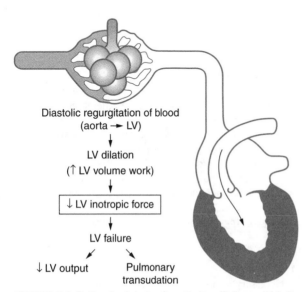

FIGURE 8-4. Pathophysiology of aortic insufficiency. LV, left ventricle.

Key Avoids
Refer to "Avoids" for mitral insufficiency.

Medical Therapy
- Necessary in presence of dysrhythmias

Anticoagulation
- Not indicated

Anesthetic Issues
- Epidural acceptable

Labor and Delivery
- Reserve cesarean section for usual obstetric indications, not demonstrated to improve outcomes.

Mitral Valve Prolapse

- One of the most common cardiac issues during pregnancy.
- Most women are asymptomatic but may have palpitations.
- Pregnancy tolerated well.
- No changes in antenatal or intrapartum management recommended.

Mechanical Heart Valves

Key Points
- Prevention of valve thrombosis poses the primary management challenge in pregnancy. Patients with mechanical valve prostheses require lifelong anticoagulation. Warfarin is the recommended anticoagulant in the nonpregnant population.
- Nonmechanical tissue valves do not significantly increase risk for thromboembolism and do not require anticoagulation unless other risk factors (ie, atrial fibrillation) are present.
- Patients with any of the following are considered high risk for thrombosis:[18]
  - Any mechanical mitral valve.
  - A mechanical aortic valve with any of the following risk factors: atrial fibrillation, previous thromboembolism, ejection fraction <30%, a hypercoagulable state, older generation thrombogenic valves, or multiple valves.

- Older more thrombogenic valves include aortic caged-ball or tilting disc valves (ie, Lillehei Kaster, Omniscience, Starr Edwards).
- The 10-year survival for patients with mechanical valves is 70%. Pregnancy does not appear to shorten expected survival.[19]

Recommended Workup and Clinical Findings
- Echocardiogram to establish location and type of valve and exclude thrombosis. Evaluation of left ventricular dysfunction is also important.
- ECG to establish baseline and exclude atrial fibrillation. Findings are variable like aortic caged-ball or tilting disc valves (eg, Lillehei Kaster, Omniscience, Starr Edwards).
- Auscultation can reveal a variety of findings based on the type and location of the valve. Clicking of the valve may be audible.

Potential Complications
- Maternal mortality risk approximately 3%.[20]
- Valve failure may occur independent of pregnancy.
- Thrombosis of the valve is primary concern.
- Over- and under-anticoagulation can pose risks for maternal and fetal complications.
- Rates of pregnancy loss are increased, particularly with warfarin use.

Key Avoids

Avoids: mechanical valves on anticoagulation

---

1. Avoid warfarin beyond 6 weeks gestation to avoid development of warfarin embryopathy.
2. Avoid insufficient anticoagulation.
3. Avoid continuing anticoagulation intrapartum.
4. Avoid waiting too long to resume anticoagulation postpartum (4-6 h).
5. Avoid resuming warfarin alone postpartum. Include UFH or LMWH until therapeutic.

Medical Therapy
- Anticoagulation addressed below.
- Treat atrial dysrhythmias if present.

Anticoagulation
- Anticoagulation decisions are tailored to patient's risk factors and preference as well as compliance.

- The 2008 Eighth American College of Chest Physicians (ACCP) guidelines for anticoagulation are summarized below:[21]

Option 1: High-dose LMWH therapy throughout gestation. Start enoxaparin 1 mg/kg q 12 h. Goal anti-Xa level 4 h postinjection is ~1 (0.7-1.2) U/mL.

Option 2: High-dose UFH throughout gestation. UFH subcutaneously q 12 h. Goal anti-Xa level mid interval is 0.35-0.7 U/mL or goal mid interval aPTT ≥ 2 times control.

Option 3: Either of the above regimens through completed week 12, then change to warfarin until ~36 wk or close to delivery. Goal INR ~3 (2.5-3.5). UFH or LMWH can then be resumed until delivery.

Option 4: Coumadin throughout gestation until close to delivery. Given increase in fetal complications, this regimen should be considered only for patients at highest risk (prior thromboembolism, older generation prosthesis at mitral location).

LMWH: low molecular weight heparin, UFH: unfractionated heparin

---

- Daily low-dose aspirin may be added to patients at significant increased risk for thrombosis.

Anesthetic Issues
- Epidural acceptable but must be coordinated with last dose of anticoagulation to minimize the risk of epidural hematoma.
- High-dose LMWH should be discontinued 24 hours prior to epidural placement.
- If the patient is on higher doses of UFH, document normal aPTT before placing epidural.[22]

Labor and Delivery
- Reserve cesarean section for usual obstetric indications, not demonstrated to improve outcomes. Operative delivery poses increased risk of bleeding related to need for anticoagulation.
- Consider switch to UFH at 36 weeks or before delivery. Discontinue UFH 4 to 6 hours before delivery and resume anticoagulation 4 to 6 hours postpartum.
- Start LMWH or UFH 4 to 6 hours postpartum. Start warfarin same day. Continue UFH or LMWH until warfarin therapeutic 24 to 48 hours or minimum 72 hours.

■ CONGENITAL CARDIAC LESIONS

Intracardiac communications in the form of atrial and ventricular septal defects as well as patent ductus arteriosus, allow for shunting of blood across the defect. As a result, the heart must contend with larger volumes and additional demands. Over time this can lead to ventricular dysfunction, overdistension of the atria, cardiac failure or pulmonary overload, and pulmonary hypertension. Flow is typically in a left-to-right direction. As the pulmonary pressures increase, shunting can change direction and become right to left, as with Eisenmenger syndrome which is addressed later. The shunt is described by the direction of flow as well as the proportion of pulmonary to systemic (right-to-left) flow.

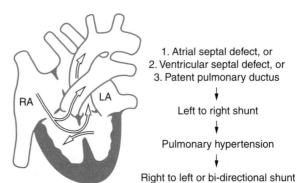

1. Atrial septal defect, or
2. Ventricular septal defect, or
3. Patent pulmonary ductus

↓

Left to right shunt

↓

Pulmonary hypertension

↓

Right to left or bi-directional shunt

FIGURE 8-5. Pathophysiology of Eisenmenger syndrome. RA, right atrium; LA, left atrium.

Atrial Septal Defect (ASD)

Key Points

- Secundum ASD is the most common defect seen in pregnancy.
- ASD size and flow across the shunt can worsen in adults. Spontaneous closure is rare in adults.[23]
- Pregnancy is generally well tolerated.
- Pregnancy does not change indications for closure. Patients with symptoms (paradoxical emboli, exercise intolerance, fatigue, heart failure, dysrhythmias) or pulmonary to systemic shunt flow ratio >2:1 are candidates for closure of the defect.

Recommended Workup and Clinical Findings

- Echocardiogram to evaluate size of defect, severity of shunting, and measure pulmonary artery pressures. Pregnancy may falsely elevate echocardiogram estimates of pulmonary artery pressures.[24]
- ECG: Partial right bundle branch block, right axis deviation, and sometimes right ventricular hypertrophy.
- Auscultation: Systolic ejection murmur at left sternal border and wide fixed split second heart sound.

Potential Complications

- Patients with a large defect and significant left-to-right shunt may develop atrial arrhythmias (atrial fibrillation) and congestive heart failure in pregnancy.
- Pulmonary hypertension may be present and may lead to Eisenmenger syndrome (covered in later section). Demonstrated in Fig 8-5.
- Paradoxical emboli: Emboli originating in lower extremities and pelvis or from the defect may travel across defect to brain, causing stroke.

Medical Therapy

- Necessary in presence of dysrhythmias

Anticoagulation

- Not indicated. Role of anticoagulation for patients with history of paradoxical embolus and unrepaired defect is unclear. VTE prophylaxis is recommended for patients at prolonged bed rest or perioperatively.

Anesthetic Issues

- Epidural acceptable

Labor and Delivery

- Reserve cesarean for usual obstetric indications, not demonstrated to improve outcome.

Ventricular Septal Defect (VSD)

Key Points

- Common in childhood, but most close spontaneously or have been surgically repaired by adulthood.
- Smaller VSDs (<0.5 cm) restrict flow across the lesion and carry lower risk for Eisenmenger syndrome if unrepaired into adulthood. Larger lesions (>1 cm) allow for more equal flow between the left and right heart and are more likely associated with increased pulmonary pressures and Eisenmenger syndrome in the adult. See Fig 8-5.
  - Because most larger lesions have been repaired by adulthood, pregnancy is generally well tolerated.

Recommended Workup and Clinical Findings

- Echocardiogram to determine size of the lesion, direction of shunt flow, estimation of pulmonary artery pressures, and performance of the ventricles.

- ECG: Usually normal, may demonstrate left or right ventricular hypertrophy.
- Auscultation: Holosystolic thrill and murmur at left sternal border.

Potential Complications
- Similar to ASD
- Congestive heart failure or dysrhythmias possible with large lesions

Key Avoids

> **Avoids: ASD, VSD, and PDA**
>
> 1. Avoid hypertension (increase in systemic vascular resistance increases left-to-right shunt).
> 2. Avoid decrease in pulmonary vascular resistance (increases left-to-right shunt).
> 3. Avoid supraventricular arrhythmias, tachycardia (may increase left-to-right shunt).
> 4. If pulmonary hypertension is present, avoid increase in pulmonary vascular resistance (metabolic acidosis, excess catecholamines, hypoxemia, nitrous oxide, hypercarbia, pharmacologic vasoconstrictors, and lung hyperinflation) and hypotension. Both may worsen right-to-left shunt and lead to Eisenmenger syndrome.

Medical Therapy
- Necessary in presence of dysrhythmias

Anticoagulation
- Not indicated. Refer to comments on ASD.

Anesthetic Issues
- Epidural acceptable in absence of pulmonary hypertension or known Eisenmenger syndrome

Labor and Delivery
- Reserve cesarean for usual obstetric indications, not demonstrated to improve outcome

Patent Ductus Arteriosus (PDA)

Key Points
- Most cases are diagnosed and corrected in childhood.
- Uncommon lesion in pregnancy.
- Small PDA usually asymptomatic and tolerated well in pregnancy.
- Large PDAs are associated with risks of ventricular overload and pulmonary hypertension similar to ASD and VSD.

Recommended Workup and Clinical Findings
- Echocardiogram to evaluate diameter and length of patent ductus and to calculate the pulmonary to systemic shunt ration. Ratios >2.2 to 1 are considered large.
- ECG: Usually normal, may demonstrate left or right ventricular hypertrophy.
- Auscultation: Grade 3/6 continuous systolic and diastolic murmur in infraclavicular region (Gibson murmur).

Potential Complications
- Similar to ASD and VSD. See Fig 8-5.

Key Avoids
Refer to table in VSD section.

Medical Therapy
- Necessary in presence of dysrhythmias

Anticoagulation
- Not indicated. Refer to comments on ASD and VSD.

Anesthetic Issues
- Epidural acceptable in absence of pulmonary hypertension or known Eisenmenger syndrome

Labor and Delivery
- Reserve cesarean for usual obstetric indications, not demonstrated to improve outcome

Secondary Pulmonary Hypertension and Eisenmenger Syndrome

Key Points
Figure 8-5 is a diagram of Eisenmenger syndrome due to ASD, VSD, or PDA.

- Secondary pulmonary hypertension results from excess flow into the pulmonary circulation from chronic left-to-right (systemic-to-pulmonary) shunting across an intracardiac communication (most commonly ASD, VSD, PDA).
- Pulmonary pressures may exceed systemic pressures. When this happens, flow across the shunt reverses to right-to-left. The result is decreased pulmonary perfusion, hypoxemia, and worsening pulmonary hypertension as a result of hypoxemia. This reversal defines Eisenmenger syndrome.
- Mortality rates are high. Pregnancy termination should be discussed with the patient.
- Fetal loss rates approach 75%.

Recommended Workup and Clinical Findings
- In patients with suspected secondary pulmonary hypertension, the following evaluation is recommended:[25]
  - Pulse oximetry, including finger and toe oximetry, with and without administration of supplemental oxygen.
  - Electrocardiogram may show ventricular hypertrophy with associated ST-T wave changes or a right atrial abnormality.
  - Chest x-ray abnormalities include dilatation of the central pulmonary arteries, abrupt termination of peripheral pulmonary artery branches (pruning), and right heart enlargement.
  - Complete blood count and nuclear lung scintigraphy.
  - Transthoracic and transesophageal echocardiography, cardiovascular magnetic resonance imaging (CMRI), or computed tomography (CT).
- Cyanosis and clubbing as well as poor exercise tolerance are typical findings.
- Polycythemia is common.

Potential Complications
- Decreased systemic vascular resistance of pregnancy leads to worsening of the right-to-left shunt, worsening hypoxemia and death in 30% to 50% of patients.
- Death usually occurs in the first week postpartum.
- Most common causes of death are due to worsening and intractable hypoxemia, volume depletion, preeclampsia, and thromboembolism.

Key Avoids

Avoids: secondary pulmonary hypertension and Eisenmenger syndrome

1. Avoid hypotension (decrease in systemic vascular resistance causes massive right-to-left shunting, bypassing pulmonary circulation leading to severe hypoxemia and worsening pulmonary hypertension).
2. Avoid excessive blood loss and volume depletion (causes hypotension by decrease in venous return).
3. Avoid increase in pulmonary vascular resistance (ie, hypoxemia, hypercarbia, metabolic acidosis, excess catecholamines).
4. Avoid myocardial depressant drugs.
5. Avoid iron deficiency.
6. Avoid high altitude.
7. Avoid exercise.

Medical Therapy
- Pulmonary artery vasodilators are recommended.[26]

Anticoagulation
- Pulmonary artery thrombosis is common in nonpregnant patients (21%-70%) and is more likely to occur in women.[27,28] Prophylactic anticoagulation should be considered in patients who continue the pregnancy.

Anesthetic Issues
- Epidural is contraindicated. Narcotic-only epidural may be acceptable.

Labor and Delivery
- Outcomes appear to be similar with cesarean or vaginal delivery. Mortality rates for any surgery in nonpregnant patients with Eisenmenger syndrome are high (19%).[29]
- Continuous pulse oximetry and supplemental oxygen to keep oxygen saturations at or above 90%.
- Avoid air embolism: meticulous attention to IV infusions.

Coarctation of Aorta

Key Points
- Rarely seen in pregnancy, as most are corrected in childhood.
- Classic presentation in adults is hypertension.
- Most common site is distal to the left subclavian artery, so hypertension will be measured equally in both arms. The femoral pulse is delayed compared to the brachial pulse, and the lower extremity pressures are low.
- Surgical repair is recommended for adults with a "peak to peak" gradient >20 mm Hg (the difference between the peak pressure distal and proximal to the narrowing).[30]
- Postrepair, patients remain at risk for complications including re-coarctation, aortic aneurysm and dissection, and hypertension.
- Thirty to forty percent of patients will also have a bicuspid aortic valve.
- Ten percent of patients will also have intracranial aneurysms (versus 2% in the general population).
- All patients should have magnetic resonance angiography of the thoracic aorta and intracranial vessels performed at least once.[31]

Recommended Workup and Clinical Findings
- Echocardiogram to identify severity of the narrowing, evaluate left ventricular function and exclude additional cardiac defects.

- ECG is usually normal, may show left ventricular hypertrophy.
- Auscultation: may be normal. Various murmurs are possible based on presence of associated anomalies and size of collateral vessel development.

Potential Complications
- Adults with uncorrected coarctation (native) are likely to have hypertension and coronary artery disease and are at risk for dissection and heart failure. This may be exacerbated by pregnancy.

Key Avoids

> **Avoids: aortic coarctation**
>
> ---
>
> 1. Avoid excessive blood loss (causes hypotension by decrease in venous return).
> 2. Avoid myocardial depressant drugs.
> 3. Avoid bradycardia.
> 4. Avoid Valsalva efforts.

Medical Therapy
- Treat systemic hypertension as needed.

Anticoagulation
- Not indicated

Anesthetic Issues
- Epidural acceptable

Labor and Delivery
- Cesarean delivery rates are higher primarily due to perceived risk of intracranial hemorrhage or aortic dissection.
- Vaginal delivery may be accomplished with attention to controlling pain and blood pressure fluctuations, maintaining adequate cardiac preload and minimizing Valsalva efforts at delivery.

Tetralogy of Fallot

Key Points
- Tetrad of findings:
  - Ventricular septal defect
  - Overriding aorta
  - Right ventricular outflow obstruction
  - Right ventricular hypertrophy

- Most patients undergo intracardiac repair in first year of life.
- Major long-term issues postrepair include right ventricular dysfunction and failure, tricuspid regurgitation, atrial and ventricular dysrhythmias, and sudden cardiac death.[32]
- Patients may also have persistent intracardiac shunting, pulmonary hypertension, aortic root dilation, or aortic valve incompetence.
- Most common cause of death is sudden cardiac death and heart failure. Mortality rates approximately 1% annually 25 years post procedure.

Recommended Workup and Clinical Findings
- Echocardiogram to establish cardiac anatomy, evaluate valvular and right ventricular function, assess pulmonary hypertension, and measure aortic root diameter.
- Electrocardiogram will be variable depending on the type of correction performed. Important to establish baseline and exclude atrial and ventricular dysrhythmias.

Potential Complications
- Spontaneous fetal loss rates increased.
- Patients with surgically corrected Tetralogy of Fallot (TOF) generally tolerate pregnancy well. However, patients with evidence of right ventricular dysfunction, severe pulmonary regurgitation, pulmonary hypertension, and hypoxemia are at increased risk for cardiac complications. These include dysrhythmias, cardiac failure, worsening cyanosis, pulmonary edema, and pulmonary embolus.[32]
- Patients with persistent intracardiac shunts are at additional risk. Refer to sections on VSD, ASD, and PDA.

Medical Therapy
- Antidysrhythmic therapy as needed.
- Patients may already be on diuretic therapy, beta blockers, or antihypertensive medications.

Anticoagulation
- Not indicated

Anesthetic Issues
- Epidural acceptable if an intracardiac shunt is not present.

Labor and Delivery
- Cesarean delivery is common and typically performed due to perceived cardiac risk. Data are lacking to demonstrate improved outcomes compared to vaginal delivery.

The Marfan Syndrome

Key Points

- Autosomal dominant condition. Eighty percent will have cardiac effects of the disease.
- Aneurysmal dilation and dissection of the aorta account for the majority of the morbidity and mortality with the Marfan syndrome.
- Sixty to eighty percent of adults with the Marfan syndrome will have aortic root dilation with or without aortic regurgitation.
- Risk of aortic rupture or dissection during pregnancy is ~10% if aortic root diameter >4 cm.[33]
- Rupture and dissection can occur even with normal aortic dimension (<1%). Because of this risk, all women with the Marfan syndrome should be counseled against pregnancy and termination discussed if the patient becomes pregnant.[34]
- Aortic root diameter >4.5 cm is an indication for preconception repair if patient desires pregnancy. The risk for dissection is decreased but not eliminated following surgical correction.
- Pregnancy may hasten rate of aortic root dilation in patients with aortic root >4 cm.[35]

Recommended Workup and Clinical Findings

- Echocardiogram to establish size of aortic root. This should be followed serially even if the baseline diameter is normal.
- The Marfan syndrome is associated with other clinical abnormalities including: joint hypermobility, ectopia lentis, pectus excavatum, arm span exceeds height, scoliosis, and arachnodactyly.

Potential Complications

- Aortic root dissection and rupture are the most significant risks of pregnancy.

Key Avoids

> **Avoids: the Marfan syndrome**
>
> 1. Avoid hypertension.
> 2. Avoid tachycardia.
> 3. Avoid Valsalva.

Medical Therapy

- Labetalol or metoprolol is required for all patients to maintain heart rate <110 bpm after submaximal exercise and <90 bpm resting.

Anticoagulation

- Not indicated

Anesthetic Issues

- Epidural acceptable and may be recommended to minimize tachycardia due to pain and avoid urge for Valsalva during delivery.

Labor and Delivery

- Avoid tachycardia—consider continuous beta blocker.
- Assisted second stage to minimize Valsalva effort. Avoid pushing in labor.
- Cesarean may benefit patients with aortic root diameter >4 cm, aortic root dissection, or heart failure.[36]

Peripartum Cardiomyopathy

Key Points

- Criteria for diagnosis of peripartum cardiomyopathy
  - Classic:
    - Development of cardiac failure in last month or within 5 months postpartum
    - Absence of an identifiable cause for cardiac failure
    - Absence of recognizable heart disease prior to last month of pregnancy
  - Additional:
    - Left ventricular systolic dysfunction: ejection fraction <45%, shortening fraction <30%, and left ventricular end-diastolic dimension >2.7 cm/m^2 body surface area.[37]
- Ninety percent of cases occur in first 2 months postpartum.
- Half of deaths occur in first 6 weeks postpartum.
- High rate of recurrence in subsequent pregnancies even with apparent recovery of cardiac function. Consider stress echocardiogram to evaluate cardiac function before subsequent pregnancies. Patients with incomplete recovery (ejection fraction <50%) have a high rate of decompensation and should be counseled against future pregnancies.
- Recommend low salt diet (<4 g/d), fluid restriction (<2 L/d) and activity limitation.

Recommended Workup and Clinical Findings

- Echocardiogram: refer to key points. Establish baseline and repeat every trimester or with worsening symptoms.
- Electrocardiogram is nonspecific, possibly atrial fibrillation.

- Chest x-ray will demonstrate cardiomegaly and pulmonary edema.
- Patients will typically present with shortness of breath, orthopnea, fatigue, and leg edema.
- B-type natriuretic peptide (BNP) will be markedly elevated.

Potential Complications

- Worsening cardiac failure and pulmonary edema. Patients with an initial ejection fraction of <25% are at greatest risk for subsequent cardiac transplantation.[38]
- Failure to normalize cardiac function within 6 months postpartum carries mortality rate of 85% by 5 years.
- Cause of death commonly dysrhythmias, progressive cardiac failure, or thromboembolic phenomena.

Key Avoids

> **Avoids: cardiomyopathy**
>
> 1. Avoid hypertension.
> 2. Avoid excessive fluid.
> 3. Avoid increasing cardiac demand.

Medical Therapy

- Goals of therapy:
  - Reduce preload: diuretic therapy (ie, furosemide 20-40 mg po qd).
  - Reduce afterload: vasodilator therapy (ie, hydralazine 25-100 mg po qd, amlodipine 5-10 mg po qd; postpartum use enalapril 5 mg bid).
  - Improve contractility: digoxin 0.25-0.5 mg po qd.
  - Reduce myocardial oxygen requirement: Goal HR 80 to 100 bpm (metoprolol 25-100 mg po qd, carvedilol 3.25 to 25 mg po qd).
- Pentoxifylline (Trental®) 400 mg po tid may reduce inflammation and reduce mortality risk.[39,40]

Anticoagulation

- Consider in presence of significant ventricular dilation or atrial dysrhythmia.

Anesthetic Issues

- Epidural acceptable and will decrease preload and afterload. Also minimizes tachycardia from pain.

Labor and Delivery

- Reserve cesarean for usual obstetric indications, not demonstrated to improve outcome.
- Consider assisted second stage if significant cardiac dysfunction.

Acute Myocardial Infarction (MI)

Key Points

- Rare event but risk increased by pregnancy.
- Three major risk factors: age >30, hypertension, diabetes.
- Eighty percent occur in antepartum or postpartum period.
- Findings with acute MI: atherosclerosis 40%, coronary artery dissection 27%, coronary thrombus 21%, normal coronary artery 13%-29%.[41,42]
- Diagnosis established with elevated troponin (and/or elevated CKMB levels) plus abnormal ECG. Most associated with ST segment elevation (STEMI).

Recommended Workup and Clinical Findings

- Echocardiogram to exclude unrecognized structural cardiac abnormality, evaluate ventricular function.
- Electrocardiogram to establish diagnosis: ST segment elevation or depression, Q wave abnormalities.
- Lab workup should include: troponin, CBC with platelet count, PT and INR, aPTT, electrolytes, magnesium, BUN, creatinine, blood glucose, and serum lipid profile.

Potential Complications

- Cardiac arrest possible. Prepare for possibility of perimortem cesarean section.
- Maternal mortality from in-hospital MI 5% to 7%.[43,44]
- Cardiac failure or dysrhythmias.

Medical Therapy

- Management algorithm once acute MI suspected: (Goal is completion of MONA in <10 minutes).

  M: Morphine sulfate 2-4 mg IV
  O: Oxygen nasal cannula or mask
  N: Nitroglycerin sublingual 0.5 mg q 5 min × 3
  A: Aspirin 160-325 mg chewed

- Follow with 12-lead ECG (repeat in 5-10 minutes if MI suspected and initial ECG normal).
- If ECG shows ST elevation or new left bundle branch block, treat as acute MI in consultation with cardiologists:
  - Beta blockers
  - IV nitroglycerin
  - IV heparin

- Antiplatelet therapy (clopidogrel)
- Morphine IV to treat pain
- Antithrombin therapy
- Consider reperfusion therapy in consultation with cardiologist
- If viable fetus, monitor fetal heart rate throughout therapy.

Anticoagulation
- See above.

Anesthetic Issues
- Epidural recommended to reduce afterload and to minimize pain and subsequent tachycardia.

Labor and Delivery
- Expert opinion recommends postponing delivery until 2 to 3 weeks postinfarct to minimize additional cardiac demands.[42]
- If vaginal delivery attempted, consider assisted second stage to minimize cardiac work.
- Delivery route should be individualized. Cesarean delivery may be associated with increased mortality risk.[45]
- Avoid hypertension or tachycardia.
- Avoid methergine and prostaglandins as they may cause coronary vasoconstriction.

REFERENCES

1. Berg CJ, Atrash HK, Koonin LM, Tucker M. Pregnancy-related mortality in the United States, 1987-1990. *Obstet Gynecol*. 1996 Aug;88(2):161-167.

2. Berg CJ, Chang J, Callaghan WM, Whitehead SJ. Pregnancy-related mortality in the United States, 1991-1997. *Obstet Gynecol*. 2003 Feb;101(2):289-296.

3. El-Solh AA, Grant BJ. A comparison of severity of illness scoring systems for critically ill obstetric patients. *Chest*. 1996 Nov;110(5):1299-1304.

4. Loverro G, Pansini V, Greco P, Vimercati A, Parisi AM, Selvaggi L. Indications and outcome for intensive care unit admission during puerperium. *Arch Gynecol Obstet*. 2001 Nov;265(4):195-198.

5. Mabie WC, Sibai BM. Treatment in an obstetric intensive care unit. *Am J Obstet Gynecol*. 1990 Jan;162(1):1-4.

6. Mahutte NG, Murphy-Kaulbeck L, Le Q, Solomon J, Benjamin A, Boyd ME. Obstetric admissions to the intensive care unit. *Obstet Gynecol*. 1999 Aug;94(2):263-266.

7. Naylor DF Jr, Olson MM. Critical care obstetrics and gynecology. *Crit Care Clin*. 2003 Jan;19(1):127-149.

8. Tang LC, Kwok AC, Wong AY, Lee YY, Sun KO, So AP. Critical care in obstetrical patients: an eight-year review. *Chin Med J (Engl)*. 1997 Dec;110(12):936-941.

9. Zeeman GG, Wendel GD Jr, Cunningham FG. A blueprint for obstetric critical care. *Am J Obstet Gynecol*. 2003 Feb;188(2):532-536.

10. Hsieh TT, Chen KC, Soong JH. Outcome of pregnancy in patients with organic heart disease in Taiwan. *Asia Oceania J Obstet Gynaecol*. 1993 Mar;19(1):21-27.

11. Clark SL. Structural cardiac disease in pregnancy. In: Clark SL, Cotton DB, Phelan JP, eds. *Critical Care Obstetrics*. Oradell, NJ: Medical Economics Books; 1987:92.

12. Siu SC, Sermer M, Colman JM, et al. Prospective multicenter study of pregnancy outcomes in women with heart disease. *Circulation*. 2001 Jul 31;104(5):515-521.

13. Dye TD, Gordon H, Held B, Tolliver NJ, Holmes AP. Retrospective maternal mortality case ascertainment in West Virginia, 1985 to 1989. *Am J Obstet Gynecol*. 1992 Jul;167(1):72-76.

14. de SM. Maternal mortality from heart disease in pregnancy. *Br Heart J*. 1993 Jun;69(6):524.

15. Siu SC, Colman JM, Sorensen S, et al. Adverse neonatal and cardiac outcomes are more common in pregnant women with cardiac disease. *Circulation*. 2002 May 7;105(18):2179-2184.

16. Wilson W, Taubert KA, Gewitz M, et al. Prevention of infective endocarditis: guidelines from the American Heart Association: a guideline from the American Heart Association Rheumatic Fever, Endocarditis, and Kawasaki Disease Committee, Council on Cardiovascular Disease in the Young, and the Council on Clinical Cardiology, Council on Cardiovascular Surgery and Anesthesia, and the Quality of Care and Outcomes Research Interdisciplinary Working Group. *Circulation*. 2007 Oct 9;116(15):1736-1754.

17. Reimold SC, Rutherford JD. Clinical practice. Valvular heart disease in pregnancy. *N Engl J Med*. 2003 Jul 3;349(1):52-59.

18. Douketis JD, Berger PB, Dunn AS, et al. The perioperative management of antithrombotic therapy: American College of Chest Physicians Evidence-Based Clinical Practice Guidelines (8th ed.). *Chest*. 2008 Jun;133(6 Suppl):299S-339S.

19. North RA, Sadler L, Stewart AW, McCowan LM, Kerr AR, White HD. Long-term survival and valve-related complications in young women with cardiac valve replacements. *Circulation*. 1999 May 25;99(20):2669-2676.

20. Chan WS, Anand S, Ginsberg JS. Anticoagulation of pregnant women with mechanical heart valves: a systematic review of the literature. *Arch Intern Med*. 2000 Jan 24;160(2):191-196.

21. Bates SM, Greer IA, Pabinger I, Sofaer S, Hirsh J. Venous thromboembolism, thrombophilia, antithrombotic therapy, and pregnancy: American College of Chest Physicians Evidence-Based Clinical Practice Guidelines (8th ed.). *Chest.* 2008 Jun;133(6 Suppl):844S-886S.

22. Neal JM, Bernards CM, Hadzic A, et al. ASRA Practice Advisory on Neurologic Complications in Regional Anesthesia and Pain Medicine. *Reg Anesth Pain Med.* 2008 Sep;33(5):404-415.

23. McMahon CJ, Feltes TF, Fraley JK, et al. Natural history of growth of secundum atrial septal defects and implications for transcatheter closure. *Heart.* 2002 Mar;87(3):256-259.

24. Penning S, Robinson KD, Major CA, Garite TJ. A comparison of echocardiography and pulmonary artery catheterization for evaluation of pulmonary artery pressures in pregnant patients with suspected pulmonary hypertension. *Am J Obstet Gynecol.* 2001 Jun;184(7):1568-1570.

25. Warnes CA, Williams RG, Bashore TM, et al. ACC/AHA 2008 Guidelines for the Management of Adults with Congenital Heart Disease: a report of the American College of Cardiology/American Heart Association Task Force on Practice Guidelines (writing committee to develop guidelines on the management of adults with congenital heart disease). *Circulation.* 2008 Dec 2;118(23):e714-e833.

26. Warnes CA, Williams RG, Bashore TM, et al. ACC/AHA 2008 Guidelines for the Management of Adults with Congenital Heart Disease: a report of the American College of Cardiology/American Heart Association Task Force on Practice Guidelines (writing committee to develop guidelines on the management of adults with congenital heart disease). *Circulation.* 2008 Dec 2;118(23):e714-e833.

27. Silversides CK, Granton JT, Konen E, Hart MA, Webb GD, Therrien J. Pulmonary thrombosis in adults with Eisenmenger syndrome. *J Am Coll Cardiol.* 2003 Dec 3;42(11):1982-1987.

28. Perloff JK, Hart EM, Greaves SM, Miner PD, Child JS. Proximal pulmonary arterial and intrapulmonary radiologic features of Eisenmenger syndrome and primary pulmonary hypertension. *Am J Cardiol.* 2003 Jul 15;92(2):182-187.

29. Vongpatanasin W, Brickner ME, Hillis LD, Lange RA. The Eisenmenger syndrome in adults. *Ann Intern Med.* 1998 May 1;128(9):745-755.

30. Warnes CA, Williams RG, Bashore TM, et al. ACC/AHA 2008 Guidelines for the Management of Adults with Congenital Heart Disease: a report of the American College of Cardiology/American Heart Association Task Force on Practice Guidelines (writing committee to develop guidelines on the management of adults with congenital heart disease). *Circulation.* 2008 Dec 2;118(23):e714-e833.

31. Warnes CA, Williams RG, Bashore TM, et al. ACC/AHA 2008 Guidelines for the Management of Adults with Congenital Heart Disease: a report of the American College of Cardiology/American Heart Association Task Force on Practice Guidelines (writing committee to develop guidelines on the management of adults with congenital heart disease). *Circulation.* 2008 Dec 2;118(23):e714-e833.

32. Veldtman GR, Connolly HM, Grogan M, Ammash NM, Warnes CA. Outcomes of pregnancy in women with tetralogy of Fallot. *J Am Coll Cardiol.* 2004 Jul 7;44(1):174-180.

33. Expert consensus document on management of cardiovascular diseases during pregnancy. *Eur Heart J.* 2003 Apr;24(8):761-781.

34. Bonow RO, Carabello BA, Chatterjee K, et al. ACC/AHA 2006 guidelines for the management of patients with valvular heart disease: a report of the American College of Cardiology/American Heart Association Task Force on Practice Guidelines (writing committee to revise the 1998 guidelines for the management of patients with valvular heart disease) developed in collaboration with the Society of Cardiovascular Anesthesiologists endorsed by the Society for Cardiovascular Angiography and Interventions and the Society of Thoracic Surgeons. *J Am Coll Cardiol.* 2006 Aug 1;48(3):e1-e148.

35. Meijboom LJ, Vos FE, Timmermans J, Boers GH, Zwinderman AH, Mulder BJ. Pregnancy and aortic root growth in the Marfan syndrome: a prospective study. *Eur Heart J.* 2005 May;26(9):914-920.

36. Vahanian A, Baumgartner H, Bax J, et al. Guidelines on the management of valvular heart disease: The Task Force on the Management of Valvular Heart Disease of the European Society of Cardiology. *Eur Heart J.* 2007 Jan;28(2):230-268.

37. Pearson GD, Veille JC, Rahimtoola S, et al. Peripartum cardiomyopathy: National Heart, Lung, and Blood Institute and Office of Rare Diseases (National Institutes of Health) workshop recommendations and review. *JAMA.* 2000 Mar 1;283(9):1183-1188.

38. Habli M, O'Brien T, Nowack E, Khoury S, Barton JR, Sibai B. Peripartum cardiomyopathy: prognostic factors for long-term maternal outcome. *Am J Obstet Gynecol.* 2008 Oct;199(4):415.

39. Sliwa K, Skudicky D, Candy G, Bergemann A, Hopley M, Sareli P. The addition of pentoxifylline to conventional therapy improves outcome in patients with peripartum cardiomyopathy. *Eur J Heart Fail.* 2002 Jun;4(3):305-309.

40. Sliwa K, Fett J, Elkayam U. Peripartum cardiomyopathy. *Lancet.* 2006 Aug 19;368(9536):687-693.

41. Roth A, Elkayam U. Acute myocardial infarction associated with pregnancy. *J Am Coll Cardiol.* 2008 Jul 15;52(3):171-180.

42. Roth A, Elkayam U. Acute myocardial infarction associated with pregnancy. *Ann Intern Med.* 1996 Nov 1;125(9):751-762.

43. Ladner HE, Danielsen B, Gilbert WM. Acute myocardial infarction in pregnancy and the puerperium: a population-based study. *Obstet Gynecol.* 2005 Mar;105(3):480-484.

44. James AH, Jamison MG, Biswas MS, Brancazio LR, Swamy GK, Myers ER. Acute myocardial infarction in pregnancy: a United States population-based study. *Circulation.* 2006 Mar 28;113(12):1564-1571.

45. Badui E, Enciso R. Acute myocardial infarction during pregnancy and puerperium: a review. *Angiology.* 1996 Aug;47(8):739-756.

CHAPTER 9

Maternal Sepsis

• *George R. Saade*

Sepsis, severe sepsis, and septic shock are a continuum in the systemic response to infection. Sepsis is the leading cause of mortality in intensive care units and accounts for 10% of direct maternal deaths in North America. Most deaths in sepsis are due to multiple organ dysfunction syndrome (MODS), the final stage in the sepsis spectrum. The obstetric patient is particularly vulnerable to sepsis because of the association between pregnancy and infectious complications such as pyelonephritis, chorioamnionitis, endometritis, wound infection, necrotizing fasciitis, and cholecystitis. Septic shock occurs in up to 4% of bacteremic patients, and 40% to 60% of patients in septic shock have bacteremia. The relationship between bacteremia and sepsis also depends on other contributing factors such as immune suppression, and associated medical conditions. Overall, gram-negative aerobic bacilli used to be the predominant organisms associated with sepsis. However, the incidence of infection with gram-positive organisms in patients with sepsis has increased and may now equal that of gram-negative infections.

■ DEFINITIONS

Sepsis is the development of systemic inflammatory response syndrome (SIRS, Table 9-1) in response to infection. Sepsis is called severe when there is evidence of end-organ damage. Septic shock is defined as sepsis with hypotension (systolic blood pressure <90 mm Hg or a reduction of ≥40 mm Hg from baseline) despite volume replacement (or requirement for vasopressors) along with the presence of perfusion abnormalities that may include, but are not limited to, lactic acidosis, oliguria, or an acute alteration in mental status.

■ PATHOGENESIS

Sepsis has been viewed as an uncontrolled inflammatory response to infection. This hypothesis was based on animal studies as well as measures of immune response in humans, including cytokine levels. This view has been recently challenged by the failure to decrease mortality in clinical trials of anti-inflammatory agents, and by evidence of a severely compromised immune system that is unable to eradicate the infection. The immunological response in patients with sepsis may even be biphasic, with an anti-inflammatory phase following an initial overwhelming response. The cardiovascular manifestations of sepsis are the results of alterations in peripheral vascular tone and cardiac function. The decrease in vascular tone affects both the arterial and venous systems, and is believed to be due to an increase in smooth muscle relaxants such as nitric oxide. Microvascular changes such as endothelial cell swelling, fibrin deposition, and aggregation of circulating cells also contribute to the abnormal blood flow seen in patients with sepsis. Cardiac output depends on the intravascular volume status of the patient. In the early stages of septic shock, cardiac output may be decreased because of hypovolemia and low cardiac filling. Cardiac output increases after fluid replacement. Myocardial dysfunction is seen in most patients with septic shock and affects both the right and left ventricles. Myocardial depressants include many of the cytokines as well as nitric oxide.

■ MANAGEMENT

The general management guidelines for a patient with sepsis are outlined in Table 9-2. The following discussion will concentrate on the overall principles for the management of sepsis, mostly septic shock. The details of each management option (central hemodynamic monitoring, drug pharmacology, fetal effects, etc) are covered in the different chapters pertaining specifically to these issues. A number of studies have shown that implementation of sepsis protocols for early identification and management improve outcomes.

■ TABLE 9-1. Definition of Systemic Inflammatory Response Syndrome

- Temperature >38°C or <36°C
- Respiratory rate >20 breaths per minute or $PaCO_2$ <32 mm Hg
- Pulse >90 bpm
- White blood cell count >12,000/cc, or <4000/cc, or bands >10%

At least two of the above are required.

■ TABLE 9-3. Most Common Sources for Infection in Obstetrical Patients

- Reproductive tract
- Urinary
- Wound infection
- Chorioamnionitis
- Cholecystitis
- Respiratory

During the initial evaluation, a search for the source of the infection should take into account the most common sources in a pregnant or postpartum woman (Table 9-3). Testing may include chest x-ray to exclude pneumonia, abdomino-pelvic CT scan or MRI to search for abscesses, myometrial necrosis, and pyometria, as well as amniocentesis to exclude intra-amniotic infection. Diagnosis of infection relies on clinical suspicion and a search for an infectious agent. Collections identified by radiology should be aspirated and drained under guidance, and samples sent for Gram and fungal staining and culture. Purulent wounds or those with spreading cellulitis should prompt swabbing for culture. When infection is suspected in contaminated or dirty abdominal wounds, anaerobic infections should be assumed irrespective of the culture results. Blood cultures should be taken as soon as possible after the onset of fever or chills. According to the recommendations of the International Sepsis Forum, blood for culture should be obtained by fresh venipuncture. The skin

■ TABLE 9-2. General Treatment Guidelines for Sepsis

- Broad spectrum antibiotics
- Aggressive fluid replacement guided by CVP or pulmonary artery catheter (wedge pressure 12-18 mm Hg)
- Blood products as needed (anemia, DIC)
- Vasopressors and inotropes
- Removal of infection source
- Ventilatory support
- Supportive care (DVT prophylaxis, nutritional support, stress ulcer prophylaxis, hemofiltration)
- Immunological therapy
- Delivery as last resort (unless chorioamnionitis)

should be swabbed twice with either 70% isopropyl alcohol or iodine-containing solution. About 10 to 30 mL of blood should be inoculated in each culture bottle, and priority is given to the aerobic bottle if the volume of blood obtained is insufficient. The needle used for venipuncture should be changed prior to inoculation of the blood into the culture bottles. About two to three sets of blood cultures should be obtained for each suspected episode of bacteremia. In critically ill patients, the source of sepsis is frequently iatrogenic such as caused by a central venous catheter (CVC), urinary indwelling catheter, or ventilator. Specific techniques and procedures should be followed to obtain and interpret cultures from these sources. These include culture of blood aspirated from the CVC, quantitative cultures of the CVC tip, and culture from the CVC insertion site. A sample of secretions aspirated via the endotracheal tube should be sent for Gram staining and for bacterial and fungal culture. Pleural effusions greater than 10 mm should be aspirated, cultured, and sent for Gram and fungal stainings. Unless contraindicated, bronchoscopy should be performed whenever ventilator-associated pneumonia is suspected. A policy of routine screening of hospitalized patients for *Candida* colonization is not recommended. Among septic patients, however, invasive fungal infection is more likely in those patients who are heavily colonized. Blood cultures should be obtained from septic patients colonized by *Candida* at two or more sites.

Early administration of antibiotics reduces mortality and morbidity in septic patients. The patient should be started empirically on broad-spectrum antibiotics. For pregnancy-related infections, a combination of penicillin, aminoglycoside, and either clindamycin or metronidazole for anaerobes should cover most possible organisms. Alternatively, a carbapenem or a third- or fourth-generation cephalosporin may be used in nonneutropenic patients. Aztreonam and fluoroquinolones do not have adequate activity against gram-positive bacteria and therefore are not recommended for initial empirical treatment. Vancomycin should be used for suspected methicillin-resistant *Staphylococcus* infection (catheter-related infection, or centers where methicillin-resistant staphylococci predominate). Antifungal agents should not be used as routine empirical therapy. In situations where immune suppression, or other conditions conducive to fungal infection, may have contributed to the initial inciting event, coverage with amphotericin or equivalent antimicrobials should be considered. Fluconazole is as effective as amphotericin B, and less toxic in nonneutropenic patients. However, amphotericin B should be used as first-line therapy in neutropenic septic patients until identification and susceptibility are determined. The initial and subsequent choice of antimicrobials should always be predicated by allergy history, renal and liver function, culture results, and hospital- or community-specific microbial sensitivity testing. It is also important to remember that cultures may be falsely negative or yield incomplete information as some organisms may not be detected. This is especially true in obstetrically related infections which tend to be poly-microbial.

Hemodynamic support in sepsis is one of the central components of the management. The goal is to restore tissue perfusion and normalize cellular metabolism. Volume replacement, most often with fluid alone, is sometimes sufficient to reverse hypotension, restore hemodynamic stability, and improve oxygen delivery. Volume replacement should be titrated according to blood pressure (maintain a systolic blood pressure of at least 90 mm Hg or a mean arterial pressure of 60 to 65 mm Hg), heart rate, and urine output (≥0.5 mL/kg/h). Boluses of 250 to 1000 mL of crytalloids over 5 to 15 minutes are recommended. Oncotic pressure decreases in pregnancy, with further decrease in malnourished or preeclamptic women. Combined with the propensity for capillary leak in sepsis, the gestational decrease in oncotic pressure predisposes pregnant or postpartum women for pulmonary edema. The initial fluid boluses can be guided by the overall subjective assessment of the patient's intravascular volume status (prior fluid replacements and losses), intravascular oncotic pressure (nutritional status, conditions decreasing oncotic pressure, etc), and clinical measures of pulmonary function (oxygen saturation, auscultation, etc). If hypotension persists despite the initial attempts, further volume expansion should be guided by central venous pressure (maintained at 8 to 12 mm Hg) or pulmonary capillary wedge pressure (maintained at 12 to 16 mm Hg), the latter being

more appropriate than the former in cases where central venous pressure may not reflect left ventricular end-diastolic pressures (eg, preeclampsia) or when the central venous pressure is elevated. If central monitoring is indicated, then the use of a catheter with the capability to measure venous oxyhemoglobin saturation can be very useful in guiding further management. Systemic oxygen delivery depends on cardiac output and the oxygen-carrying capacity of the blood. Increases in cardiac output can be proportional to the degree of intravascular volume expansion, while increases in the oxygen-carrying capacity can be achieved by increasing the hemoglobin. The recommended hemoglobin concentration in patients with septic shock is 9 to 10 mg/dL.

Vasopressors are required when the fluid and red blood cell replacement fail to restore adequate organ perfusion (Table 9-4). The choice between the different vasopressors depends on the balance between cardiac and peripheral vascular effects. Dopamine and epinephrine are more likely to increase heart rate than norepinephrine and phenylephrine. Dopamine and norepinephrine raise both blood pressure and cardiac index. Overall, recent data suggest that norepinephrine is the best choice for a vasopressor because of less tachycardia, no interference with the hypothalamic-pituitary axis, and a likely survival advantage over other vasopressors. In septic shock, norepinephrine is a more potent vasopressor than dopamine and increases cardiac output, renal blood flow, and urine output. Despite the negative effect of sepsis on cardiac function, most patients have increased cardiac output especially following intravascular volume expansion, with or without norepinephrine. If cardiac output remains low-normal or decreased, then inotropic support is required, with dobutamine being the most appropriate choice (start at 2.5 μg/kg/min and increase by 2.5 μg/kg/min every 30 minutes to achieve a cardiac index of 3 or more). In the presence of hypotension, dobutamine should be used in combination with a

■ **TABLE 9-4. Dose of Agents Used as Vasopressors in Septic Shock**

Dopamine	10-25 μg/kg/min
Norepinephrine	1-50 μg/min
Epinephrine	1-10 μg/min
Phenylephrine	40-180 μg/min
Vasopressin	0.01-0.04 U/min

vasopressor, preferably norepinephrine. Finally, vasopressin can be added if organ perfusion remains abnormal despite high doses of vasopressors and inotropes. Doses should be limited to 0.01 to 0.04 U/min in order to prevent splanchnic and coronary artery ischemia, as well as decreased cardiac output. Routine intravenous bicarbonate therapy for anion gap acidosis and supranormal oxygen delivery (increasing oxygen delivery to higher than normal values) are no longer recommended. Early recognition of septic shock in patients with infection is critical in order to initiate aggressive and timely cardiovascular management, since the response in the initial few hours has a tremendous bearing on outcome.

The source of infection should be eliminated as soon as the patient's condition permits. Debridement of infected and devitalized tissue is indicated in cases of wound infection or fasciitis. Ultrasound evaluation of the endometrial cavity can be used to determine the presence of retained products and need for curettage. If well-defined and accessible, intra-abdominal or pelvic abscesses detected on CT scan or MRI can be initially managed by percutaneous drainage, either for definitive treatment or as a temporizing measure while optimizing the patient's condition in preparation for laparotomy. Laparotomy should be reserved for not well-defined collections, presence of dead tissue that requires debridement, or failure of initial percutaneous drainage. In postpartum patients, the radiologist should be alerted to the possibility of myometrial necrosis, which can be detected on CT scan or MRI, and requires hysterectomy. Amniocentesis may be required to exclude chorioamnionitis in septic patients who are still pregnant, and who have no other obvious source as delivery would be required if intra-amniotic infection is confirmed by low amniotic fluid glucose concentration and Gram staining. Since pregnant and postpartum women are prone to cholelithiasis, cholecystitis should be excluded and cholecystectomy be entertained if present. Similarly, pyelonephritis associated with urinary obstruction should be treated with stenting and drainage.

According to the recommendations of the International Sepsis Forum, early endotracheal intubation and mechanical ventilation should be used in severe sepsis or septic shock. Noninvasive positive-pressure ventilation should be avoided. Indications for mechanical ventilation include severe tachypnea (respiratory rate >40 bpm), muscular respiratory failure (use of accessory muscles), altered mental status, and severe hypoxemia despite supplemental oxygen. Permissive hypercapnia through reduced tidal volume

ventilation (6 mL/kg ideal body weight to maintain end-inspiratory plateau pressures at <30 cm H_2O), and prone positioning are a few strategies that can be used in complicated cases. The respiratory management of patients with acute lung injury/acute respiratory distress syndrome (complicates 18% to 40% of cases) is discussed in detail in Chap 12.

There are a number of therapies that fall into the supportive category in critically ill patients in general, and septic obstetrical patients in particular. Examples of such therapies include prophylaxis for thromboembolism, nutritional support, stress ulcer prophylaxis, and hemofiltration for renal insufficiency. Sepsis and pregnancy are predisposing factors for thromboembolism and deep vein thrombosis prophylaxis is recommended. Either low-dose unfractionated heparin (5000 units three times per day) or low molecular weight heparin can be used. If the patient has a contraindication to heparin (coagulopathy, active bleeding, allergy), then mechanical devices should be substituted. Nutritional support is recommended in septic patients. This topic is dealt with in more detail elsewhere. In summary, enteral nutrition is the preferred method, with parenteral nutrition as a second choice. The American College of Chest Physicians and the American Society of Parenteral and Enteral Nutrition have issued specific recommendations for septic patients (Table 9-5; not specific to obstetrical patients). The efficacy of antacids, sucralfate or histamine-2 receptor antagonists in prevention of stress ulcer bleeding has been confirmed in numerous trials of critically ill patients.

The popularity of certain additional therapies has waxed and waned over time, while others are still in the

---

■ TABLE 9-5. Guidelines for Nutritional Support in Septic Patients

- Daily caloric intake: 25-30 kcal/kg usual body weight
- Protein: 1.3-2.0 g/kg/d
- Glucose: 30%-70% of total nonprotein calories, to maintain serum glucose <225 mg/dL
- Lipids: 15%-30% of total nonprotein calories (with reduction in polyunsaturated fatty acid)

Established by the American College of Chest Physicians and the American Society of Parenteral and Enteral Nutrition consensus conferences.

experimental phase. Corticosteroids are, currently, the favored immunological therapy. Corticosteroids should be reserved for refractory septic shock, and should not be used in sepsis without shock or with mild shock. Low dose (or stress dose) hydrocortisone (100 mg three times per day) for 5 to 10 days followed by tapering according to hemodynamic status is one treatment option. Corticosteroids should be started within the first few hours of septic shock and high doses should not be used. Recombinant activated protein C (rhAPC; drotrecogin alpha) was recently approved by the FDA for the treatment of patients in septic shock or those with severe sepsis at the highest risk for mortality (APACHE II ≥25). The anticoagulant and profibrinolytic effects of rhAPC target the consumptive coagulopathy and the associated activation of inflammatory cascade in patients with sepsis. rhAPC also has direct anti-inflammatory properties. The benefits of rhAPC should be weighed against the risk of bleeding. Caution is advised in the use of rhAPC in patients with an INR >3 or platelet count <30,000 cells/mm³. It should be noted that a recent Cochrane review found that there is insufficient evidence to support the use of rhAPC in sepsis; moreover there is an increased risk of internal bleeding associated with its use. Intensive insulin therapy to maintain blood glucose between 80 and 100 mg/dL has been shown to reduce the death rate from multiple organ failure in patients with sepsis. If intensive insulin therapy is used, frequent monitoring of blood glucose is recommended to prevent hypoglycemic brain injury secondary to overzealous treatment. Granulocyte colony-stimulating factor should not be used in nonneutropenic patients, and hemofiltration should not be used without renal indications. Other therapies that have been tried, but which should not be used for the treatment of sepsis unless additional studies show a clear benefit, include ibuprofen, prostaglandins, pentoxifyilline, N-acetylcysteine, selenium, antithrombin III, immunoglobulins, and growth hormone.

The effect of pregnancy on the critically ill patient and vice versa is discussed elsewhere. Pregnant septic patients are at risk for utero-placental insufficiency and preterm labor. The decision for continuous fetal heart rate monitoring and/or tocolysis should take into account the gestational age and the patient's condition. A non-reassuring fetal heart rate pattern or contractions frequently resolve with correction of maternal hypoxemia and acidosis of short-term duration. Longer periods of maternal hypoxemia and acidosis, however, may result in permanent fetal damage or progression into active labor and may require delivery. In the absence of chorioamnionitis, labor, or non-reassuring fetal status, the decision for delivery should also be based on gestational age and the patient's condition. If respiratory and cardiovascular functions continue to deteriorate despite aggressive management, then decompression of a gravid uterus after 28 weeks' gestation may improve venous return and lung volumes.

SUGGESTED READINGS

The Acute Respiratory Distress Syndrome Network. Ventilation with lower tidal volumes as compared with traditional tidal volumes for acute lung injury and the acute respiratory distress syndrome. *N Engl J Med.* 2000;342:1301-1308.

Astiz ME, Rackow EC. Septic shock. *Lancet.* 1998;351:1501-1505.

Bernard GR, Vincent JL, Laterre PF, et al. Efficacy and safety of recombinant human activated protein C for severe sepsis. *N Engl J Med.* 2001;344:699-709.

Bollaert PE, Bauer P, Audibert G, et al. Effects of epinephrine on hemodynamics and oxygen metabolism in dopamine-resistant septic shock. *Chest.* 1990;98:949-53.

Bone RC, Sibbald WJ, Sprung CL. The ACCP-SCCM consensus conference on sepsis and organ failure. *Chest.* 1992;101:1481-3.

Brun-Buisson C, Doyon F, Carlet J, et al. Incidence, risk factors, and outcome of severe sepsis and septic shock in adults: a multicenter prospective study in intensive care units. *JAMA.* 1995;274:968-74.

Cook DJ, Reeve BK, Guyatt GH, et al. Stress ulcer prophylaxis in critically ill patients: resolving discordant meta-analyses. *JAMA.* 1996;275:308-14.

Cooper MS, Stewart PM. Corticosteroid insufficiency in acutely ill patients. *N Engl J Med.* 2003;348-727.

Dellinger RP. Cardiovascular management of septic shock. *Crit Care Med.* 2003;31:946-955.

Hack CE, Zeerleder S. The endothelium in sepsis: source of and a target for inflammation. *Crit Care Med.* 2001;29:S21-7.

Hinds C, Watson D. Manipulating hemodynamic and oxygen transport in critically ill patients. *N Engl J Med.* 1995;333:1074-5.

Hotchkiss RS, Karl IE. The pathophysiology and treatment of sepsis. *N Engl J Med.* 2003;348:138-150.

The International Sepsis Forum. Recommendations for the management of patients with severe sepsis and septic shock. *Intensive Care Med.* 2001;27:S1-S134.

Mabie WC, Barton JR, Sibai B. Septic shock in pregnancy. *Obstet Gynecol.* 1997;90:533-561.

Marshall JC. Inflammation, coagulopathy, and the pathogenesis of multiple organ dysfunction syndrome. *Crit Care Med.* 2001;29(Suppl):S99-S106.

Martin C, Papazian L, Perrin G, et al. Norepinephrine or dopamine for the treatment of hyperdynamic septic shock? *Chest.* 1993;103:1826-31.

Martin GS, Mannino DM, Eaton S, et al. The epidemiology of sepsis in the United States from 1979 through 2000. *N Eng J Med.* 2003;348:1546-1554.

Rangel-Frausto MS, Pittet D, Costigan M, et al. The natural history of the systemic inflammatory response syndrome (SIRS). *JAMA.* 1995;273:117-23.

Rivers EP, Ahrens, T. Improving Outcomes for Severe Sepsis and Septic Shock: Tools for Early Identification of At-Risk Patients and Treatment Protocol Implementation. *Crit Care Clin.* 2008;23:S1–S47

Rivers E, Nguyen B, Havstad S, et al. Early goal-directed therapy in the treatment of severe sepsis and septic shock. *N Engl J Med.* 2001;345:1368-1377.

Sharma S, Kumar A. Septic shock, multiple organ failure, and acute respiratory distress syndrome. *Curr Opin Pulm Med.* 2003;9:199-209.

Vincent JL, de Carvalho FB, De Backer D. Management of septic shock. *Ann Med.* 2002;34:606-613.

Wheeler AP, Bernard GR. Treating patients with severe sepsis. *N Engl J Med.* 1999;340:207-214.

Wojnar MM, Hawkins WG, Lang CH. Nutritional support of the septic patient. *Crit Care Clin.* 1995;11:717.

Yu M, Levy MM, Smith P, et al. Effect of maximizing oxygen delivery on morbidity and mortality rates in critically ill patients: a prospective, randomized, controlled study. *Crit Care Med.* 1993;21:830-8.

CHAPTER 10

Thyroid and Other Endocrine Emergencies

• *Michael A. Belfort*

■ THYROID AND OTHER ENDOCRINE EMERGENCIES

This chapter will address several common endocrine emergencies that may be seen in pregnant women. While most endocrine conditions can become emergencies if ignored or untreated, the intention of this chapter is not to exhaustively review endocrine complications in pregnancy; rather, the conditions that might realistically be faced in an ICU situation have been highlighted. These include thyrotoxicosis and thyroid storm, hypothyroidism and myxedema coma, Addisonian crisis, pheochromocytoma, primary hyperalderonism, and diabetes insipidus. Diabetes mellitus and ketoacidosis have been dealt with elsewhere.

Thyroid Disease

Thyroid disease is the second most common endocrine condition affecting women of reproductive age. It is now common for obstetricians to care for women who enter pregnancy with an established thyroid deficiency or overactivity state. Since pregnancy in and of itself affects thyroid function, even women who are well-controlled prepregnancy may become uncontrolled requiring continued monitoring and adjustment. In addition, it is important to remember that the developing fetus may be at significant risk from circulating maternal antibodies that are no longer an issue for the mother. Despite the fact that hyperthyroidism is uncommon during pregnancy (0.2% of pregnancies), and thyroid storm is considered rare, vigilance is important because of the potential for significant morbidity and mortality in these conditions.

Definitions

Thyrotoxicosis is a generic term referring to a clinical and biochemical state resulting from over production of, and exposure to, thyroid hormone. The most common cause of thyrotoxicosis in pregnancy is **Graves disease**. This disorder is an autoimmune condition characterized by production of thyroid-stimulating immunoglobulin (TSI) and thyroid-stimulating hormone binding inhibitory immunoglobulin (TBII) that act on the thyroid stimulating hormone (TSH) receptor to mediate thyroid stimulation or inhibition, respectively.

Thyroid storm is characterized by an acute, severe exacerbation of hyperthyroidism.

Hypothyroidism results from inadequate thyroid hormone production and **myxedema coma** is an extreme form of hypothyroidism.

Thyroiditis is caused by an autoimmune inflammation of the thyroid gland and may occur for the first time postpartum. It is usually painless and may present as de novo hypothyroidism, transient thyrotoxicosis, or as initial hyperthyroidism followed by hypothyroidism within 1 year postpartum.

Physiology

Thyroxine (T_4) is the major secretory product of the thyroid. The majority of circulating T_4 is converted in the peripheral tissues to triiodothyronine (T_3), the biologically active form of this hormone. T_4 secretion is under the direct control of the pituitary thyroid-stimulating hormone (TSH). The cell surface receptor for TSH is similar to the receptors for luteinizing hormone (LH) and human chorionic gonadotrophin (hCG). T_4 and T_3 are transported in the peripheral circulation bound to thyroxine-binding globulin (TBG), transthyretin (formerly called prealbumin), and albumin. Less than 0.05% of plasma T_4 and less than 0.5% of plasma T_3 are unbound and able to interact with target tissues. Routine T_4 measurements reflect total serum concentration and may be factitiously altered by increases or decreases in concentrations of circulating proteins. Plasma concentrations of TBG increase 2.5-fold by 20 weeks' gestation, due to reduced hepatic clearance and an estrogen-induced change in the structure of TBG that prolongs the serum half-life. This TBG alteration causes significant changes in many of the thyroid test results in pregnancy. There is a 25% to 45% increase in serum total T_4 (TT_4) from a pregravid level of 5 to 12 mg% to 9 to 16 mg%. Total T_3 (TT_3) increases by about 30% in the first trimester and by 50% to 65% later. In order to maintain the homeostasis of free T_4, the thyroid gland produces more thyroxine until the new steady state has been reached, around mid gestation. Thereafter, changes in peripheral thyroid hormone metabolism require persistently increased T_4 production to maintain normal serum free T_4 concentrations. TSH levels are transiently depressed in the first trimester due to hCG elevation, but increase to normal in the second and third trimesters. Pregnancy affects other changes in the thyroid system and ultimately the interpretation of thyroid function tests (Table 10-1).

Fetal Effects
The fetal hypothalamic-pituitary-thyroid axis develops independently of the maternal thyroid function. The fetus

begins concentrating iodine between 10 and 12 weeks' gestation. By 20 weeks gestation, the fetal pituitary TSH is functional. The human placenta acts as a significant barrier to circulating T_4, T_3, and TSH. Despite this, in cases of congenital hypothyroidism there is still sufficient passage of maternal thyroid hormones across the placenta (cord levels 25%-50% of normal) to prevent overt hypothyroidism at birth. Immunoglobulin G (IgG) autoantibodies, iodine, thyrotropin-releasing hormone (TRH), and antithyroid medications (PTU, methimazole) can readily cross the placenta and interfere with fetal thyroid activity. Fetuses of women being treated with antithyroid drugs are at risk for hypothyroidism and goiter and should be closely monitored. Targeted ultrasound for fetal growth abnormalities and thyroid size should be performed serially. Antepartum fetal heart rate monitoring and occasionally percutaneous fetal blood sampling (if ultrasound reveals an obvious goiter) should also be entertained. Since IgG autoantibodies can cross the placenta, it is important that women with a prior history of Graves disease are tested for thyroid stimulating immunoglobulin (TSI) and thyroid stimulating hormone binding inhibitory immunoglobulin (TBII).

Hyperthyroidism

The causes of hyperthyroidism in pregnancy are listed in Table 10-2. Hyperthyroidism occurs in 0.2% of pregnancies and Graves disease accounts for more than 90% of these cases. Autoantibodies against TSH receptors (thyroid-stimulating antibody [TSAb]—formerly known as LATS [long-acting thyroid stimulator]) act as TSH agonists, thereby stimulating increased production of thyroid hormone. The clinical presentation of mild hyperthyroidism is similar to the symptoms of normal pregnancy

■ TABLE 10-1. Thyroid Function Changes during Pregnancy

Normal hypothalamic-pituitary-thyroid axis
First trimester TSH depression due to hCG, normalized thereafter
First trimester: 0.24-2.99
Second trimester: 0.46-2.95
Third trimester: 0.43-2.78

Increased renal iodide clearance (increased glomerular filtration rate)
Goiter-minimal in regions of iodine sufficiency; 30% increase in size in regions with dietary iodine deficiency
Increased serum TBG; decreased T_3 resin uptake
Increased total serum T_4 and total serum T_3
Normal serum free T_4 and free T_3

■ TABLE 10-2. Causes of Hyperthyroidism during Pregnancy

Graves disease
Toxic multinodular goiter (rare in the reproductive age group)
Toxic adenoma
Hyperemesis gravidarum
Trophoblastic disease
Thyroiditis (chronic, subacute, viral)
Exogenous thyroid hormone

(fatigue, increased appetite, vomiting, palpitations, tachycardia, heat intolerance, increased urinary frequency, insomnia, emotional lability) and may confound the diagnosis. More specific symptoms and signs highly suggestive of hyperthyroidism include tremor, nervousness, frequent stools, excessive sweating, brisk reflexes, muscle weakness, goiter, hypertension, and weight loss. Graves ophthalmopathy (stare, lid lag and retraction, exophthalmos) and dermopathy (localized or pretibial myxedema) are diagnostic. The disease usually gets worse in the first trimester but moderates later in pregnancy. Untreated hyperthyroidism poses considerable maternal and fetal risks including IUGR, preterm delivery, severe preeclampsia, and heart failure (Table 10-3).

Fetal and Neonatal Implications

Perinatal risks include IUGR, prematurity, cardiac dysrhythmias, and intrauterine death. Fetal thyrotoxicosis should be considered in any pregnancy with Graves disease. Neonates of women with thyrotoxicosis are at risk for immune mediated hypothyroidism and hyperthyroidism secondary to autoantibodies that may cross the placenta (Graves disease and chronic autoimmune thyroiditis). TBII can cause transient neonatal hypothyroidism and TSI can result in neonatal hyperthyroidism. The incidence is low (<5%) because thioamide treatment frequently decreases the titers of these antibodies. Maternal autoantibodies are cleared slowly in the neonate sometimes resulting in delayed presentation of neonatal Graves disease. Neonates of women with prior Graves disease who have been treated with surgery or radioactive iodine and who do not need thioamide therapy during pregnancy remain at significant risk for neonatal Graves disease because of the persistence of the thyrotropic antibodies.

Laboratory Diagnosis

Laboratory diagnosis of hyperthyroidism is confirmed with a suppressed serum TSH in the setting of elevated free T_4 levels (or FTI) without the presence of a nodular goiter or thyroid mass. In rare circumstances, the serum total T_3 may demonstrate greater (or earlier) elevation than T_4 (T_3 toxicosis).

Hyperthyroidism may also result from elevated serum levels of hCG, as seen with trophoblastic diseases and hyperemesis gravidarum. In these circumstances, treatment is seldom required, since the disease spontaneously resolves after the trophoblastic tissue is evacuated or vomiting is resolved. Biochemical hyperthyroidism is seen in up to 66% of women with severe hyperemesis gravidarum (undetectable TSH level or elevated FTI, or both) but this usually resolves by 18 weeks. If therapy is needed, efforts should be directed toward uncovering an underlying thyroid condition since clinical hyperthyroidism (as opposed to biochemical hyperthyroidism) is extremely unusual with hyperemesis gravidarum. Cardiac decompensation in pregnancy usually occurs only in poorly controlled hyperthyroid patients with anemia, infection, or hypertension. Reversible dilated cardiomyopathy, congestive cardiac failure, and ventricular fibrillation have been reported with thyroid storm. The hemodynamic changes associated with hyperthyroidism during pregnancy are outlined in Table 10-4.

β-adrenergic blockade is theoretically contraindicated with congestive heart failure, since adrenergic stimulation of the heart is the major compensating mechanism against cardiac failure. The negative inotropic effect imposed by β-adrenergic blockade may depress myocardial contractility. These drugs, however, are very effective for treating atrial fibrillation and supraventricular

---

■ TABLE 10-3. Fetal and Maternal Risks with Untreated Hyperthyroidism	
Fetal	**Maternal**
Spontaneous abortion	Preeclampsia
Prematurity	Maternal heart failure
Low birth weight	Infection
Fetal/neonatal	Anemia
thyrotoxicosis	Thyroid storm

■ TABLE 10-4. Hemodynamic Changes with Hyperthyroidism
Increased stroke volume and cardiac output
Increased pulse rate
Reduced peripheral vascular resistance
Increased blood volume
Impaired myocardial contractility
Electrocardiographic changes:
Left ventricular hypertrophy (15%)
Atrial fibrillation (21%)
Wolff-Parkinson-White syndrome

tachycardia that may accompany hyperthyroidism. Thus, cautious use of β-blocker therapy is recommended, since congestive heart failure during pregnancy is often rate related. Utilization of a pulmonary artery catheter is an important adjunct to the effective and safe use of β-blocker therapy in these critical situations. Other helpful therapeutic modalities include diuretic therapy, digoxin, and bed rest. Cardiac dysfunction may linger for months after restoration of normal thyroid function.

Treatment of Hyperthyroidism during Pregnancy

The primary objective of treatment is to effectively control thyroid dysfunction until after delivery. Protecting the fetus from the effects of the disease and the side effects of the medical regimen is a secondary yet important objective. Basic treatment options are outlined in Table 10-5.

Observation alone may be a reasonable treatment plan for mild clinical disease without cardiovascular compromise. For overt disease, antithyroid medications are the mainstay of treatment. Propylthiouracil (PTU) and methimazole (Tapazole) are two of the thioamide agents currently available in the United States. In Europe, the methimazole derivative carbimazole is used. Since carbimazole is rapidly metabolized to methimazole, these drugs are essentially the same. Both methimazole and PTU effectively block intrathyroid hormone synthesis, but PTU also blocks extrathyroid conversion of T_4 to T_3. Both agents readily cross the placenta and may inhibit fetal thyroid function. Methimazole was believed to be approximately four times more bioavailable to fetal tissue than PTU and has also been associated with aplasia cutis in infancy. For these two reasons, PTU has become the preferred medication for treating hyperthyroidism in pregnancy in the United States. Both of these beliefs have recently been disputed with studies showing no differences in mean umbilical cord TSH or FT_4 levels between PTU and methimazole treated neonates and no increased incidence of cutis aplasia. Twice daily doses of 150 to 200 mg

PTU or a dosage of 100 mg tid will usually control hyperthyroidism within 4 to 8 weeks. Lack of response is usually due to noncompliance and may require hospitalization. The goal of treatment is to use the smallest dose that maintains maternal free T_4 levels at or just above the upper limit of normal. Clinical and laboratory follow-up (TSH, free T_4, free T_3) should occur every 2 to 4 weeks. Most women (90%) will have a significant improvement within 2 to 4 weeks. Rapid improvement necessitates a decrease in dosage. Improvement commonly occurs in the second trimester, and as many as 40% of mothers may discontinue therapy. It may, however, be reasonable to continue giving small doses to ameliorate the risks of fetal thyrotoxicosis imposed by transplacental passage of TSAb and to reduce the general overall incidence of thyroid storm during labor and delivery.

Baseline white blood cell (WBC) and liver function tests should be obtained before initiating antithyroid therapy, since hyperthyroidism itself may also cause liver enzyme elevations and leukopenia. The incidence of agranulocytosis with thioamides is about 0.1 to 0.4%. This is usually heralded by a fever and sore throat and these symptoms should precipitate immediate discontinuation of the drug and checking for leukopenia. Antithyroid medications should also be discontinued if liver function values become extremely abnormal. These medications may be restarted during the postpartum period as disease activity dictates but the clinician should be aware that treatment with other thioamides carries a high risk for cross reaction. Other major side effects of thioamides, which include a lupus-like syndrome, thrombocytopenia, hepatitis/hepatic infarction, and vasculitis occur in less than 1% of patients. Minor side effects include rash, argthralgias, nausea, anorexia, fever, and a loss of taste or smell may occur in up to 5% of cases. Breast-feeding is permissible while taking PTU because little is passed into breast milk with standard doses. Breast-feeding is also acceptable with methimazole therapy despite the fact that it is present in a higher ratio than PTU in breast milk.

β-adrenergic blockers may be used as adjunctive therapy to control the symptoms of tremor and palpitations until the thioamides decrease thyroid hormone levels. Propranolol is the most commonly used β-blocker for this purpose. Relative contraindications to the use of β-adrenergic blockers include obstructive lung disease, heart block, heart failure, and insulin use. Although unusual, there may

■ TABLE 10-5. Treatment Options for Hyperthyroidism
Observation
Antithyroid medications
β-adrenergic blocking agents
Thyroid surgery

be adverse fetal effects such as bradycardia, growth restriction, and neonatal hypoglycemia. It is advisable to minimize the duration of β-adrenergic blocker therapy during gestation.

Subtotal thyroidectomy is reserved for patients with severe antithyroid drug side effects or failed medical suppression of thyroid function. To minimize pregnancy complications, surgery is usually performed during the second trimester. Preoperatively, hyperthyroidism should be controlled with antithyroid medication for 7 to 10 days, a β-adrenergic blocker (propranolol, 20 mg, 3-4 times daily, and inorganic iodide (Lugol solution, three drops twice daily) for 4 to 5 days. The latter two can be discontinued 48 hours postoperatively. Iodide must be used cautiously to minimize the risk of severe fetal hypothyroidism and goiter.

Radioactive iodine administration is contraindicated during pregnancy because of the risk of fetal thyroid ablation. It is recommended that women avoid pregnancy or breast-feeding for 4 months after I-131 therapy. This agent readily crosses the placenta and may cause permanent damage to the fetal thyroid if used after 10 to 12 weeks of gestation. Inadvertent use of I-131 in very early pregnancy (up to 10 weeks) is usually not associated with any long-term fetal/neonatal thyroid side effects.

Thyroid Storm

Thyroid storm is a rare but potentially fatal hypermetabolic complication of hyperthyroidism characterized by cardiovascular compromise (tachycardia out of proportion to the fever, dysrhythmia, cardiac failure), hyperpyrexia, and central nervous system changes (restlessness, nervousness, changed mental status, confusion, and seizures) (Table 10-6). Thyroid storm is estimated to occur in 1% to 2% of pregnancies complicated by hyperthyroidism. This rare but devastating complication is usually seen in patients with poorly controlled hyperthyroidism complicated by additional physiologic stressors such as infection, surgery, thromboembolism, preeclampsia, and parturition. Precipitating events for thyroid storm are presented in Table 10-7. Diagnosis can be difficult and if delayed the patient may lapse into shock and/or coma. The laboratory profile of the mother with thyroid storm reveals leukocytosis, elevated hepatic enzymes, and occasionally hypercalcemia. Thyroid function test results are consistent with hyperthyroidism (elevated FT_4/FT_3 and depressed TSH) but do not always correlate with the severity of the

■ TABLE 10-6. Diagnosis of Thyroid Storm

Hypermetabolism

Fever above 100°F
Perspiration
Warm, flushed skin

Cardiovascular

Tachycardia
Atrial fibrillation
Ventricular fibrillation
Congestive heart failure
Reversible dilated cardiomyoapthy

Central nervous system

Irritability
Agitation
Tremor
Mental status change (delirium, psychosis, coma)

Gastrointestinal

Nausea, vomiting
Diarrhea
Jaundice

Supporting laboratory evidence

Leukocytosis
Elevated liver function values
Hypercalcemia
Low TSH, high free T_4 and/or T_3

■ TABLE 10-7. Common Precipitants of Thyroid Storm

Acute surgical emergency
Induction of anesthesia
Diabetic ketoacidosis
Pulmonary embolism
Noncompliance with antithyroid medications
Myocardial infarction
Infection
Hypertension/preeclampsia
Labor and delivery
Severe anemia

thyroid storm. Treatment should, however, be initiated on the suspicion of the condition and the clinician should not wait for laboratory confirmation before starting therapy. Management is best accomplished in an obstetric intensive care unit. Table 10-8 reviews basic supportive adjunctive care for patients in thyroid storm. The basic goals of therapy are to:

1. Reduce the synthesis and release of thyroid hormone
2. Remove thyroid hormone from the circulation and increase the concentration of TBG
3. Block the peripheral conversion of T_4 to T_3
4. Block the peripheral actions of thyroid hormone
5. Treat the complications of thyroid storm and provide support
6. Identify and treat the potential precipitating conditions

To these ends the following drugs are available: (1) propylthiouracil and methimazole, both of which inhibit iodination of tyrosine (leading to reduced synthesis of thyroid hormones), and block peripheral conversion of T_4 to T_3. These drugs alone can reduce the T_3 concentration by 75%. (2) For thyroid storm Lugol iodine, SSKI (saturated solution of potassium iodide), sodium iodide, orografin, and lithium carbonate. These drugs function by blocking the *release* of stored hormone by inhibiting the proteolysis of thyroglobulin. One of the side effects of such agents is to initially increase the *production* of thyroid hormone, and it is therefore very important to *start propylthiouracil prior to giving iodides*. The mainstay of therapy are glucocorticoids which should be started as soon as the condition is recognized and act by blocking the *release* of stored hormone (as do iodides), and by blocking *peripheral conversion* of T_4 to T_3 (as do the thioamides). Specifics of the medical therapy are detailed below:

1. Oral PTU (or by nasogastric tube if necessary) with a 300- to 600-mg loading dose followed by 150 to 200 mg orally every 4 to 6 hours.
2. Iodide initiated 1 to 2 hours after PTU administration:
   a. Oral saturated solution of potassium iodide (SSKI) to block T_4 release (two to five drops orally every 8 hours)
   b. Intravenous (IV) sodium iodide, 500 to 1000 mg every 8 hours
   c. Oral Lugol iodine solution (eight drops every 6 hours)
   d. Oragrafin (62% iodine) can be used if other solutions are not available. Three grams given orally will suppress thyroid hormone release for 2 to 3 days.
   e. Oral lithium carbonate, 300 mg every 6 hours (therapeutic level = 1 meq/L)
3. Adrenal glucocorticoids: This may be in the form of dexamethasone, 2 mg intravenously or intramuscularly every 6 hours for four doses (or hydrocortisone, 300 mg/d IV or prednisone, 60 mg/d orally).
4. Propranolol (20 to 80 mg orally or by nasogastric tube every 4 to 6 hours or 1 to 2 mg/min IV for 5 minutes for a total of 6 mg, followed by 1 to 10 mg every IV for 4 hours) is effective for controlling tachycardia. If the patient has a history of severe bronchospasm reserpine or guanethidine may be used:
   a. Reserpine, 1 to 5 mg IM every 4 to 6 hours
   b. Guanethidine, 1 mg/kg orally every 12 hours
5. Phenobarbital, 30 to 60 mg orally every 6 to 8 hours as needed to control restlessness.
6. Iodides and glucocorticoids may be discontinued after initial clinical improvement.
7. Plasmapheresis or peritoneal dialysis to remove circulating thyroid hormone is an extreme measure reserved for patients who do not respond to conventional therapy.
8. An algorithm for the management of thyroid storm is presented in Fig 10-1.

Hypothyroidism

Most cases of hypothyroidism in pregnancy are the result of a primary thyroid dysfunction or are iatrogenic from prior thyroid surgery or radioactive iodine. A few cases are caused by hypothalamic abnormalities. The most common causes of hypothyroidism in pregnant or postpartum women are Hashimoto disease (chronic thyroiditis or chronic autoimmune thyroiditis), subacute thyroiditis,

---

■ **TABLE 10-8. Supportive Adjunctive Care for the Patient in Thyroid Storm**

Intravenous fluids and electrolytes
Cardiac monitoring
Consideration of pulmonary artery catheterization (central hemodynamic monitoring to guide β-blocker therapy during hyperdynamic cardiac failure)
Cooling measure: blanket, sponge bath, acetaminophen
Oxygen therapy (consider arterial line to follow serial blood gases)
No salicylates (increased T_4)
Nasogastric tube if patient is unable to swallow (may be the only avenue for PTU administration)

| Admit Patient to an Obstetric Intensive Care Unit (Consult Endocrinology, Maternal-Fetal Medicine, and Neonatology) |

Initiate supportive measures: send CBC, electrolytes, liver functions, glucose and renal functions; do not intervene on behalf of the fetus until maternal stabilization is accomplished. Use position changes, cooling measures, fluids and oxygen therapy to help improve oxygen delivery to the fetus.
1. Start electronic fetal monitoring if the fetus is potentially viable
2. Intravenous fluids/electrolyte replacement
3. Cardiac monitoring (continuous ECG [obtain 12-lead at onset])
4. Cooling measure (cooling blanket, sponge bath, acetaminophen)
5. Oxygen therapy (pulse oximetry, obtain maternal blood gas at onset)
6. Nasogastric tube if patient is unable to swallow

Give agents to reduce synthesis of the thyroid hormones: PTU (propylthiouracil) followed by iodides to block T_4 release (IV sodium iodide or oral Lugols):
1. PTU orally or via nasogastric cut, 300-600 mg loading dose followed by 150-300 mg q6h
2. 1 h after instituting PTU give:
   a. Sodium iodide, 500 mg q8-12h
   or
   b. Oral Lugol's solution, 30-60 drops daily in divided doses
   c. Iodides may be discontinued after initial improvement.

Give agents to control maternal tachycardia:
1. Propranolol, 1-2 mg/min IV or dose sufficient to slow heart rate to 90 bpm; or 40-80 mg po q4-6h
2. Consider a pulmonary artery catheter to help guide.

Give adrenal glucocorticoids to inhibit peripheral conversion of T_4 to T_3. Consider any of the following options as appropriate:
1. Hydrocortisone, 100 mg IV q8h or
2. Prednisone, 60 mg po everyday or
3. Dexamethasone, 2 mg IV or IM every 6 h
4. Glucocorticoids may be discontinued after initial improvement.

Plasmapheresis or peritoneal dialysis (to remove circulating thyroid hormones) should be considered when patient fails to respond to conventional management.

If conventional therapy unsuccessful:
1. Consider subtotal thyroidectomy (during second trimester pregnancy) or radioactive iodine (postpartum)

FIGURE 10-1. Management algorithm for thyroid storm.

thyroidectomy, radioactive iodine therapy and iodine deficiency, and drugs that interfere with thyroid function (Table 10-9). Hashimoto disease is the most common etiology in developed countries and is characterized by production of antithyroid antibodies. These include thyroid antimicrosomal and antithyroglobulin antibodies. Hashimoto disease may be associated with thyroid enlargement (as is iodine deficiency which is rare in the United States). Hashimoto disease is more common in patients with diabetes mellitus; in one study of 100 diabetic women, 20% of patients with type-I diabetes also had Hashimoto disease. Subacute thyroiditis is not associated with goiter. Goiter is generally thought to be a sign of compensatory TSH production in the face of low circulating thyroxine. On a worldwide basis the most common cause of hypothyroidism is iodine deficiency. Patients

■ **TABLE 10-9. Causes of Hypothyroidism during Pregnancy**

Primary thyroid dysfunction

Hashimoto disease (chronic thyroiditis, chronic
  autoimmune thyroiditis)
Subacute thyroiditis
Circulating TSH receptor blocking antibody

Hypothalamic dysfunction

Iatrogenic
Prior thyroid surgery (thyroidectomy)
Radioactive iodine therapy
Iodine deficiency[a]
Relative hypothyroidism and goitrogenesis

[a]Iodine deficiency does not usually cause overt hypothyroidism
(unless very severe deficiency) and more commonly presents with
compensatory goiter development and relative hypothyroidism.

■ **TABLE 10-10. Symptoms and Signs of Severe Hypothyroidism**

Hypometabolism

Cold intolerance and low body temperature
Failure to increase body temperature in the face of
  infection
Cool, dry skin
Coarse hair, loss of hair
Large tongue and hoarse voice
Periorbital edema and nonpitting edema of hands
  and feet
Postpartum amenorrhea and galactorrhea

Cardiovascular and respiratory

Gestational hypertension
Decreased pulse pressure with predominant increase
  in diastolic pressure
Slow heart rate and respiration
Enlarged tonsils, nasopharynx, and larynx
Lungs may be congested, consolidated and there
  may be pleural effusions
Pericardial effusion

Central nervous system

Parasthesias
Lethargy and fatigue
Irritability and inability to concentrate (may develop
  confusion, stupor, obtundation, seizures and coma
  in severe myxedema)
Delayed deep tendon reflexes

Gastrointestinal

Constipation
Distended abdomen associated with ileus or ascites

Supporting laboratory evidence

Increased TSH
Decreased T_4 and free T_4
Presence of antithyroid antibodies
Hyponatremia, low serum osmolality, elevated serum
  creatinine, hypoglycemia, elevated CK (skeletal
  muscle usually)
Electrocardiogram—sinus bradycardia, low-amplitude
  QRS complexes, prolonged QT interval, flattened or
  inverted T waves

recently arrived in the United States from a region where iodine deficiency is endemic and who have features of hypothyroidism, as well as those with malnutrition, should be considered as candidates for iodine replacement.

The symptoms of hypothyroidism are common to all of the underlying etiologies (Table 10-10). Patients complain of constipation, cold intolerance, cool, dry skin, coarse hair, irritability, and inability to concentrate. Of note, however, is a significant overlap with complaints common to euthyroid pregnant women, making the clinical diagnosis difficult. The presence of paresthesias may be helpful, as it is an early symptom in approximately 75% of patients with hypothyroidism. The presence of delayed deep tendon reflexes is also suggestive of hypothyroidism. In addition, signs of gross myexedma, including a low body temperature, large tongue, hoarse voice, and periorbital edema, are not found in normal pregnancy, and their presence should prompt an immediate evaluation for hypothyroidism. Patients may complain of excessive fatigue. Gestational hypertension is common. Postpartum amenorrhea and galactorrhea associated with hyperprolactinemia may be indicative of hypothyroidism.

Fetal and Neonatal Implications
Laboratory diagnosis, an elevated TSH in association with a low serum free T_4 concentration, is the most sensitive indicator of primary hypothyroidism. Because TBG is elevated in pregnancy, the total serum T_4 level may not be as low as would be expected, and may appear inappropriately

high in the setting of an elevated TSH. Positive thyroid autoantibodies support the diagnosis of hypothyroidism, particularly in the absence of a past history of thyroidectomy or radioactive iodine therapy. Elevated serum cholesterol concentration is useful in nonpregnant patients but is not helpful in pregnancy, since serum cholesterol concentration increases by up to 60% above prepregnancy values during gestation.

Treatment of Hypothyroidism during Pregnancy

Once a diagnosis of hypothyroidism is made in a pregnant patient, full replacement doses of T_4 should be instituted, regardless of the degree of thyroid function. This will minimize further fetal exposure to a hypothyroid environment. Therapy can be titrated rapidly in young pregnant women with no other comorbid conditions starting with 0.1 mg of T_4 daily for 3 to 5 weeks. Thereafter, dosage adjustments can be made depending on the thyroid function test results. Since T_4 has a long half-life it can be given once a day. With adequate treatment, the serum TSH concentration should decrease to values below 6 U/mL within 4 weeks, and the serum free T_4 concentration should increase to normal values for pregnancy in the same timespan. The optimal range for TSH during pregnancy is <3.0 U/mL. It is important to note that normal total serum T_4 concentrations in pregnancy are higher than the normal range for nonpregnant women due to an increase in thyroxine binding and increases in serum TBG concentration. The free T_4 concentration is ideally in the upper range of normal value. If the values do not return to normal, the dose of T_4 should be increased by 0.05 mg increments. The serum TSH concentration may take longer to return to normal values.

■ MYXEDEMA COMA

Myxedema coma represents the extreme expression of severe hypothyroidism and is considered a medical emergency with a 20% mortality rate. It is very rare in pregnancy and usually affects older patients. It is characterized by hypothermia, hypotension, hypoventilation, hyponatremia, and bradycardia. Primary objectives in treating myxedema coma are restoration of normal thyroid hormone levels, correction of electrolyte disturbances, and identification and treatment of any underlying infection. Because of the inherently high mortality rate, treatment should be started immediately and should include appropriate supportive therapy and corticosteroids to prevent adrenal insufficiency (Table 10-11). Possible precipitating

■ **TABLE 10-11. Treatment of Myxedema Coma**

Endotracheal intubation and ventilation if there is hypercapnia or hypoxia

Ordinary warming (normal blankets)—avoid external rewarming devices

Intravenous fluids and electrolytes and inotropic supportive therapy if required

Intravenous sodium may be needed if serum sodium <120 meq/L

Cardiac monitoring

ECG

Troponin and CPK levels to rule out myocardial infarction

Blood pressure monitoring

Corticosteroids

Draw baseline cortisol level

100 mg hydrocortisone every 8 h until baseline cortisol level is known, then titrate accordingly

Levothyroxine sodium (synthroid, levoxyl) intravenously (nasogastric tube if IV administration not possible— oral dose is 30%-50% more than the IV dose)

Slow bolus IV dose 300-500 µg

Daily IV doses of 75-100 µg

Daily oral does of 50-200 µg once patient is ambulatory

Liothyronine (cytomel, triostat) T_3 replacement in young patients with low cardiovascular risk (more likely than T_4 to cause arrhythmias)

10 µg IV every 8 h

Panculture and emperic antibiotic therapy until culture results are known

factors should also be identified and treated. Levothyroxine sodium may be given via a nasogastric tube, but the preferred route of administration is intravenous. A bolus dose of levothyroxine sodium is given as quickly as possible to increase the peripheral pool of T_4. This should usually be between 300 and 500 µg. Although such a dose is usually tolerated well, rapid intravenous administration of large doses of levothyroxine sodium should be cautiously undertaken in patients with cardiac compromise. Clinical judgment in this situation may dictate smaller intravenous doses of levothyroxine sodium. The initial dose is followed by daily intravenous doses of 75 to 100 µg until the patient is stable and oral administration is feasible. Normal T_4 levels are usually achieved within 24 hours, followed by progressive increases in T_3. Improvement in cardiac output, blood pressure, temperature, and mental status generally occur within 24 hours, with further improvement in the other manifestations of hypothyroidism in 4 to 7 days.

■ ACUTE ADRENAL INSUFFICIENCY IN PREGNANCY

Acute adrenocortical insufficiency or Addisonian crisis can occur in pregnancy when a patient with chronic adrenal insufficiency is stressed, or in one who is undiagnosed. Normal levels of total and free cortisol, urinary free cortisol, and ACTH in pregnancy are shown in Table 10-12. It may also result from an obstetric complication that results in DIC, such as severe preeclampsia or eclampsia, abruptio placentae, amniotic fluid embolus, or postpartum hemorrhage. In such cases bilateral massive adrenal hemorrhage may occur and constitute an acute emergency. This condition usually presents with nausea, vomiting, abdominal pain, and shock, and is frequently fatal. Early recognition and treatment are paramount to avoiding a bad outcome. A similar presentation has been noted in the third trimester of pregnancy or in the postpartum period in association with acute pyelonephritis,

gram-negative bacillemia, and fulminant meningococcal infection (Waterhouse-Friderichsen syndrome). Therapy for acute adrenocortical insufficiency in pregnancy should include an initial intravenous bolus of 200 mg hydrocortisone succinate (Solu-Cortef) followed by 100 mg in 1 L of normal saline solution given over 30 minutes. One hundred milligrams of hydrocortisone succinate should be placed in each subsequent liter of normal saline infused, until the patient is adequately hydrated. This may take up to 5 L. Hypoglycemia may be prevented by instituting a 50-gm glucose infusion. Since the patient will receive up to 600 mg of hydrocortisone succinate with this protocol, no added mineralocorticoid is required.

Pheochromocytoma in Pregnancy

Pheochromocytoma is a rare endocrine tumor. When associated with pregnancy, it can be very dangerous for both the mother and the fetus. The main sign of the disease is hypertension, which is common in pregnancy, and can be easily mistaken for pregnancy-induced hypertension. Differentiation from preeclampsia should, however, be straightforward since the edema, proteinuria, and hyperuricemia found in preeclampsia are absent in pheochromocytoma. Plasma and urinary catecholamines may be modestly elevated in preeclampsia and other serious pregnancy complications requiring hospitalization, though they remain

■ TABLE 10-12. Normal Plasma Total and Free Cortisol, Urinary Free Cortisol and ACTH Levels in Normal Pregnancy		
	Nonpregnant	**Third trimester**
Total cortisol		
09.00 h	11.34 ± 3.5 mg/mL	36.0 ± 7 mg/mL
	324 ± 100 nmol/L	1029 ± 200 nmol/L
24.00 h	3.6 ± 2.6 mg/mL	23.5 ± 4.34 mg/mL
	103 ± 76 nmol/L	470 ± 124 nmol/L
Plasma-free cortisol		
09.00 h	0.63 ± 0.3 mg/mL	1.33 ± 0.4 mg/mL
	18 ± 9 nmol/L	32 ± 12 nmol/L
24.00 h	0.2 ± 0.14 mg/mL	0.59 ± 0.17 mg/mL
	6 ± 4 nmol/L	17 ± 5 nmol/L
Urinary-free cortisol	4.7-9.5 mg/d	82.4-244.8 mg/d
	13-256 nmol/d	229-680 nmol/d
Plasma ACTH	15-70 pg/mL	20-120 pg/mL
	3.3-15.4 pmol/L	4.4-26.4 pmol/L

normal in mild preeclampsia and pregnancy-induced hypertension. Catecholamine levels may, however, be two to four times the normal level after an eclamptic seizure and this can be confusing.

An unrecognized pheochromocytoma can be lethal because a fatal hypertensive crisis may be precipitated by anesthesia or even normal delivery. As the uterus enlarges and an actively moving fetus compresses the adrenal neoplasm, maternal complications such as severe hypertension, hemorrhage into the neoplasm, hemodynamic collapse, myocardial infarction, cardiac arrhythmias, congestive heart failure, and cerebral hemorrhage may occur. Extraadrenal tumors, which occur in 10%, such as in the organ of Zuckerkandl at the aortic bifurcation, are particularly prone to hypertensive episodes with changes in position, uterine contractions, fetal movement, and Valsalva maneuvers. Unrecognized pheochromocytoma is associated with a maternal mortality rate of 50% at induction of anesthesia or during labor. A recent review of 41 pregnant women with known pheochromocytoma by Ahlawat et al, however, showed a much lower maternal mortality rate of 4% and a fetal mortality rate of 11%. Antenatal diagnosis of pheochromocytoma reduced the maternal mortality rate to 2%. These mortality rates are significantly lower than those of prior studies and can be attributed to increased awareness of the condition and more reliable testing modalities (Table 10-13).

There is minimal placental transfer of catecholamines. Adverse fetal effects, such as hypoxia, are a result of catecholamine-induced uteroplacental vasoconstriction

and placental insufficiency, as well as maternal hypertension, hypotension, or vascular collapse. Pheochromocytoma can also occur as part of multiple endocrine neoplasia type 2 (MEN 2) in association with medullary carcinoma of the thyroid gland and parathyroid adenomas. Identification of the *RET* protooncogene mutations that cause MEN 2 can be used to screen family members of MEN 2 kindred and to monitor those who are at risk. The women at risk should be monitored very closely during pregnancy. Patients with MEN 2A are more likely to have paroxysmal hypertension and have higher rates of bilateral neoplasms than those with sporadic pheochromocytoma. Examination for associated evidence for MEN 2 may be difficult in pregnancy, with the expected pregnancy alterations in calcium, PTH, and calcitonin. Clinical thyroid examination should be assisted by fine needle aspiration of any suspicious nodules so that overt medullary carcinoma can be treated immediately.

Most pregnant patients with pheochromocytoma will initially complain of symptomatic hypertension that is severe and fluctuating, and which is often associated with severe headache, perspiration, palpitation, and tachycardia (Table 10-13). Other possible signs and symptoms include arrhythmias, postural hypotension, chest or abdominal pain, visual disturbance, convulsions, or sudden collapse. Symptoms may occur or worsen during pregnancy because of the increased vascularity of the tumor and mechanical factors such as pressure from the expanding uterus or fetal movement. The coexistence of diabetes mellitus, possible hyperthyroidism, and myocardial infarction are important and should prompt a search for pheochromocytoma. Individuals with neurofibromatosis, von Hippel-Lindau disease, or retinal angiomatosis should also be screened for pheochromocytomas prior to pregnancy since these conditions are associated with an increased risk of pheochromocytoma.

The diagnosis is confirmed by an accurate 24-hour urine collection for both epinephrine, norepinephrine, and their metabolites. The assays should preferably be performed on specimens collected during or after a hypertensive episode. Laboratory diagnosis of pheochromocytoma is unchanged from the nonpregnant state since catecholamine metabolism is not altered by pregnancy per se. If possible, methyldopa and labetalol should be discontinued prior to the investigation as these agents may interfere with the quantification of the catecholamines and VMA. Provocative testing should be avoided because of the increased risk of maternal and fetal mortality.

■ TABLE 10-13. Symptoms and Signs of Pheochromocytoma
Symptomatic hypertension
Severe and fluctuating
Dyspnea
Dizziness
Severe headache
Perspiration
Palpitations and tachycardia
Arrhythmias
Postural hypotension
Chest or abdominal pain
Visual disturbances
Convulsions
Cardiovascular collapse

Efforts to localize the tumor should be made once a biochemical diagnosis is made. MRI and ultrasound are the preferred methods for localization of tumors in pregnant patients because they avoid exposing the fetus to ionizing radiation. Metaiodobenzylguanidine scans are contraindicated in pregnancy, but may be necessary if other tumor localization methods fail.

Initial medical management involves an α-blockade with phenoxybenzamine, phentolamine, prazocin, or labetalol (Table 10-14). All of these agents are well tolerated by the

---

■ TABLE 10-14. Management of Pheochromocytoma

Pharmacologic control of hypertension and tachycardia
α-adrenergic receptor blockade
Phenoxybenzamine
   Start at 10 mg bid and gradually increase (10 mg every other day) to maximum dosage (20-40 mg bid/tid)
   or until patient develops orthostatic hypotension
Phentolamine
   Only given parenterally (5-10 mg IM or IV) and is reserved for emergency or preoperative situations
Prazosin
   Start at 1 mg po bid/tid and increase to a maximum daily dose of 6-15 mg given in divided doses (bid/tid)
Labetalol
   Start 100 mg po bid and increase by 100 mg bid every 2 wk until blood pressure controlled; maximum dose is
    2400 mg/d. When discontinuing labetalol taper dose over 1-2 wk
   In an emergency labetalol can be given IV—start with 20 mg IV over 2 min and increase by 20 mg every 10 min
    until blood pressure is controlled or a maximum dose of 300 mg is reached
   Labetalol can also be given as a continuous infusion of 2 mg/min until blood pressure is controlled and then
    switched to oral dosing with 200-400 mg every 6-12 h
Nitroprusside
   Start at 0.25 μg/kg/min IV infusion and titrate to control blood pressure. The maximum recommended infusion
    rate is 10 μg/kg/min
Metyrosine may be used if hypertension is still uncontrolled
β-blockade
   Reserved for tachycardia or arrhythmia, and predominantly adrenaline-secreting tumors. Selective and short
    acting agents are preferred:
   Metoprolol
   • 50-200 mg po bid
   Atenolol
   • Start at 50 mg po everyday and increase after 10-14 d to a maximum of 100 mg/d
   Propranolol
    Only to be used after adequate α-blockade has been instituted
    Start 40 mg po bid and increase every 3-7 d to a maximum of 480 mg daily in divided doses (bid)
Fluid management
Surgical management
Timing depends on
• Medical control
• Tumor size
• Risk of malignancy
• Stage of pregnancy (best in second trimester)
• laparoscopy vs laparotomy

Third trimester
• C/S after confirmation of lung maturity with adrenalectomy Or
• vaginal delivery and laparoscopic removal of tumor postpartum

fetus, but phenoxybenzamine is considered the preferred agent as it provides long-acting, stable, noncompetitive blockade. Placental transfer of phenoxybenzamine occurs, but is generally safe. If hypertension remains inadequately controlled, metyrosine has also been used successfully to reduce catecholamine synthesis in a pregnancy complicated by malignant pheochromocytoma, but may potentially adversely affect the fetus. β-blockade is reserved for treating maternal tachycardia or arrhythmias which persist after complete α-blockade and volume repletion. β-blockade without prior α-blockade is contraindicated because the unopposed α-adrenergic activity may lead to vasoconstriction and hypertensive crisis. Propranolol has been successfully used after appropriate α-blockade in pregnancy. β-blockers may be associated with fetal bradycardia and intrauterine fetal growth restriction when used early in pregnancy. All of these potential fetal risks are small compared to the risk of fetal wastage from unblocked high maternal levels of catecholamines. Hypertensive emergencies should be treated with phentolamine or nitroprusside. The definitive treatment of pheochromocytoma is surgical removal of the tumor(s) and this should ideally be accomplished before 24 weeks of gestation, and only after achieving adequate α-blockade. Successful laparoscopic excision of a pheochromocytoma has been described in the second trimester of pregnancy. After 24 weeks of gestation, uterine size makes abdominal exploration and access to the tumor difficult and it is generally recommended that surgery be delayed until fetal maturity is reached. To that end, steroid therapy may be used to hasten fetal lung maturity. Once delivery is entertained, adequate α-blockade should be instituted and elective cesarean delivery may be performed, followed immediately by adrenal exploration. Cesarean section is recommended for delivery based on the work of Schenker and Granat who reported higher maternal mortality rates with vaginal delivery (31%) compared to cesarean delivery (19%). Labor may result in uncontrolled release of catecholamines secondary to pain and uterine contractions. Severe maternal hypertension may lead to placental ischemia and fetal hypoxia. However, in the well-blocked patient, vaginal delivery may be possible if cesarean section is not possible, as long as there is intensive pain management with epidural anesthesia, avoidance of mechanical compression, passive descent, and instrumental delivery.

There is no available information regarding the impact of maternal use of phenoxybenzamine on the nursing neonate. Malignant pheochromocytoma may recur in pregnancy. Life-long monitoring is necessary in all patients, with extra caution in those who are pregnant.

■ PRIMARY HYPERALDOSTERONISM

Primary hyperaldosteronism is a rare cause of hypertension in pregnancy. Occasionally this hypertension can be severe, and confusing with preeclampsia. In addition, the degree of hypertension can be variable and can significantly worsen in the first 6 weeks of the postpartum period.

Patients with classic hyperaldosteronism present with hypertension, hypokalemia, and elevated urine potassium levels. Before biochemical diagnosis, hypokalemia should be corrected because low potassium levels may suppress aldosterone. When making the diagnosis, potassium replacement should be initiated, all diuretics should be discontinued for at least 2 weeks, and high doses of β-blockers should be reduced because they reduce renin production. Calcium channel blockers should not be used for at least 2 to 3 hours before testing.

The measurement of plasma aldosterone levels may not be useful in the diagnosis of hyperaldosteronism in pregnant women because of the physiological increase in aldosterone levels in pregnancy. The levels measured during normal pregnancy are often within the primary hyperaldosteronism range. Pregnant women may have less urinary potassium wasting than patients with primary hyperaldosteronism because of the antagonizing effects of progesterone. Another factor that may complicate the diagnosis during pregnancy is the increase in plasma renin levels in normal pregnancy. In primary hyperaldosteronism, plasma renin levels are usually decreased, and in pregnancy the decrease may be attenuated. Outside of pregnancy salt-loading studies are desirable to confirm the autonomous secretion of aldosterone, but during pregnancy there are concerns about volume overload, worsening of hypokalemia, and the lack of specific reference ranges for pregnancy. One test that can be used in pregnancy involves prolonged positioning of the patient in an upright posture. This usually causes a modest increase in plasma renin activity. However, if there is primary hyperaldosteronism, the renin activity remains suppressed.

Ultrasonography and MRI are the preferred imaging methods in pregnant women for localizing the tumor, but if necessary, any appropriate imaging modality should be used to confirm the presence of a tumor.

If an adrenal adenoma is detected, the preferred treatment is unilateral adrenalectomy. Cases of successful adrenalectomy in the second trimester have been reported. Early delivery may need to be considered in the third trimester since spironolactone and angiotensin-converting enzyme inhibitors are generally avoided in pregnancy. The goals of therapy are to reduce blood pressure and replace potassium, and while α-methyl dopa, β-blockers, and calcium channel blockers can be used, they have variable success rates.

■ DIABETES INSIPIDUS

Diabetes insipidus in pregnancy is caused by either an abnormality of vasopressin secretion, an abnormality of vasopressin action, or vasopressin degradation. The presenting features are polydipsia, polyuria, and dehydration. Three types of diabetes insipidus can be found in pregnancy: central, nephrogenic, and transient vasopressin resistant (Table 10-15).

Central Diabetes Insipidus

Central diabetes insipidus is caused by decreased production of vasopressin by the paraventricular nuclei of the hypothalamus. It complicates 1 in 15,000 deliveries. The

■ TABLE 10-15. Causes of Diabetes Insipidus in Pregnancy

Type of DI	Cause
Central	• Pregnancy worsening of prior DI • CNS tumor, eg, prolactinoma • Granuloma, eg, sarcoid • Histiocytosis X • Aneurysm • Lymphocytic hypophysitis • Sheehan syndrome
Nephrogenic	• X-linked abnormality of vasopressin V2 receptor
Transient vasopressin resistant	• Increased vasopressinase activity due to decreased vasopressinase degradation due to hepatic disease (eg, acute fatty liver, HELLP syndrome, or hepatitis)

most common presentation is that of a woman who has central diabetes insipidus before conception, arising from a pituitary tumor or another invasive disease such as histiocytosis X. Central diabetes insipidus often worsens during pregnancy due to an increase in the clearance of endogenous vasopressin by placental vasopressinase. Vasopressinase concentration increases during pregnancy in proportion to the placental weight. It is metabolized by the liver, thus its activity is increased in liver disease. Subclinical central diabetes insipidus may be unmasked for the first time during pregnancy, because of the need for vasopressin release, low serum osmolality, and increased clearance of vasopressinase. During pregnancy 60% of established cases of central diabetes insipidus worsen, but 25% improve, and 15% remain the same.

The diagnosis of central diabetes insipidus during pregnancy has been seen following development of Sheehan syndrome and as a result of the enlargement of a prolactinoma, histiocytosis X, and lymphocytic hypophysitis. It has also been reported as a complication of ventriculoperitoneal shunt during pregnancy.

The diagnosis of central diabetes insipidus that occurs for the first time during pregnancy requires modification of the standard water deprivation test. Nonpregnant patients normally need to lose up to 5% of their total body weight before the induced dehydration adequately stimulates vasopressin release. Such dehydration can be dangerous in pregnancy and should not be used. The use of DDAVP as a test of urinary concentrating ability has been described and is currently the preferred method. Maximum urine osmolality over 11 hours after administration of DDAVP is assessed. Any value greater than 700 mosmol/kg is considered normal.

The treatment of central diabetes insipidus in pregnancy is with DDAVP, 2 to 20 µg intranasally twice daily. This treatment can be given parenterally after cesarean section, but intravenous dosing is 5- to 20-fold more potent than the intranasal spray and the dose should be adjusted accordingly. DDAVP is not degraded by vasopressinase and no further adjustment is needed in patients with increased vasopressinase activity. Transfer of DDAVP to breast milk is minimal, and breast-feeding is not contraindicated. Treatment of central maternal diabetes insipidus with DDAVP throughout pregnancy does not pose a risk to the infant.

Labor proceeds normally in women with central diabetes insipidus, and surges of oxytocin can be detected during labor and the puerperium. This suggests that women with central diabetes insipidus, although they are vasopressin deficient, still secrete oxytocin normally. Lactation is not impaired.

Nephrogenic Diabetes Insipidus

Nephrogenic diabetes insipidus is a rare X-linked disorder. At least six mutations in this gene have been identified and direct mutation analysis can now be used for carrier detection and early prenatal diagnosis. Nonpregnant women with nephrogenic diabetes insipidus are usually treated with thiazide diuretics or chlorpropamide. Chlorpropamide stimulates vasopressin release and enhances its action on the renal tubule, but it may cause fetal hypoglycemia and neonatal diabetes insipidus, and therefore should not be used in pregnancy. Thiazide diuretics are the treatment of choice for nephrogenic diabetes insipidus during pregnancy.

Transient Vasopressin-Resistant Diabetes Insipidus

Transient vasopressin-resistant diabetes insipidus is probably the most common form of diabetes insipidus seen in pregnancy. It is caused by increased vasopressinase activity due to either increased placental production of the enzyme or decreased hepatic vasopressinase metabolism as a result of liver damage. Transient disturbances of liver function may be seen in acute fatty liver of pregnancy, preeclampsia, HELLP syndrome, and hepatitis.

The treatment of transient vasopressin-resistant diabetes insipidus in pregnancy requires DDAVP because DDAVP is not degraded by vasopressinase. Electrolyte and fluid balance should be closely monitored during the postpartum period. The symptoms of transient vasopressin-resistant diabetes insipidus resolve in a few days to a few weeks after delivery, when hepatic function returns to normal.

■ SHEEHAN SYNDROME

Severe hemorrhage, shock, or prolonged hypotension during or after delivery may lead to postpartum pituitary necrosis or the Sheehan syndrome. This condition is rare (1:10,000 deliveries) and its pathogenesis is still unclear. It is believed to be the result of spasm in the arterial supply to the anterior lobe of the pituitary gland leading to ischemia and edema and ultimate necrosis and thrombosis in the portal sinuses and capillaries. A second theory as to the etiology is based on the development of DIC and intrapituitary bleeding. Sheehan syndrome usually involves only anterior pituitary function because the posterior pituitary and hypothalamus are supplied by the inferior hypophyseal artery and the circle of Willis, which makes them less vulnerable to ischemic necrosis. In rare cases, however, some women with Sheehan syndrome may develop partial or overt diabetes insipidus due to reduced vasopressin (antidiuretic hormone; ADH) secretion. There is frequently poor correlation between the severity of the postpartum hemorrhage and the occurrence of Sheehan syndrome and patients suspected of this complication should be investigated regardless of the severity of their postpartum/intrapartum bleed.

The presentation of Sheehan syndrome is highly variable. It is estimated that 95% to 99% of the anterior pituitary gland needs to be destroyed before the characteristic postpartum failure of lactation, secondary amenorrhea, loss of axillary and pubic hair, genital and breast atrophy, increasing signs of secondary hypothyroidism, and adrenocortical insufficiency occur. The most specific early postpartum sign will be failure of lactation. Since mineralocorticoid secretion is not impaired, there are usually no electrolyte disturbances. However, hyponatremia has been reported in conjunction with Sheehan syndrome and appears to be on the basis of inappropriate ADH secretion (SIADH).

Less extensive pituitary destruction (50%-95%) is associated with an atypical form of the disease with loss of one or more trophic hormones. Postpartum diagnosis of Sheehan syndrome requires dynamic provocative testing of both anterior and posterior lobes of the pituitary gland. The anterior pituitary gland function is best assessed with pituitary hormone response to standard stimulatory tests in conjunction with pituitary imaging with axial CT or MRI. Posterior pituitary function in Sheehan syndrome can be studied with plasma vasopressin response to either osmotic stimuli during 5% hypotonic saline infusion or following a water deprivation test. Spontaneous recovery from hypopituitarism due to postpartum hemorrhage has also been reported.

SUGGESTED READINGS

Aboul-Khair SA, Crooks J, Turnbull AC, et al. The physiological changes in thyroid function during pregnancy. *Clin Sci.* 1964;27:195.

Ahlawat SK, Jain S, Kumari S, et al. Pheochromocytoma associated with pregnancy: case report and review of the literature. *Obstet Gynecol Surv.* 1999;54(11):728-737.

Azizi F. Effect of methimazole treatment of maternal thyrotoxicosis on thyroid function in breast-feeding infants. *J Pediatr.* 1996;128:855.

Azizi F, Khoshniat M, Bahrainian M, et al. Thyroid function and intellectual development of infants nursed by mothers taking methimazole. *J Clin Endocrinol Metab.* 2000;85: 3233-3238.

Baron F, Sprauve ME, Hiddleston JF, et al. Diagnosis and surgical treatment of primary hyperaldosteronism in pregnancy. *Obstet Gynecol.* 1995;86:644.

Black JA. Neonatal goiter and mental deficiency: the role of iodides taken during pregnancy. *Arch Dis Child.* 1963;38:526.

Burrow G. Thyroid function and hyperfunction during gestation. *Endocrinol Rev.* 1993;14:194-202.

Burrow GN, Fisher DA, Larsen PR. Maternal and fetal thyroid function. *N Engl J Med.* 1994;331:1074.

Cheong HI, Park HW, Ha IS, et al. Six novel mutations in the vasopressin V2 receptor gene causing nephrogenic diabetes insipidus. *Nephron.* 1997;75:431.

Daly MJ, Wilson CM, Dolan SJ, Kennedy A, McCance DR. Reversible dilated cardiomyopathy associated with post-partum thyrotoxic storm. *QJM.* 2009;102:217-219. Epub 2009 Jan 13.

Davis L, Lucas M, Hankins G, et al. Thyrotoxicosis complicating pregnancy. *Am J Obstet Gynecol.* 1989;160:63.

Derksen RHWV, van der Wiel A, Poortman J, et al. Plasma exchange in the treatment of severe thyrotoxicosis in pregnancy. *Eur J Obstet Gynecol Reprod Biol.* 1984;18:139.

Devoe LD, O'Dell BE, Castillo RA, et al. Metastatic pheochromocytoma in pregnancy and fetal biophysical assessment after maternal administration of alpha-adrenergic, beta-adrenergic, and dopamine antagonists. *Obstet Gynecol.* 1986;68(Suppl 3):15S.

Durr JA, Hoggard JG, Hunt JM, et al. Diabetes insipidus in pregnancy associated with abnormally high circulating vasopressinase activity. *N Engl J Med.* 1982;316:1070.

Easterling T, Schmucker B, Carlson K, et al. Maternal hemodynamics in pregnancies complicated by hyperthyroidism. *Obstet Gynecol.* 1991;78:348.

Endocrine Society. Management of thyroid dysfunction during pregnancy and postpartum. *J Clin Endcrinol Metab.* 2007;92(Suppl 8):S1-S47

Falterman CJ, Kreisberg R. Pheochromocytoma: clinical diagnosis and management. *South Med J.* 1982;75:321.

Finkenstedt G, Gasser RW, Hofle G, et al. Pheochromocytoma and sub-clinical Cushing's syndrome during pregnancy: diagnosis, medical pre-treatment and cure by laparoscopic unilateral adrenalectomy. *J Endocrinol Invest.* 1999;22:551.

Freier DT, Eckhauser FE, Harrison TS. Pheochromocytoma. *Arch Surg.* 1980;115:388.

Freier DT, Thompson NW. Pheochromocytoma and pregnancy: the epitome of high risk. *Surgery.* 1993;114:1148.

Glinoer D. The regulation of thyroid function in pregnancy: pathways of endocrine adaptation from physiology to pathology. *Endocrine Rev.* 1997;18:404-433.

Glinoer D, De Nayer P, Bourdoux P, et al. Regulation of maternal thyroid during pregnancy. *J Clin Endocrinol Metab.* 1990;71:276-287.

Glinoer D, Solo M, Bourdoux P, et al. Pregnancy in patients with mild thyroid abnormalities: maternal and neonatal repercussions. *J Clin Endocrinol Metab.* 1991;73:421-427.

Goodwin T, Montoro M, Mestman J, et al. The role of chorionic gonadotropin in transient hyperthyroidism of hyperemesis gravidarum. *J Clin Endocrinol Metab.* 1992;75:1333.

Gurlek A, Cobankara V, Bayraktar M. Liver tests in hyperthyroidism: effect of antithyroid therapy. *J Clin Gastroenterol.* 1997;24:180-183.

Haddow JE, Palomaki GE, Allan WC, et al. Maternal thyroid deficiency during pregnancy and subsequent neuropsychological development of the child. *N Engl J Med.* 1999;341:549-555.

Hall R, Richards C, Lazarus J. The thyroid and pregnancy. *Br J Obstet Gynaecol.* 1993;100:512.

Hammond TG, Buchanan JG, Scoggins BA, et al. Primary hyperaldosteronism in pregnancy. *Aus NZ J Med.* 1982;12: 537.

Harper MA, Murnaghan GA, Kennedy L, et al. Pheochromocytoma in pregnancy: five cases and a review of the literature. *Br J Obstet Gynaecol.* 1989;96:594.

Hime MC, Williams DJ. Osmoregulatory adaptation in pregnancy and its disorders. *J Endocrinol.* 1992;132:7.

Huchon DJR, Van Ziji JAWM, Campbell-Brown BM, McFadyen IR. Desmopressin as a test of urinary concentrating ability in pregnancy. *J Obstet Gynecol.* 1982;2:206.

Ingbar SH. Management of emergencies, IX. Thyrotoxic storm. *N Engl J Med.* 1966;274:1252.

Isely W, Dahl S, Gibbs H. Use of esmolol in managing a thyrotoxic patient needing emergency surgery. *Am J Med.* 1990;89:122.

Jialal I, Desai RK, Rajput MC. An assessment of posterior pituitary function in patients with Sheehan syndrome. *Clin Endocrinol.* 1987;27:91.

Jordan RM. Myxedema coma. Pathophysiology, therapy, and factors affecting prognosis. *Med Clin North Am.* 1995;79(1): 185-194.

Kageyama Y, Hirose S, Terashi K, et al. A case of postpartum hypopituitarism associated with hyponatremia and congestive heart failure. *Jpn J Med.* 1988;27:337.

Kalff V, Shapiro B, Lloyd R, et al. The spectrum of pheochromocytoma in hypertensive patients with neurofibromatosis. *Arch Intern Med.* 1982;142:2092.

Kallen BA, Carlsson SS, Bergen BK. Diabetes insipidus and the use of desmopressin during pregnancy. *Eur J Endocrinol.* 1995;132:144-146.

Khunda S. Pregnancy and Addison's disease. *Obstet Gynecol.* 1972;39:431.

Kothari A, Bethune M, Manwaring J, et al. Massive bilateral pheochromocytomas in association with von Hippel Lindau syndrome in pregnancy. *Aust NZ J Obstet Gynaecol.* 1999;39:381.

Lau P, Permezel M, Dawson P, et al. Pheochromocytoma in pregnancy. *Aust N Z J Obstet Gynaecol.* 1996;36:472.

Laurberg P, Nygaard B, Glinoer D, Grussendorf M, Orgiazzi J. Guidelines for TSH-receptor antibody measurements in pregnancy: results of an evidence-based symposium organized by the European Thyroid Association. *Eur J Endocrinol.* 1998;139:584-586.

Laurel MT, Kabadi UM. Primary hyperaldosteronism. *Endocrine Practice.* 1997;3:47.

Leung A, Millar L, Koonings P, et al. Perinatal outcome in hypothyroid pregnancies. *Obstet Gynecol.* 1993;81:349.

Levin N, McTighe A, Abdel-Aziz MIE. Extra-adrenal pheochromocytoma in pregnancy. *Maryland State Med J.* 1983;32:377.

Liaw YF, Huang MJ, Fan KD, et al. Hepatic injury during propylthiouracil therapy in patients with hyperthyroidism. *Ann Intern Med.* 1993;118:424-428.

MacGillivray I. Acute suprarenal insufficiency in pregnancy. *BMJ.* 1951;2:212.

Mandel SJ, Brent GA, Larsen PR. Review of antithyroid drug use during pregnancy and report of a case of aplasia cutis. *Thyroid.* 1994;4:129.

Maragliano G, Zuppa AA, Florio MG, et al. Efficacy of oral iodide therapy on neonatal hyperthyroidism caused by maternal Graves' disease. *Fetal Diagn Ther.* 2000;15(2):122-126.

Mazzaferri EL. Evolution and management of common thyroid disorders in women. *Am J Obstet Gynecol.* 1997;176:507.

Momotani N, Noh JY, Ishikawa N, Ito K. Effects of propylthiouracil and methimazole on fetal thyroid status in mothers with Graves' hyperthyroidism. *J Clin Endocrinol Metab.* 1997;82:3633-3636.

Momotani N, Yamashita R, Yoshimoto M, et al. Recovery from foetal hypothyroidism: evidence for the safety of breast-feeding while taking propylthiouracil. *Clin Endocrinol.* 1989;31:591.

Monturo MN, Collea JA, Frasier SN, et al. Successful outcome of pregnancy in women with hypothyroidism. *Ann Intern Med.* 1981;94:31.

Moodley J, McFadyen ML, Dilraj A, et al. Plasma noradrenaline and adrenaline levels in eclampsia. *S Afr Med J.* 1991;80:191.

Ohyama T, Nagasaki A, Kakai A, et al. Spontaneous recovery from hypopituitarism due to postpartum hemorrhage. *Horm Metab Res.* 1989;21:320.

Oishi S, Sato T. Pheochromocytoma in pregnancy: a review of the Japanese literature. *Endocrine J.* 1994;41:219.

Pederson EB, Rasmussen AB, Christensen NJ, et al. Plasma noradrenaline and adrenaline in preeclampsia, essential hypertension in pregnancy and normotensive pregnant control subjects. *Acta Endocrinol (Copenh).* 1982;99:594.

Prihoda J, Davis L. Metabolic emergencies in obstetrics. *Obstet Gynecol Clin North Am.* 1991;18:301.

Rubin PC. Beta-blockers in pregnancy. *N Engl J Med.* 1983;18:73.

Saarikoski S. Fate of noradrenaline in the human fetoplacental unit. *Acta Physiol Scand.* 1974;421:1.

Safa AM, Schumacher OP, Rodriguez-Antunez A. Long-term follow-up results in children and adolescents treated with radioactive iodine (131I) for hypothyroidism. *N Engl J Med.* 1975;292:167.

Sandstrom B. Antihypertensive treatment with the adrenergic beta-receptor blocker metoprolol during pregnancy. *Gynecol Invest.* 1978;9:195.

Santeiro ML, Stromquist C, Wyble L. Phenoxybenzamine placental transfer during the third trimester. *Ann Pharmacother.* 1996;30:1249.

Schenker JG, Granat M. Pheochromocytoma and pregnancy—an updated appraisal. *Aust NZ J Obstet Gynaecol.* 1982;22:1.

Sheehan HL. Postpartum necrosis of the anterior pituitary. *J Path Bacteriol.* 1937;45:189.

Sheps SG, Jiang NS, Klee GC. Diagnostic evaluation of pheochromocytoma. *Endocrinol Metab Clin North Am.* 1988;17:397.

Sitar D, Abu-Bakare A, Gardiner R. Propylthiouracil disposition in pregnant and postpartum women. *Pharmacology.* 1982;25:57.

Soler NG, Nicholson H. Diabetes and thyroid disease during pregnancy. *Obstet Gynecol.* 1979;54:318.

Solomon GC, Thiet M, Moore F, et al. Primary hyperaldosteronism in pregnancy. *Obstet Gynecol.* 1996;41:255.

Thorpe-Beeston J, Nicolaides K, Felton C, et al. Maturation of the secretion of thyroid hormone and thyroid-stimulating hormone in the fetus. *N Engl J Med.* 1991;324:531.

Uhrig JD, Hurley RM. Chlorpropamide in pregnancy and transient neonatal diabetes insipidus. *Can Med Assoc J.* 1983;128:368.

Usta IM, Barton JR, Amon EA, et al. Acute fatty liver of pregnancy: an experience in the diagnosis and management of fourteen cases. *Am J Obstet Gynecol.* 1994;171:1342.

Van Dijke CP, Heydendael RJ, De Kleine MJ. Methimazole, carbimazole, and congenital skin defects. *Ann Intern Med.* 1987 Jan;106(1):60-61.

Vaquero E, Lazzarin CD, Valensise H, et al. Mild thyroid abnormalities and recurrent spontaneous abortion: diagnostic and therapeutical approach. *Am J Reprod Immunol.* 2000;43:204-208.

Vitug AC, Goldman JM. Hepatotoxicity from antithyroid drugs. *Hormone Res.* 1985;21:229-234.

Wartofsky L. Myxedema coma. In: Werner SC, Ingbar SH, Braverman LE, Utiger RD, eds. *Werner & Ingbar's the Thyroid: A Fundamental and Clinical Text.* 8th ed. Philadelphia, PA: Lipincott Williams & Wilkins; 2000:843-847.

Wing DA, Millar LK, Koonings PP, Montoro MN, Mestman JH. A comparison of propylthiouracil versus methimazole in the treatment of hyperthyroidism in pregnancy. *Am J Obstet Gynecol.* 1994;170:90-95.

Diabetic Ketoacidosis in Pregnancy

• *Michael R. Foley and Ravindu P. Gunatilake*

Despite recent advances in the evaluation and medical treatment of diabetes in pregnancy, diabetic ketoacidosis (DKA) remains a matter of significant concern. The fetal loss rate in most contemporary series has been estimated to range from 10% to 25%. Fortunately, since the advent and implementation of insulin therapy, the maternal mortality rate has declined to 1% or less. In order to favorably influence the outcome in these high-risk patients, it is imperative that the obstetrician/provider be familiar with the basics of the pathophysiology, diagnosis, and treatment of diabetic ketoacidosis in pregnancy.

■ PATHOPHYSIOLOGY

DKA is characterized by hyperglycemia and accelerated ketogenesis. Both a lack of insulin and an excess **of glucagon and other counter-regulatory hormones significantly contribute to these problems and their resultant clinical manifestations. In a nutshell, glucose normally enters the cell secondary to the presence of insulin. The cell then may use glucose for nutrition and energy production. When insulin is lacking, glucose fails to enter the cell. The cell responds** to this starvation by facilitating the release of counter-regulatory hormones including glucagon, catecholamines, and cortisol. These counter-regulatory hormones are responsible for providing the cell with an alternative substrate for nutrition and energy production. By the process of gluconeogenesis, fatty acids from adipose tissue are broken down by hepatocytes to ketones (acetone, acetoacetate, and β-hydroxybutyrate = ketone bodies), which are then utilized by the cells of the body for nutrition and energy production (see

Fig 11-1). The lack of insulin also contributes to increased lipolysis and decreased reutilization of free fatty acids, thereby providing more substrate for hepatic ketogenesis. A basic review of the *biochemistry of diabetic ketoacidosis* is presented in Fig 11-1.

■ MATERNAL CONCERNS

Now that we have an understanding of how and why ketone bodies are produced during diabetic ketoacidosis, what are the maternal consequences resulting from excessive ketogenesis? In general, ketone bodies are considered to be moderately strong acids. In response to the fall in pH in most body fluids created by an accumulation of these acids, the body reacts physiologically to correct the resultant metabolic acidosis. The respiratory rate and depth increase (Kussmaul respirations) in an attempt to blow off carbon dioxide, initiating a corrective trend towards compensatory respiratory alkalosis. Serum bicarbonate levels decline and as a result the anion gap becomes abnormally elevated. In addition to increasing fatty acid production, poor glucose utilization results in severe hyperglycemia. Untreated hyperglycemia leads to marked glycosuria, initiating a significant osmotic diuresis. As a result, dehydration, electrolyte depletion, and if left untreated, cardiac failure, and death may follow.

A vicious cycle is created by an increase in dehydration-mediated serum hyperosmolarity and catabolism, propagated by Kussmaul respiration, leading to a further production of glucose counter-regulatory hormones, lipolysis, and subsequent hyperketonemia. An algorithm for this clinical pathophysiologic response is presented in Fig 11-2.

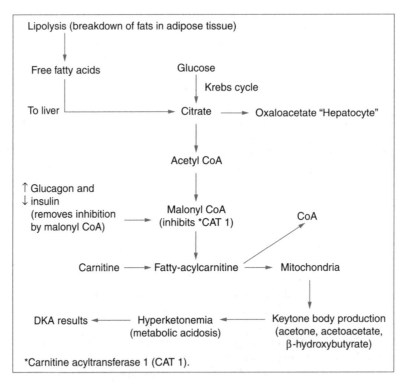

FIGURE 11-1. Basic biochemistry of diabetic ketoacidosis. (*Adapted from Berkowitz RL, ed.* Critical Care of the Obstetric Patient. *New York, NY: Churchill Livingstone; 198:416.*)

■ FETAL CONCERNS

The fetus appears to be at significant risk of sudden intrauterine death during an episode of maternal diabetic ketoacidosis. The mechanism for this sudden death is not completely understood; however, it appears to be related to a combination of factors. Alterations in fetal fluid and electrolyte balance, poor uterine perfusion resulting from maternal hypovolemia, and increased acid load in the form of fatty acids and lactate, all favor a reduction in fetal oxygenation and metabolic acid clearance. When caring for a patient in DKA who is carrying a potentially viable fetus, careful fetal monitoring should be judiciously utilized. Often, signs of fetal stress become apparent reflecting the

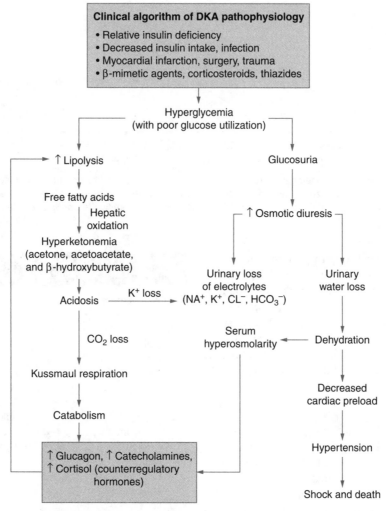

FIGURE 11-2. Metabolic alterations in diabetic ketoacidosis. (*Modified from Hagay ZJ, Reece EA. Diabetes mellitus in pregnancy. In: Reece EA, Hubbins JC, Mahoney MJ, et al, eds.* Medicine of the Fetus and the Mother. *Philadelphia, PA: J.B. Lippincott; 1992: 982-1020.*)

degree of maternal metabolic derangement. Decreased variability and late decelerations in the fetal heart tracing as well as abnormal umbilical artery Doppler values are among the changes that can be observed. Delivery of a compromised baby should be prudently delayed until the mother is metabolically stable. Correction of maternal metabolic abnormalities generally results in a rapidly improved fetal condition. Therefore, efforts should be directed at improving maternal deficits reserving emergency operative intervention for unresponsive persistent fetal compromise.

■ DIAGNOSIS OF DKA

In pregnancy, DKA may occur at a lower plasma glucose value as compared to the nonpregnant patient. DKA has been observed at plasma glucose levels as low as 180 mg/dL. It appears that a relative insulin resistance of pregnancy combined with a greater tendency toward ketosis reduces the threshold for DKA during pregnancy. The insulin resistance during pregnancy is related to an increased production of placental hormones, insulinase, and cortisol (Fig 11-3).

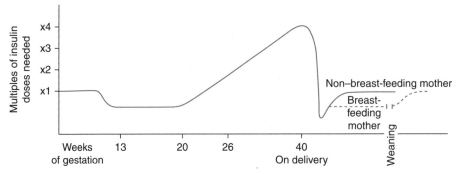

FIGURE 11-3. Changing insulin needs during pregnancy caused by properties of placental hormones and enzyme (insulinase) and cortisol. (*Adapted from Bobak IM, Jensen MD, Zalar MK. Maternity and Gynecologic Care: The Nurse and the Family. 4th ed. St. Louis, MO: C.V. Mosby;1989:783.*)

The maternal and fetal concerns resulting from DKA emphasize the importance of a rapid and reliable diagnosis. Following the axiom that laboratory tests should be utilized only to verify or nullify a clinical suspicion, the diagnosis of DKA should be based on clinical examination and supported by an evaluation of biochemical parameters. Table 11-1 summarizes the clinical presentation, the biochemical definition, and additional laboratory findings associated with diabetic ketoacidosis.

■ TREATMENT OF DKA

Diabetic ketoacidosis during pregnancy is a medical emergency. The patient should be admitted to an intensive care facility and consultations obtained from Maternal-Fetal Medicine, Endocrinology, and Neonatology. A detailed history and physical examination should be performed to search for underlying precipitating factors for DKA such as noncompliance with insulin administration, insulin pump malfunction, or infection (urine, skin, lungs, dental, and amniotic cavity). Glucocorticoid administration in the setting of preterm labor has also been implicated in hyperglycemia leading to DKA. Remember that any process that results in dehydration, starvation, or a catabolic state (stress) with insulin antagonism predisposes the patient to DKA. Defining the underlying etiology is also a priority not only for the treatment of the current episode of DKA, but also for preventing a future recurrence.

Fetal monitoring should be initiated if there is a potentially viable fetus (see Chap 24). Intervention on behalf of the fetus should be withheld until the maternal metabolic condition is stabilized. Oxygen therapy and maternal position changes, however, should be initiated to help improve

■ TABLE 11-1. Diagnostic and Biochemical Parameters of DKA

Clinical features

General	Neurologic
Malaise	Lethargy
Drowsiness	Coma
Weakness	Respiratory
Dehydration	Kussmaul respirations
Polyuria	Tachypnea
Polydipsia	Cardiovascular
Fruity breath	Tachycardia
Gastrointestinal	Hypotension
Nausea	
Vomiting	
Abdominal pain	
Ileus	

Biochemical definition (memory aid)

Diabetic → Glucose ≥180 mg/dL
Keto → Serum acetone or β-hydroxybutyrate is ≥1:2
Acidosis → Arterial pH ≤7.3, HCO_3^- ≤15, and anion gap $[Na^+ - (Cl^- + HCO_3^-)] > 12$

Additional laborary findings

Glycosuria	Leukocytosis
Ketonuria	Elevated CPK
Metabolic acidosis	Elevated amylase
Hyperosmolality	Elevated transaminases
Hypokalemia	Elevated BUN
Hypomagnesemia	Elevated creatinine
Hypophosphatemia	

fetal perfusion while correcting maternal biochemical and plasma volume abnormalities (see Chap 22). A detailed flow sheet including a comprehensive recording of serial laboratory values, at appropriate time intervals, should be started at bedside to facilitate patient assessment following therapy. The use of invasive hemodynamic monitoring should be reserved for the patient with severe renal compromise in an effort to properly guide rehydration while avoiding iatrogenic pulmonary edema. Other less invasive measures such as the initiation of an arterial line to follow serial arterial blood gases, a Foley catheter to monitor strict urinary output, and continuous peripheral pulse oximetry should be initiated as an early adjunct to beginning therapy. The basic premise for the treatment of diabetic ketoacidosis in the pregnant patient is the simultaneous correction of fluid and electrolyte imbalance and treatment of hyperglycemia and acidosis (see Fig 11-4).

■ TREATMENT OF HYPOVOLEMIA

Hypovolemia during diabetic ketoacidosis results primarily from hyperglycemia-induced osmotic diuresis (see Fig 11-2). Since the restoration of intravascular volume improves perfusion and augments systemic insulin delivery to peripheral tissues, repletion of the circulating intravascular volume is the number one treatment priority. The estimated total water deficit is calculated to be 100 mL/kg of actual body weight (4-10 L deficit). Once renal competence is established (urinary output of at least 0.5 cc/kg/h), fluid replacement may be initiated. Keeping in mind that many of the patients encountered with DKA during pregnancy may have preexisting renal compromise (class F DM), a baseline evaluation of serum BUN and creatinine would be prudent to avoid fluid overload in a patient with markedly reduced creatinine clearance. Most authorities recommend isotonic normal saline as the intravenous fluid of choice for volume replacement instead of lactated Ringer solution. The reason behind this recommendation is that the use of hypotonic solutions (0.45 NS [normal saline]or lactated Ringer) as initial treatment can lead to a rapid decline in plasma osmolarity which may lead to cellular swelling and resultant cerebral edema. Therefore, the recommended approach is to utilize isotonic NS and replace 75% of the total calculated fluid deficit within the first 24 hours of therapy. The remaining 25% of the deficit is replaced over the remainder of the patient's hospitalization. At our institution, 1 L of isotonic NS is given over the first hour, and 500 cc NS per hour is given over second and third hours. Isotonic NS, therefore, is used for the first 3 hours of therapy. Crystalloid infusions such as Plasmalyte are increasingly aining favor for initial volume resuscitation in the presence of severe hypovolemia associated with DKA. Thereafter, however, lactated Ringer or 0.45 NS is given at a rate of 250 cc/h until 75% of the total deficit is replaced over the first 24 hours. Lactated Ringer solution is utilized to avoid further iatrogenic contributions to the fall in serum pH since the pH of lactated Ringer is 6.5 compared to a pH of 5.0 for isotonic NS. In addition, the sodium load with isotonic saline may create hypernatremia fostering the recommendations to switch from isotonic saline to a more hypotonic solution (lactated Ringer or 0.45 NS) when the patient's serum sodium increases above 150 to 155 mEq/L (see Table 11-2).

■ INSULIN THERAPY

Intravenous insulin administration is the mainstay treatment for the pregnant patient in diabetic ketoacidosis. An initial intravenous loading dose of 0.1 U/kg (8-10 units is a good starting point) followed by a constant infusion of 0.1 U/kg/h effectively inhibits lipolysis and ketogenesis leading to suppression of hepatic glucose output with resultant lower serum glucose levels. The insulin infusion is prepared by adding 100 units of regular insulin to 100 mL of NS (1 cc = 1unit). Alternatively, 0.4 U/kg may be administered as a subcutaneous (SC) or intramuscular (IM) bolus until parenteral (IV) access is achieved. However, the subcutaneous and intramuscular routes are fraught with unreliable insulin absorption due to poor perfusion associated with the hypovolemic state. Serum glucose levels should be measured every 1 to 2 hours during insulin infusion. General principles of an intravenous insulin infusion are listed in Table 11-3.

The intravenous insulin infusion should be titrated to reduce the serum glucose at a rate of less than or equal to 60 to 75 mg/dL/h to avoid rapid changes in the serum osmolarity which may precipitate cerebral edema and risk cerebellar pontine myelinolysis. A good rule of thumb is that if the plasma glucose does not decrease by 10% in the first hour or 20% by the second hour of therapy; repeat the intravenous loading dose or double the current continuous infusion rate. As the patient's blood glucose approaches 250 mg/dL, add 5% dextrose to the IV infusion and reduce the hourly insulin infusion by one half (0.05-0.1 U/kg/h). Maintain serum glucose levels between 150 and 200 mg/dL while hypovolemia and electrolyte abnormalities are corrected. Be aware that while monitoring serum ketones in response to insulin administration,

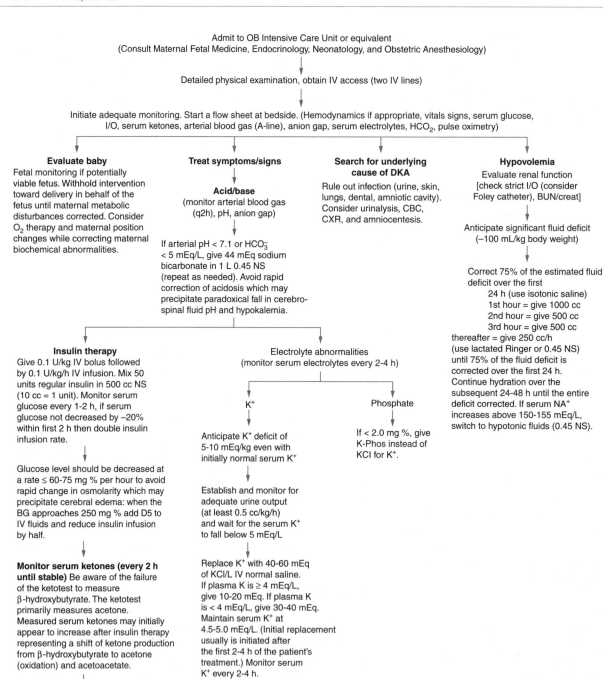

FIGURE 11-4. Treatment algorithm for diabetic ketoacidosis.

■ TABLE 11-2. Common Intravenous Fluids

1 L	Glu (gm)	Na (mEq)	Cl (mEq)	K (mEq)	Ca (mEq)	Lactate (mEq)	pH
>5% Dextrose/water	50	0	0	0	0	0	3.5-6.5
0.9% NaCl normal saline	0	154	154	0	0	0	5.0
Lactated Ringer	0	130	109	4	3	28	6.5

a paradoxical increase in serum acetone should be anticipated. While β-hydroxybutyrate (BHB) is the predominant ketone in DKA, the ketotest primarily measures serum acetone. During insulin therapy, the overall production of ketones clearly diminishes and there is a shift of ketone production from β-hydroxybutyrate to acetone (oxidation) and acetoacetate. This phenomenon results in the apparent paradoxical worsening of ketoacidemia at the onset of insulin therapy. When testing is available, BHB should be measured directly in lieu of the ketotest and the anion gap should be used to assess response to therapy. The intravenous insulin infusion should be continued until the serum bicarbonate (18-31 mEq/L) and anion gap (<12) normalize. Table 11-4 and Fig 11-5 summarize the mechanics of changing from an intravenous insulin infusion to subcutaneous insulin or subcutaneous insulin

pump, respectively. Table 11-5 provides additional helpful information regarding the insulin sensitivity factor.

■ POTASSIUM ADMINISTRATION

The anticipated potassium deficit in a pregnant patient with DKA is 5 to 10 mEq/kg. Potassium replacement, however, is most often delayed for the first 2 to 4 hours of therapy since the initial serum potassium is usually normal to mildly elevated and adequate diuresis has yet to be established. Once fluid and insulin therapy have been instituted and corrections of the metabolic acidosis are underway, serum potassium may precipitously fall as a result of urinary loss and intracellular shift. When the patient's plasma potassium has fallen below 5 mEq/L and an adequate diuresis has been established (at least 0.5 cc/kg/h),

■ TABLE 11-3. General Principles of Intravenous Insulin Infusion

1. Use *regular* insulin when mixing the infusion.
2. Pump monitor the infusion rate.
3. Clearly label the insulin infusion line with units of insulin per volume.
4. Intravenous insulin is compatible with both magnesium sulfate and pitocin.
5. To compensate for insulin binding to the plastic tubing, gently mix the insulin in the bag and thoroughly flush the tubing with insulin before beginning administration.
6. Obtain blood samples from the patient's arm opposite the infusion.
7. Monitor the patient's blood glucose hourly during insulin infusion
8. Have injectable dextrose 50% and dextrose 10% (500 mL) available at bedside for treatment of hypoglycemia.
9. Do not preload with glucose containing solutions before regional anesthesia (ie, epidural) or as a bolus infusion to improve a nonreassuring fetal heart rate tracing.
10. Before discontinuing intravenous infusion, give subcutaneous or intramuscular insulin to prevent rebound hyperglycemia.

Regular insulin half-life

- Intravenous regular insulin: 5-min half-life
- Intramuscular regular insulin: 2-h half-life
- Subcutaneous regular insulin: 4-h half-life

■ TABLE 11-4. Managing the Conversion: Intravenous to Subcutaneous Insulin After Resolution of DKA

1. The patient should be tolerant of a full diet.
2. Calculate the total number of insulin units administered over 24 h following stabilization (normalization of anion gap).

Total units/day

	Before Breakfast	*Distribution*
	2/3 of total units/day ⟶	2/3 Neutral protamine Hagedorn (NPH)[a] 1/3 Lispro
	Before Dinner	
	1/3 of total units/day ⟶	1/2 Neutral protamine Hagedorn (NPH)[a] 1/2 Lispro

Example
Insulin infusion 2 U/h × 24 h (stabilized)
Total insulin/24 h = 48 units

AM 2/3 × 48 = 32 ⟶ 2/3 as NPH = 21 units NPH
1/3 as Lispro = 11 units Lispro
PM 1/3 × 48 = 16 ⟶ 1/2 as NPH = 8 units NPH
1/2 as Lispro = 8 units Lispro

Insulin	Onset	Peak (maximum effect)	Duration
Lispro	15 min	30-90 min	2-4 h
Regular	1 h	2-3 h	4-5 h
NPH	2 h	8 h	24 h

[a]NPH may be given at bedtime instead of at dinner if hypoglycemia occurs at 3 AM.

■ TABLE 11-5. Helpful Hints for the Insulin Pump

The insulin sensitivity factor
How much of a reduction in blood glucose should you expect for each 1.0 unit of insulin delivered to the patient?

The 1500 rule

$$\text{Insulin sensitivity factor} = \frac{1500}{\text{Total daily insulin}}$$

Example
If your patient receives a total daily insulin of 50 units

$$\frac{1500}{50} = 30 \text{ mg/dL blood glucose drop per 1.0 unit of insulin}$$

To correct this patient's blood glucose to 100 mg/d:

$$\frac{\text{Patient's blood glucose} - 100}{30} = \text{Supplemental units of insulin}$$

**Total daily insulin requirement
(after stabilization)**

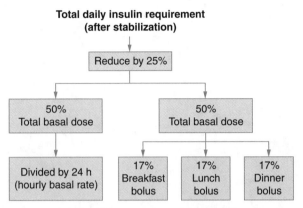

FIGURE 11-5. Transition to subcutaneous insulin pump.

then potassium administration should be initiated. The recommended method of potassium replacement is summarized as follows:

1. Mix 40 to 60 mEq KCl/L in isotonic saline.
2. If plasma K^+ is

    ≥ 4 mEq/L, give 10 to 20 mEq

    <4 mEq/L, give 30 to 40 mEq

3. Replace K^+ cautiously, monitoring urinary output and serum K^+ frequently (every 2-4 hours).
4. Do not exceed K^+ supplementation to greater than 20 mEq/h due to concern for cardiotoxicity/arrhythmias.
5. Replace entire K^+ deficit over the span of the patient's entire hospitalization.
6. Alternatively, in the face of DKA-induced maternal phosphate deficiency (<2 mg/dL), K_2PO_4 (K-Phos) may be given as potassium replacement instead of KCL.

■ BICARBONATE THERAPY

The use of sodium bicarbonate therapy in patients with severe DKA remains a controversial practice and should be used carefully. Recent studies of pregnant patients with DKA have failed to show an improvement in outcomes among those receiving bicarbonate therapy. Bicarbonate is usually reserved for those patients who have an arterial pH of <6.9-7.0 and/or a HCO_3^- <5 mEq/L. Rapid undiluted correction of metabolic acidosis with sodium

bicarbonate is unwarranted and may lead to severe hypokalemia, hypernatremia, impaired oxygen delivery, and a paradoxical fall in cerebrospinal fluid pH. Administration of one ampule (44 mEq sodium bicarbonate) diluted in 1000 mL of 0.45 NS is a reasonable dose in a patient with severe acidemia (pH <7.0). The total deficit of bicarbonate may be calculated (obtain base deficit on arterial blood gas):

Bicarbonate (mEq) regained to fully correct metabolic acidosis

$$= \frac{\text{Base deficit (mEq/L)} \times \text{patient weight (kg)}}{4}$$

Since oxygen hemoglobin affinity is augmented in the presence of an alkalotic shift of the oxygen-hemoglobin disassociation curve to the left, it is prudent not to fully correct the patient's metabolic acidosis, ensuring better oxygen delivery to the fetus.

Please refer to Table 11-4 for an algorithmic summary of the treatment of diabetic ketoacidosis in pregnancy.

SUGGESTED READING

Coustan, DR. Diabetic ketoacidosis. In: Richard L Berkowitz, ed. *Critical Care of the Obstetric Patient.* New York, NY: Churchill Livingstone; 1983:Chapter 15.

Diabetic ketoacidosis and nonketotic hyperosmolarity. In: Robert H Demling, Robert F Wilson, eds. *Decision Making in Surgical Critical Care.* Philadelphia, PA: B.C. Kecker; 1988:216.

Hagay ZJ. Diabetic ketoacidosis in pregnancy: etiology, pathophysiology, and management. *Clin Obstet Gynecol.* 1994; 37:39-49.

Kitabchi AE, Umpierrez GE, Murphy MB, et al. Management of hyperglycemic crises in patients with diabetes. *Diabetes Care.* 2001;24:131-153.

Landon MB, Catalano PM, Gabbe SG. Diabetes mellitus complicating pregnancy. In: Steven G Gabbe, Jennifer R Neibyl, Joe Leigh Simpson, eds. *Obstetrics: Normal and Problem Pregnancies.* 5th ed. New York, NY: Churchill Livingstone; 2007.

Reece AE, ed. Metabolic disorders in pregnancy. *Clin Obstet Gynecol.* 1994;37(1).

Winkler CL, Davis LE. Endocrine emergencies: diabetic ketoacidosis, In: Gary A. Dildy III , Belfort, George R. Saade, Steven L Clark, Gary DV Hankins, and Jeffrey P. Phelan, eds. *Critical Care Obstetrics.* 4th ed. Boston, MA: Blackwell Scientific Publications; 2004:Chapter 32.

CHAPTER 12

Respiratory Emergencies During Pregnancy

• *Alfredo F. Gei and Victor R. Suarez*

Respiratory complications during pregnancy are not unusual and can be life threatening. A careful interview and physical examination, a chest x-ray, and an arterial blood analysis are the most useful interventions in the evaluation of these conditions.

Understanding of the cardiorespiratory changes during pregnancy is essential for the diagnosis and treatment of emergencies in normal pregnant women and in women with underlying cardiopulmonary diseases.

■ BASIC SCIENCE

Oxygen is the basis of every aerobic reaction in our organism. The procurement and delivery of oxygen is a vital process that the pregnant woman has to perform for herself and her unborn child. Nature has ensured satisfactory mechanisms of exchange of oxygen with air and delivery of it to her unborn child (and adapting body) through complex anatomic (Table 12-1) and physiologic changes (Table 12-2).

Respiration involves two different but interrelated phenomena: ventilation and oxygenation. The evaluation of these processes lies in the interpretation of arterial blood gases variables: Pco_2 and Po_2 (Figs 12-1 and 12-2).

Respiration requires that O_2 be obtained from an extracorporeal source (atmosphere or ventilator), then transferred across the alveolar-endothelial barrier, transported to the different organs in the periphery, and subsequently utilized in aerobic metabolism.

At term, there is a small (200-400 mL, 4%) decrease in total lung capacity. Vital capacity (VC) does not change significantly. Functional residual capacity (FRC) consistently decreases 300-500 mL (17%-20%). Changing from a sitting to a supine position at term causes a further decrease (25%) in FRC. This may increase closure of small airways, especially in obese patients in the supine or lithotomy position.

■ BASIC PHYSIOLOGIC OXYGENATION CONCEPTS

- **O_2 content.** The content of oxygen in arterial blood is the sum of that bound to hemoglobin (Hb) and that dissolved in plasma (normally about 1.5%). The main factor that determines the extent of O_2 binding to hemoglobin (saturation) is the Pao_2 (hemoglobin-oxygen dissociation curve). The shape of the curve indicates that unless the steep part of the curve is reached (a drop of Pao_2 to <60 mm Hg), there will not be a significant deleterious effect on Hb saturation and O_2 arterial content.

- **O_2 affinity.** Several factors can change the affinity of Hb for O_2. Acidosis, fever, and increased 2,3-DPG shift the curve to the right. In the slightly acidic environment of peripheral tissues, a right shift is important to unload O_2 to the cells. Alkalosis, hypothermia, and decreased 2,3-DPG shift the curve to the left. In the slightly alkalotic environment of the pulmonary capillary, a left shift is important to load O_2 to the red blood cells. Affinity is also shifted to the left in the fetal hemoglobin.

- **O_2 delivery.** Systemic O_2 delivery is the product of arterial O_2 content (mL/L of blood) and cardiac output (mL/min).

- **O_2 consumption.** In a normal adult at rest, it is approximately 250 mL/min. During exercise it can rise to 3000 mL/min. When delivery cannot meet tissue demands, anaerobic metabolism occurs, leading to lactic acidosis.

See Chap 1.

■ TABLE 12-1. Anatomic and Physiologic Respiratory Adaptations to Pregnancy

Upper airways	• Mucosal edema and friability • Capillary engorgement *(A smaller-sized endotracheal tube may be required for intubation because of swelling of the arytenoid region of the vocal cords)*
Chest wall	• Increases in chest wall circumference (6 cm) • Elevation of the diaphragm (5 cm) • Widening of the costal angles (from 70° to 104°) • Increase in diaphragmatic excursion (1.5 cm) *(All these changes occur before significant increases in uterine size, maternal body weight, or intra-abdominal pressure)*
Respiratory musculature	• Respiratory muscle function is unchanged • Diaphragm and intercostals accessory muscles contribute equally to tidal volume during pregnancy • Maximum inspiratory and expiratory pressures are unchanged

■ TABLE 12-2. Changes in Respiratory Variables During Pregnancy

Parameter	Definition	Change in pregnancy
Respiratory rate	Number of breaths per minute	• No change
Tidal volume	Volume of air inspired and expired at each breath	• Increase up to 40% since early pregnancy; remains essentially constant for the remainder of gestation (100-200 mL)
Minute ventilation (RR × Vt)	Total amount of air (gas) inspired and expired each minute Sum of the volume of air (gas) participating in gas exchange plus the one filling the airway's dead space (ie, not participating in gas exchange)	• Increase up to 40% since early pregnancy and remains essentially constant for the remainder of gestation (100-200 mL)
Vital capacity	Maximum volume of air that can be forcibly inspired after a maximum expiration	• Unchanged
Residual volume	Volume of air remaining in the lungs after a maximum expiration	• Decreases by ~20% due to elevation of the diaphragm
Functional residual capacity (FRC)	Volume of air in lungs at resting expiratory level	• Decreases by ~20% due to elevation of the diaphragm
Inspiratory capacity	Maximum volume of air that can be inspired from resting expiratory level	• Increases 100-300 mL (5%-10%) as a result of the reduction in FRC

RR, respiratory rate.

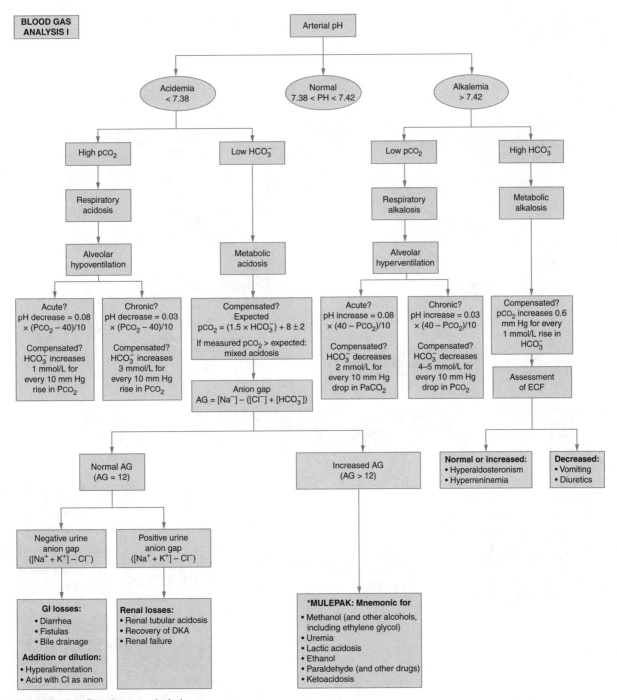

FIGURE 12-1. Blood gas analysis I.

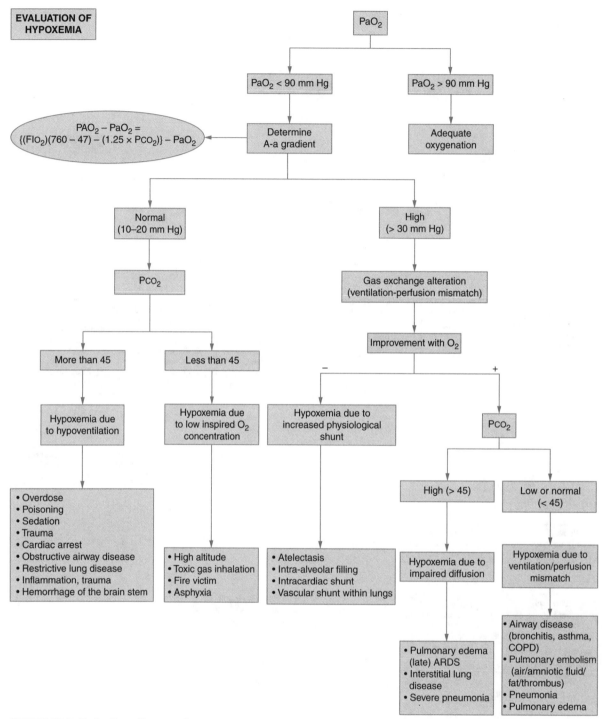

FIGURE 12-2. Evaluation of hypoxemia.

■ **TABLE 12-3. Changes in Oxygenation Variables During Pregnancy**

Parameter	Modification	Magnitude	Peak
Oxygen consumption (V_{O_2})	⇑	+20%	Term
		+40%-60%	During labor
Oxygen delivery (D_{O_2})	⇔ ⇑	700-400 mL/min	Term
Resistance of the pulmonary circulation	⇓	−34%	34 wk

■ RESPIRATORY PHYSIOLOGIC ADAPTATIONS OF PREGNANCY

Pregnancy increases O_2 consumption by 15% to 20% (Table 12-3). Half of this increase is associated with the requirements of the feto-placental unit, and the remaining half is secondary to the increased work by the maternal organs (heart, lungs, and kidneys). Increased cardiac output and minute ventilation explain how O_2 consumption increases despite no change in Pa_{O_2} and a decrease in the arteriovenous O_2 difference (increase in oxygen delivery).

Despite the favorable effects of pregnancy (progesterone is a central stimulant) on ventilation, at least half of pregnant women complain of shortness of breath (dyspnea), fatigue, and decreased exercise tolerance during gestation.

■ OXYGENATION AND ACID-BASE HOMEOSTASIS

Pregnancy is characterized by a chronically compensated respiratory alkalosis due to the hyperventilation (rather than tachypnea) state of pregnancy. Pregnancy's increase in minute ventilation (progesterone-induced hyperventilation of pregnancy) results in a decrease in Pa_{CO_2} to around 30 mm Hg. Maternal pH reflects the chronic compensated mild respiratory alkalosis. Compensation is secondary to the decline in bicarbonate concentration (secondary to increased renal excretion). The net result of these changes is facilitation of CO_2 exchange from fetus to mother.

Oxygenation is affected in at least one-fourth of pregnant women while in a supine position (lower Pa_{O_2} and larger A-a gradient). These changes are reversed when the maternal position changes to the upright state (Table 12-4).

■ **TABLE 12-4. Changes in Arterial Blood Gases During Pregnancy**

ABG variable	Nonpregnant adult	Pregnant
pH	7.35-7.43	7.40-7.47
P_{CO_2} (mm Hg)	37-40	·27-34 *(there is a compensatory increase in renal bicarbonate excretion)*
P_{O_2} (mm Hg)	103	• 106-108 (sea level) • 101-104 (third trimester) • Can drop to 90 (in the supine position during the II and III trimester)
$P(A-a)_{O_2}$ (mm Hg)	14	• 20 • +6 (supine position and III trimester)
Bicarbonate (mEq/L)	22-26	18-22
Base deficit (mEq/L)	1	3

■ CLINICAL IMPLICATIONS

- It is not surprising that pregnant women complain of symptoms suggestive of pulmonary or cardiac disease. In most instances, a careful interrogation and physical examination can establish whether these symptoms are physiologic or a possibility of a specific condition that needs to be addressed and evaluated (Fig 12-3).

- Pregnant patients are prone to
  - Hypoxemia (due to decreased FRC, increased alveolar ventilation, and increased O_2 consumption),
  - Aspiration (slow gastric emptying, functional displacement of lower esophagus)
  - Anesthetic overdose (decreased minimal alveolar concentration of anesthetics, decreased functional residual capacity, and increased alveolar

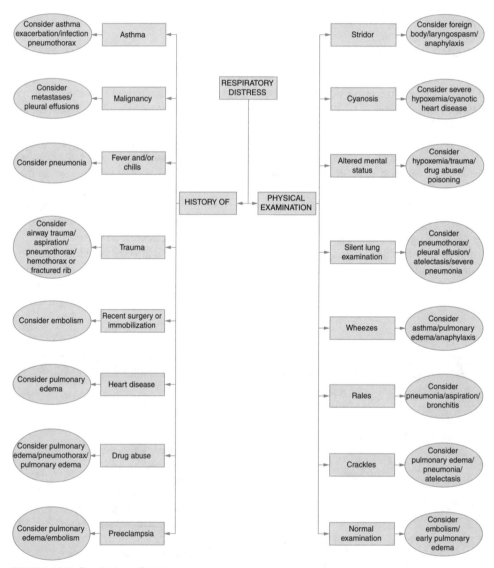

FIGURE 12-3. Respiratory distress.

ventilation). Induction and emergence of and from general anesthesia occurs more rapidly in pregnant women.

■ RESPIRATORY EMERGENCIES DURING PREGNANCY

The anatomic and physiologic changes of the cardiac (Chap 8) and respiratory systems explain why respiratory symptoms are common during pregnancy. The most frequent respiratory complaint is shortness of breath (dyspnea). Other symptoms include cough and hemoptysis. Unfortunately both benign and life-threatening conditions present with similar complaints. A careful evaluation of these symptoms will allow the practitioner to discern between pregnancy-related complaints and a more severe condition. Even when deemed benign, cardiorespiratory symptoms should be noted and evaluated prospectively in subsequent visits of the patient. Some of the conditions that can be suggested by history or physical examination are included in the Fig 12-3. Specific algorithms addressing the evaluation of dyspnea, cough, and hemoptysis (Figs 12-4, 12-5, and 12-6) are suggested.

The most frequent indications for mechanical ventilation among obstetric patients admitted to an ICU are acute respiratory failure (39%) and hemodynamic failure (38%), followed by impaired consciousness (17%) and postoperative ventilation (6%).

Leading causes of acute respiratory distress syndrome (ARDS) during pregnancy are infection, preeclampsia or eclampsia, and aspiration.

The two most helpful clinical adjuncts in the evaluation of respiratory conditions during pregnancy are:

- **Arterial blood gas interpretation.** The changes induced by the pregnant state are summarized in Table 12-4. Figures 12-1 and 12-2 illustrate the evaluation of ventilation and oxygenation through the laboratory analysis of an arterial blood sample.
- **Chest x-ray interpretation.** Table 12-5 summarizes the changes described for pregnancy. Aside from heart enlargement secondary to hypervolemia and cardiac remodeling and some cephalad flow redistribution, all other criteria used to interpret chest radiograms remain the same as in the nonpregnant state. Figure 12-7 provides a guideline for evaluation of chest x-rays and the most common pathologic processes encountered by the site of affliction. As was the case with the arterial blood gases, more than one process may coexist and affect the patient.

Several conditions specific to pregnancy and other intercurrent diseases in the pregnant woman may compromise the processes of oxygenation or ventilation. While the specific treatment of these conditions may differ, the recognition of the need for supportive respiratory therapy and the prompt institution of adequate ventilation and oxygenation support may be the dividing line between life and death.

■ RESPIRATORY FAILURE AND RESPIRATORY SUPPORT

Clinical guidelines for the recognition of respiratory failure (Table 12-6), means to provide noninvasive oxygen (Table 12-7), indications for mechanical ventilation (Table 12-8), indications for endotracheal intubation (Table 12-9), and guidelines for the initiation (Table 12-10) and discontinuation of mechanical ventilation are provided (Table 12-11). In these situations, the processes of evaluation and treatment are frequently simultaneous (Figs 12-4 and 12-8).

■ SPECIFIC CONDITIONS

In addition, an algorithm for the evaluation and treatment of acute asthma is provided (Fig 12-9) and a table with risk factors for asthma mortality included (Table 12-12). Separate tables are provided covering the general principles of management of pulmonary edema (Table 12-13), the selection of antibiotic therapy for the treatment of community acquired pneumonia (Table 12-14), the severity of community acquired pneumonia (Table 12-15), the diagnosis of ARDS (Table 12-16), and principles of management of ARDS (Table 12-17).

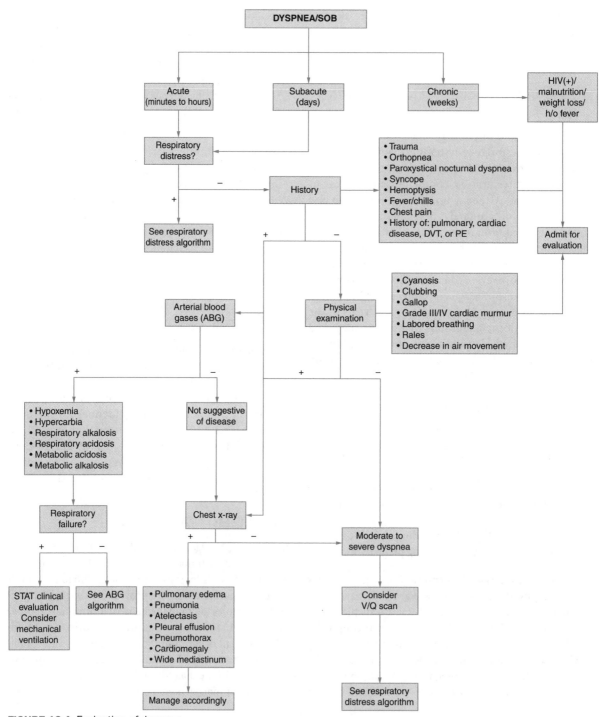

FIGURE 12-4. Evaluation of dyspnea.

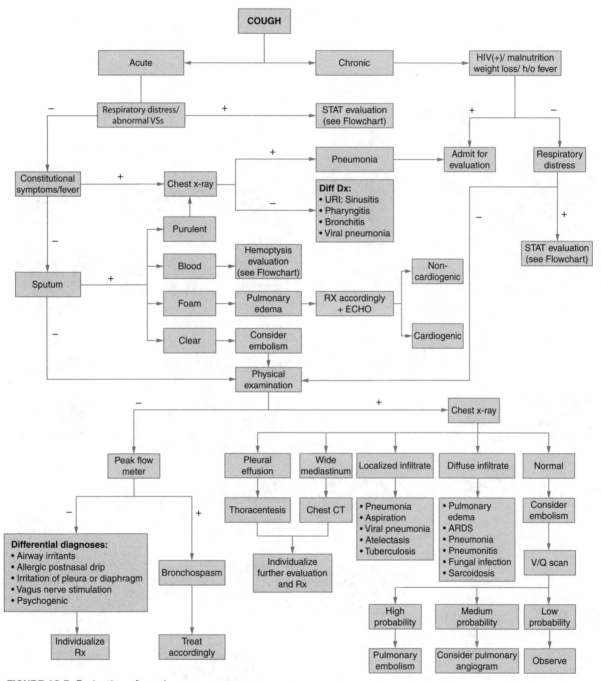

FIGURE 12-5. Evaluation of cough.

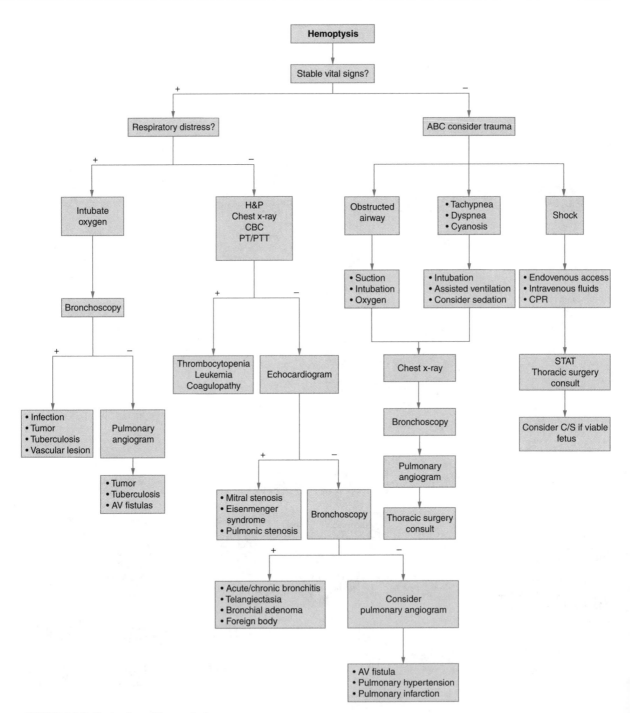

FIGURE 12-6. Evaluation of hemoptysis.

■ **TABLE 12-5. Changes in Chest X-Ray During Pregnancy**

Apparent cardiomegaly (enlarged transverse diameter)
Enlarged left atrium (lateral views)
Increased vascular markings
Straightening of left heart border
Postpartum pleural effusion (right sided)

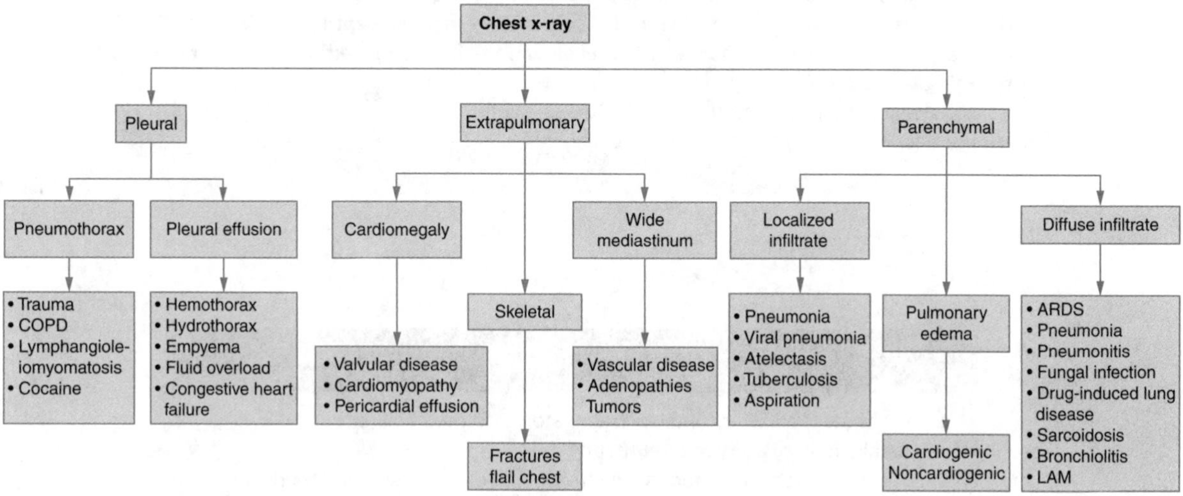

FIGURE 12-7. Evaluation of chest x-ray.

■ **TABLE 12-6. Criteria for the Diagnosis of Respiratory Failure**

Mnemonic: MOVE
1. **Mechanical**
   a. Vital capacity <15 mL/kg
   b. Maximal inspiratory force (MIF) < −25 cm H_2O
   c. Respiratory rate >35/min
2. **Oxygenation**
   a. Pao_2 <70 mm Hg with Fio_2 of 0.4
   b. $P(A-a)o_2$: >350 mm Hg with Fio_2 of 1.0
3. **Ventilation**
   a. $Paco_2$ > 55 mm Hg (if acute condition)
   b. Dead space/tidal volume (Vd/Vt) > 0.6
4. **End-inspiratory lung inflation inadequate for adequate gas exchange**

■ **TABLE 12-7.** Means to Provide Noninvasive Oxygen Therapy

Nasal cannulas
- Can provide 24%-40% oxygen with flow rates up to 6 L/min.
- Oxygen at flow rates of 4 L/min or less need not be humidified.

Simple oxygen masks
- Can provide 35%-50%, depending on fit, at flow rates from 5 to 10 L/min.
- Flow rates need to be maintained at 5 L/min or higher to avoid rebreathing exhaled CO_2 that can be retained in the mask.

Partial rebreathing mask (simple mask with a reservoir bag)
- Oxygen flow should be supplied to maintain the reservoir bag at least one-third to one-half full in inspiration.
- At flow rates of 6-10 L/min the system can provide 40%-70% oxygen.

Nonrebreathing mask (similar to the partial rebreathing mask except it has a series of one-way valves; one valve is between the mask and the bag to prevent exhaled air from returning to the bag)
- The delivered FlO_2 of this system is 60%-80%.
- There should be a minimum flow of 10 L/min.

■ **TABLE 12-8.** Indications for Mechanical Ventilation (Invasive or Noninvasive)

1. Severe respiratory or combined respiratory and metabolic acidosis
2. Sustained respiratory rate of 40/min
3. Abnormal breathing pattern suggestive of increased respiratory workload and/or respiratory muscle fatigue
4. Depressed mental status
5. Severe hypoxemia

■ **TABLE 12-9.** Indications for Endotracheal Intubation

Mnemonic: GARDD
1. **G**astro-pulmonary reflux and aspiration
2. **A**irway obstruction (present or suspected)
3. **R**espiratory arrest (actual or impending)
4. **D**epressed mental status
5. **D**ifficulty managing secretions

■ **TABLE 12-10.** Guidelines for the Initiation of Mechanical Ventilation

A. Primary goals of ventilatory support are
- Adequate oxygenation/ventilation
- Reduced work of breathing
- Synchrony between patient and ventilator
- Avoidance of high-end inspiration alveolar pressures

B. Five subsets of patients can be identified
- Normal lung mechanics and gas exchange (example: drug overdose)
  - Settings: ACV/PSV; FIo_2 of 0.5-1.0; TV: 8-15 mL/kg; RR: 8-12/min; inspiratory flow rate of 40-60 L/min; add sighs 6/h at 1.5 times Vt or PEEP of 5-7.5 cm H_2O to prevent atelectasis
- Severe airflow obstruction (example: drug overdose)
  - Settings: ACV/SIMV; FIo_2 of 0.5-1.0; TV: 5-7 mL/kg; RR: 12-15/min; inspiratory flow rate of 40-60 L/min; add PEEP if patient is triggering. Goals are to minimize alveolar overdistention (plat <30 cm H_2O) and to minimize alveolar dynamic hyperinflation auto PEEP <10 cm H_2O or end-expiratory lung volumes <20 mL/kg)
- Acute or chronic respiratory failure (example: status asthmaticus)
  - Settings: SIMV/ACV; FIo_2 of 0.4-0.6; TV: 5-7 mL/kg; RR: 24-28/min; inspiratory flow rate of 40-60 L/min
- Acute hypoxemic respiratory failure (example: ARDS)
  - Settings: ACV/PCV; FIo_2 of 1.0; TV: 5-7 mL/kg; RR: 24-28/min; minimal PEEP to keep Sao_2 of 90%. If volume is held constant, PEEP increases peak inspiratory airway pressure, a potentially undesirable effect in ARDS; PEEP levels >15 cm H_2O are rarely necessary
- Restrictive lung or chest wall disease (example: sarcoidosis)
  - Settings: FIo_2 of 0.5-1.0; TV: 5-7 mL/kg; RR: 18-24/min

C. Other recommendations
- Avoid high inspiratory peak pressures (>30 cm H_2O)
- Target pH and not pCO_2 to make changes to respiratory rate and minute ventilation
- Use PEEP in diffuse lung injury to support oxygenation and reduce the FIo_2
- Set trigger sensitivity to allow a minimal patient effort to initiate the inspiration
- In patients at risk, avoid choosing ventilator settings that limit expiratory time and cause or worsen auto-PEEP
- When poor oxygenation, inadequate ventilation, or excessively high peak inspiratory pressures are thought to be related to patient intolerance of ventilator settings and are not corrected by ventilator adjustment, consider sedation, analgesia, and/or neuromuscular blockade

■ **TABLE 12-11.** Criteria for Determining Readiness for Extubation

- Pao_2 >80 torr on FIo_2 of 0.6
- $Paco_2$ <45 torr
- Respiratory rate: <35 breaths/min
- Tidal volume: >5 mL/kg
- Vital capacity: >10 mL/kg
- Minute ventilation: <10 L/min
- Negative inspiratory force (NIF): < –20 cm H_2O
- Shallow breathing index (respiratory frequency/tidal volume): <80

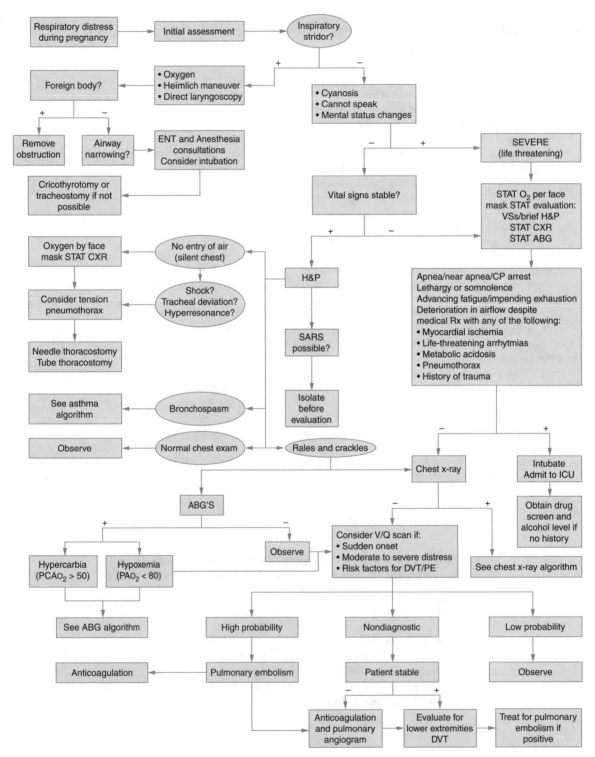

FIGURE 12-8. Evaluation of respiratory distress during pregnancy.

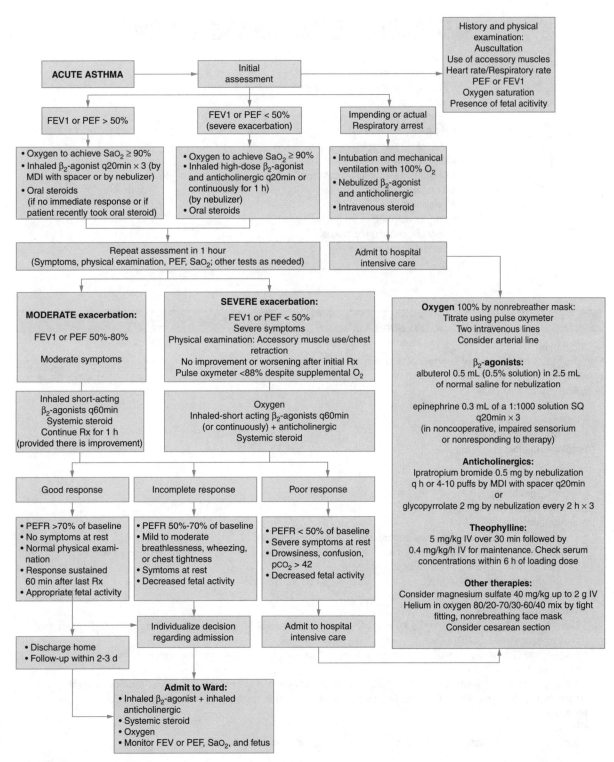

FIGURE 12-9. Evaluation of asthma.

■ TABLE 12-12. Risk Factors of Death From Asthma

- History of sudden severe exacerbations
- Prior intubations
- Prior admission to an ICU due to asthma
- >2 hospitalizations per year
- >3 ER visits for asthma
- Hospitalization or ER visit within last 30 d
- Use of >2 canisters of β_2 per month
- Current use of steroids or recent withdrawal from them
- Comorbidity (cardiovascular or COPD)
- Serious psychiatric illness
- Illicit drug use
- Poor perception of air flow or severity
- Low socioeconomic status
- Sensitivity to mold

■ TABLE 12-13. Principles of Management of Pulmonary Edema

Diagnosis
- Progressive (not sudden) shortness of breath
- Desaturation
- Tachypnea
- Occasionally hypertension
- Bilateral crackles
- S3/Gallop (not always)

Predisposing factors
- Fluid overload
- Preeclampsia
- Tocolytic treatment
- Uncontrolled hypertension

Management
- Semi-Fowler position: Elevate head and chest to improve ventilation.
- Oxygen: Administer at 10 L/min via nonrebreather face mask or with CPAP (intubation may be required).
- Continuous pulse oxymetry and cardiac monitoring.
- Establish IV access; limit intravenous fluid infusion (30-50 mL/h)
- Identify and control predisposing factor(s).

Pharmacologic therapy
- Morphine sulfate: 3-5 mg IV may be given; (avoid in the presence of altered consciousness, increased intracranial pressure, or severe COPD)
- Furosemide: 20-40 mg IV; repeat as necessary (do not use more than 120 mg/h and give slowly to prevent ototoxicity)
- Nitroglycerin: 2 in of paste to chest or 1 pill (1/150) until IV access is secured or no other therapy available
- Hydralazine: 5-10 mg IV may be considered if severe hypertension is mediating the pulmonary edema

Monitor
- Input and output
- Blood pressure and fetal heart rate monitoring if appropriate according to GA

■ **TABLE 12-14. Empirical Selection of Antibiotics for Patients with Community-Acquired Pneumonia**

Specific therapy is desirable within 8 h of onset of empirical therapy to narrow the spectrum and direct the treatment.
Hospitalized patients
I. General medical ward:
  • A respiratory fluoroquinolone (moxifloxacin, gemifloxacin, or levofloxacin)
    or
  • A β-lactam combined *plus* a macrolide *or* a respiratory fluoroquinolone

II. Intensive care unit:
  • A β-lactam (cefotaxime, ceftriaxone, or ampicillin-sulbactam)
    plus either azithromycin *or* a fluoroquinolone

  (for PCN-allergic patients, a respiratory fluoroquinolone, and aztreonam are recommended)

III. Special considerations
  • Cover for *Pseudomonas* if structural lung disease (bronchiectasis), use of steroids or prior antibiotic therapy (particularly fluoroquinolones).
    • Antipseudomonal β-lactam agents (piperacillin-tazobactam, cefepime, imipenem, or meropenem) *plus* a fluoroquinolone (ciprofloxacin or levofloxacin) *or*
    • β-Lactam agents (piperacillin-tazobactam, cefepime, imipenem, or meropenem) *plus* an aminoglycoside and azithromycin *or*
    • β-Lactam agents (piperacillin-tazobactam, cefepime, imipenem, or meropenem) *plus* an aminoglycoside and fluoroquinolone

    (for PCN-allergic patients, substitute aztreonam for the β-lactam)

  • If MRSA (increased risk if injection drug abuse, end-stage renal disease, prior influenza, or prior antibiotic therapy (particularly fluoroquinolones): Add vancomycin or linezolid.
  • If aspiration is suspected (history seizures including eclampsia, risk if injection drug abuse, end-stage renal disease, prior influenza or prior antibiotic therapy (particularly fluoroquinolones)): β-Lactam agents/β-lactamase inhibitor (piperacillin-tazobactam, ticarcillin-clavulanate, ampicillin-sulbactam, or amoxicillin-clavulanate)
  • If influenza: Oseltamivir or zanamivir.
  • If pandemic influenza: Consider in addition to oseltamivir antibacterial agents targeting *S. pneumoniae* and *S. aureus*

NOTE
Once the etiology of CAP has been identified by microbiological methods, antimicrobial therapy should be directed at that pathogen.

Source: From IDSA/ATS Guidelines for CAP in Adults. *CID.* 2007; 44 (Suppl 2):27–72.

■ **TABLE 12-15. Severity of Community-Acquired Pneumonia**

Mnemonic: SMART-COP
S: Systolic blood pressure (low)
M: Multilobal chest radiographic involvement
A: Albumin (low)
R: Respiratory rate (high)
T: Tachycardia

C: Confusion
O: Oxygenation (poor)
P: Arterial pH (low)

All factors are given 1 point with exception of : systolic blood pressure, poor oxygenation, and low ph (scored 2 points each).

A score of 3 or greater identifies patients at high risk of requiring intensive respiratory or vasopressor support.

Source: From Charles PG, Wolfe R, Whitby M, et al. SMART-COP: a tool for predicting the need for intensive respiratory or vasopressor support in community-acquired pneumonia. *Clin Infect Dis.* 2008;47:375-384.

■ **TABLE 12-16. Consensus Criteria for the Diagnosis of ARDS**

I. Acute onset
II. History compatible with specific risk factors
 • Trauma
 • Severe shock
 • Sepsis (septic abortion included)
 • Aspiration
 • Venous fluid, fat, or amniotic fluid embolism
 • Pneumonia
 • Pancreatitis
 • Blood transfusion
 • Seizures (including eclampsia)
 • Overdose
 • Drug induced
 • Eclampsia
 • Abruptio placentae
 • Dead fetus syndrome or retained products of conception
 • Diabetic ketoacidosis
III. Clinical exclusion of cardiogenic pulmonary edema (or PCWP <18 mm Hg)
IV. Respiratory distress
V. Diffuse bilateral patchy opacities in chest x-ray
VI. Pao_2/Flo_2 of <200[a]

[a]Acute lung injury: Less severe form of ARDS with a Pao_2/Flo_2 between 201 and 300.

■ **TABLE 12-17.** Principles of Treatment of ARDS

Therapeutic goals
- Adequate oxygenation
- Avoidance of barotraumas/volutrauma with treatment
- Avoidance of cardiovascular compromise

Management
- Semi-Fowler position: Elevate head and chest to improve ventilation.
- Oxygen: Administer at 10 L/min via nonrebreather face mask or with CPAP (intubation may be required).
- Continuous pulse oxymetry and cardiac monitoring.
- Establish IV access. Consider placement of arterial line and a central line.
- Identify and control predisposing factor(s).

Pharmacologic therapy: None specific available. In severe cases consult pulmonary services for consideration of nitric oxide, pulmonary vasodilatation, corticosteroids, exogenous surfactant administration, prone ventilation, or extracellular membrane oxygenation (ECMO)

Monitor
- Input and output
- Blood pressure and fetal heart rate monitoring if appropriate according to GA

Abbreviations Used

BP	Blood pressure
Hb	Hemoglobin
ICU	Intensive care unit
O_2	Oxygen
Pao_2	Arterial oxygen's partial pressure
$Paco_2$	Arterial carbon dioxide's partial pressure
$P(A-a)o_2$	Alveolar-arterial oxygen difference
PEEP	Positive end-expiratory pressure
PCN	Penicillin
SOB	Shortness of breath
Vd	Dead space
Vt	Tidal volume
Wga	Weeks of gestational age
ECF	Extracellular fluid
AG	Anion gap

SUGGESTED READING

AARC Clinical Practice Guideline. Oxygen therapy for adults in the acute care facility-2002 revision and update. *Respir Care.* 2002;47:717.

Al-Ansari MA, Hameed AA, Al-Jawder SE, et al. Use of noninvasive positive pressure ventilation during pregnancy: Case series. *Ann Thorac Med.* 2007;2:23-25.

American College of Emergency Physicians. Clinical policy for the initial approach to adults presenting with the chief complaint of chest pain, with no history of trauma. *Ann Emerg Med.* 1995;25:274.

American Thoracic Society. The diagnostic approach to acute venous thromboembolism. *Am J Respir Care Med.* 1999; 160:1043.

Bandi VD, Munnur U, Matthay MA. Acute lung injury and acute respiratory distress syndrome in pregnancy. *Crit Care Clin.* 2004;20:577-607

Bartlett JG, Dowell SF, Mandell LA, et al. Guidelines from the Infectious Diseases Society of America. Practice Guidelines for the Management of Community-Acquired Pneumonia in Adults. *CID.* 2000;31:347.

Catanzarite V, Willms D, Wong D, et al. Acute respiratory distress syndrome in pregnancy and the puerperium: causes, courses, and outcomes. *Obstet Gynecol.* 2001;97: 760-764.

Charles PG, Wolfe R, Whitby M, et al. SMART-COP: a tool for predicting the need for intensive respiratory or vasopressor support in community-acquired pneumonia. *Clin Infect Dis.* 2008;47:375-384.

Cole DE, Taylor TL, McCullough DM, et al. Acute respiratory distress syndrome in pregnancy. *Crit Care Med.* 2005;33: 269S-278S.

Crapo RO. Normal cardiopulmonary physiology during pregnancy. *Clin Obstet Gynecol.* 1999;39:3.

Deblieux PM, Summer WR. Acute respiratory failure in pregnancy. *Clin Obstet Gynecol.* 1996;39:143.

Gei AF, Vadhera RB, Hankins GDV. Embolism during pregnancy: thrombus, air and amniotic fluid. *Anesthesiology Clin N Am.* 2003;21:165.

Goodnight WH, Soper DE. Pneumonia in pregnancy. *Crit Care Med.* 2005;33:390S-397S.

Goodrum LA. Pneumonia in pregnancy. *Semin Perinatol.* 1997;21:276.

Ie S, Rubio ER, Alper B, et al. Respiratory complications of pregnancy. *Obstet Gynecol Survey.* 2001;57:39.

King TE. Restrictive lung disease in pregnancy. *Clin Chest Med.* 1992;13:607.

Lee RW. Pulmonary embolism. *Chest Surg Clin N Am.* 2002;12:417.

National Asthma Education Program: National Institute of Health. *Practical Guide for the Diagnosis and Management of Asthma.* NIH Publication A97-4053, 1997.

O'Day M. Cardiorespiratory physiological adaptation of pregnancy. *Semin Perinatol.* 1997;21:268.

Rodgers L, Dangel-Palmer MC, Berner N. Acute circulatory and respiratory collapse in obstetrical patients: a case report and review of the literature. *AANA J.* 1985;68:444.

Rowe TF. Acute gastric aspiration: prevention and treatment. *Semin Perinatol.* 1997;21:313.

Saade GR. Human immunodeficiency virus (HIV)-related pulmonary complications in pregnancy. *Semin Perinatol.* 1997;21:336.

Spiropoulos K, Prodromaki E, Tsapanos V. Effect of Body Position on Pao_2 and $Paco_2$ during Pregnancy. *Gynecol Obstet Invest.* 2004;58:22-25.

Van Hook JW. Acute respiratory distress syndrome in pregnancy. *Semin Perinatol.* 1997;21:320.

Vasquez DN, Estenssoro E, Canales HS, et al. Clinical characteristics and outcomes of obstetric patients requiring ICU admission. *Chest.* 2007;131:718-724.

Witlin AG. Asthma in pregnancy. *Semin Perinatol.* 1997;21:284.

Zimmerman JL. *Fundamental critical care support.* 4th ed. Mount Prospect, IL: Society of Critical Care Medicine; 2007.

Zlatnik MG. Pulmonary edema: etiology and treatment. *Semin Perinatol.* 1997;21:298.

CHAPTER 13

Acute Renal Failure in Pregnancy

• *Tamerou Asrat and Michael P. Nageotte*

Acute renal failure can present in multiple complicated medical conditions but is predominantly acquired in hospitalized patients. This is not a rare medical condition, with as many as 5% of all hospitalized patients having some degree of acute renal failure. With respect to the obstetrical patient, however, acute renal failure has become an uncommon complication of pregnancy in developed countries. It is estimated that the current incidence of acute renal failure (ARF) complicating pregnancy approximates 1 per 10,000 pregnant women. In three successive periods of 10 years between 1958 and 1987, Stratta and colleagues have reported a continued decrease in ARF requiring emergency renal dialysis from a rate of 1 in 3000 in 1958 to 1 in 15,000 pregnancies in 1987. They documented 81 cases of ARF in pregnancy of which 11.6 % experienced irreversible renal damage. The majority of these cases of ARF resulted from complications of either severe preeclampsia or eclampsia. Possible explanations for this dramatic trend in this subset of patients includes ready availability of prenatal care and the legalization of medical abortions as main factors responsible for this reduction in the incidence of ARF requiring dialytic support. However, in the underdeveloped countries of the world, ARF remains a frequent complication of pregnancy and has an attendant maternal mortality surpassing 50%. In these countries, ARF has a bimodal distribution with peaks in the first and third trimester, presumably reflective of the continued practice of illegal abortions, the lack of access to quality prenatal care, and the occurrence of preeclampsia or eclampsia. Whatever the explanation, acute renal failure in pregnancy can be the result of any of the disorders, which lead to severe renal dysfunction in nonpregnant patients or may result from disorders that are unique to the pregnant condition.

■ RENAL ANATOMY AND FUNCTION DURING PREGNANCY

An understanding of the dramatic changes which occur normally in renal architecture, function, and blood flow is essential to the correct diagnosis and management of renal disease in the pregnant patient. (Table 13-1)

Anatomic Changes

There is a marked increase in kidney size during pregnancy. This increase in size is primarily due to the increase in renal vascular volume and in the capacity of the collecting system. Hormonal influence is the most likely cause of the dilatation of the urinary collecting system. In addition, increased production of prostaglandin E_2 (PGE_2) which inhibits urethral peristalsis, and mechanical obstruction by the enlarging uterus and distended iliac vessels (particularly on the right side) contribute to these changes which are evident as early as the first trimester and may continue for as long as 12 weeks postpartum.

Changes in Renal Blood Flow, Glomerular Filtration Rate, and Renal Tubular Function

Substantial increases in renal blood flow occur beginning early in the first trimester. This increase in renal blood flow is caused by both an increase in cardiac output and a decrease in renal vascular resistance. Renal vasodilatation is believed to be the most important mechanism for the dramatic rise in renal blood flow. Estimates of renal vascular resistance reveal a 50% decrease by the end of the first trimester. The underlying physiologic processes and cause of this pregnancy-related renal-vasodilatation are not clearly understood. The large increases in the concentration of PGE_2 and prostacyclin (PGI_2) are believed to contribute

■ TABLE 13-1. Renal Changes in Normal Pregnancy

Alteration	Change	Clinical relevance
Increased renal size	Renal length about 1 cm greater	Postpartum decrease in size should not be mistaken for parenchymal loss
Dilation of pelves, calyces, and ureters	Resembles hydronephrosis on ultrasound or IVP	Not to be mistaken for obstructive uropathy, increased rates of upper tract infections
Increased renal hemodynamics	Increased GFR and renal plasma flow	Decreased serum creatinine and BUN; increased excretion of amino acids, protein, and glucose
Changes in acid-base metabolism	Renal bicarbonate threshold decreases	Serum bicarbonate level lower by 4-5 mEq/L
Renal water-handling	Osmoregulation altered with decreased osmotic thresholds for AVP release, and thirst	Serum osmolality decreases 10 mOsm/L during normal gestation

to this effect, but do not appear to be the only mechanism. Prolactin may be a hormonal mediator of renal vasodilatation in pregnancy. Estimation of renal plasma flow from p-aminohippuric acid clearance studies indicate an effective renal plasma flow of 809 mL/mm in the first trimester, 695 mL/mm in the last 10 weeks of pregnancy, and 482 mL/mm during the postpartum period. The most important consequence of this increase in renal blood flow during pregnancy is a dramatic rise in glomerular filtration rate (GFR). An increase in GFR of about 45% is seen as early as the end of the first trimester, and unlike renal plasma flow, this increase in GFR is maintained until term.

Despite this marked increase in GFR, the renal tubules are not only able to preserve normal sodium (Na^+) balance, but are able to achieve a cumulative Na^+ retention of 500 to 900 mEq during the course of a normal pregnancy. Further, pregnant women maintain a normal sodium balance in settings when sodium intake is either increased or decreased. Pregnant women also maintain normal water balance and retain the ability to produce appropriately concentrated or dilute urine despite a significant alteration in the thirst and argenine vasopressin release thresholds during normal pregnancy.

Similarly potassium (K^+) metabolism in pregnancy is unchanged. There is a physiologic requirement for the retention of approximately 350 mEq of potassium for the developing fetal-placental unit along with the significant expansion of maternal red cell volume. This increase in potassium retention occurs despite the dramatically elevated levels of aldosterone in the plasma of pregnant patients.

Pregnancy results in a respiratory alkalosis with a decrease of about 10 mm Hg in the arterial Pco_2. The slight respiratory alkalosis is compensated with an increased excretion of bicarbonate by the kidneys resulting in a decrease in the plasma bicarbonate level to 18 to 20 mEq/L.

These "physiologic" anatomic and functional changes seen in pregnant patients' renal systems have practical consequences. For example, dilated collecting systems make the diagnosis of an obstructive uropathy challenging. The increased GFR and tubular functions result in changes of the normal laboratory values for the commonly employed serum tests of renal function. Examples include normal blood urea nitrogen values in pregnancy average 8.7 ±1.5 mg/dL and serum creatinine levels average 0.46±0.13 mg/dL. Glucosuria is also common finding during normal pregnancy.

■ ACUTE RENAL FAILURE IN PREGNANCY

Acute Renal failure (ARF) is a syndrome characterized by the rapid (hours to weeks) decline in renal function resulting in the retention of nitrogenous waste products such as BUN and creatinine along with the inability to maintain normal fluid and electrolyte balances. Nonpregnant patients with acute renal failure are often asymptomatic but, when seen in pregnancy, ARF is rarely encountered in the absence of significant clinical findings or events complicating the gestation. ARF may complicate a host of diseases that, for purposes of diagnoses and management, are conveniently divided into three categories. (Table 13-2)

■ **TABLE 13-2.** Acute Renal Failure in Pregnancy

Differential diagnosis

Prerenal azotemia
- Hyperemesis gravidarum
- Hemorrhage from any causes

Intrarenal azotemia or acute tubular necrosis
- Preeclampsia
- HELLP syndrome
- Acute fatty liver of pregnancy
- Postpartum renal failure

Bilateral renal cortical necrosis
- Pyelonephritis

Acute interstitial nephritis
Acute glomerulonephritis
Post renal azotemia
Obstructive

1. Diseases characterized by renal hypoperfusion in which the integrity of renal parenchymal tissue is preserved (prerenal azotemia, prerenal ARF). This is the most common form of ARF, and has the best prognosis.
2. Diseases involving renal parenchymal tissue (intrarenal azotemia , or intrinsic renal ARF).
3. Diseases associated with an acute obstruction of the urinary tract (postrenal azotemia, postrenal ARF).

Most acute intrinsic renal azotemia is caused by ischemia or nephrotoxins and is classically associated with acute tubular necrosis (ATN). Thus, in clinical practice the term ATN is commonly used to denote ischemic or nephrotoxic ARF.

In prerenal ARF, impaired renal perfusion is the problem and this may be secondary to true intravascular volume depletion, decreased effective circulating volume to the kidneys secondary to impaired cardiac output, or due to agents which alter renal perfusion. Prerenal ARF may be rarely seen in the first trimester of pregnancy as a complication of severe hyperemesis gravidarum. In the second and third trimesters, severe blood loss as a complication of uterine hemorrhage in the antepartum, intrapartum, or postpartum periods is an important and not an uncommon cause of hypovolemia and subsequent ARF. It is important to remember that maternal bleeding may be concealed behind the placenta in some patients with serious placental abruption and this condition may also be accompanied by varying degrees of a consumptive coagulopathy which can further complicate the degree of renal dysfunction.

Pregnancy is associated with a higher incidence of both bladder infections and pyelonephritis. This increased incidence of both upper and lower urinary tract infections, estimated to complicate approximately 2% of all pregnancies, is believed to result from both hormonal and mechanical changes which result in stasis within the urinary collecting system. Unlike their nonpregnant counterparts, pregnant women with pyelonephritis can manifest a substantial decrease in creatinine clearance and rarely may experience some degree of transient ARF. Patients with pyelonephritis in pregnancy complicated with ARF often have evidence of chronic renal parenchymal infection and recovery following appropriate antimicrobial therapy may be incomplete.

Severe preeclampsia and eclampsia account for the majority of ARF unique to pregnancy. Renal failure is unusual even with severe disease, unless there has also been significant blood loss with hemodynamic instablility or severe disseminated intravascular coagulopathy. Usually the clinical picture of ARF seen in such patients is that of ATN and typically resolves spontaneously within the first 2 weeks postpartum. While in the short term some of these patients with preeclampsia/eclampsia-induced ATN may require dialytic support, in general even these more seriously affected patients experience complete recovery and have an excellent long-term prognosis. In those patients with ATN secondary to preeclampsia in whom the disease persists and long-term dialysis is necessary, frequently, it appears that pregnancy and/or preeclampsia have unmasked a chronic renal disorder or there has been some degree of renal cortical necrosis. When ARF develops in patients with severe preeclampsia or eclampsia, consideration should be given to effecting delivery as safely and at as expeditiously as possible since maternal condition will frequently dramatically improve postpartum.

Preeclamptic/eclamptic patients, patients who develop placental abruption with or without coagulopathy, pregnancies in which there is a prolonged intrauterine fetal demise complicated with DIC, or women experiencing an amniotic fluid embolism are at an increased risk of developing renal cortical necrosis. Renal cortical necrosis, a pathologic process which destroys the renal cortex partially or completely while sparing the medulla, is heralded by the abrupt onset of oliguria or anuria which may be accompanied by flank pain, gross hematuria, and hypotension. This triad of anuria, gross hematuria, and flank pain is unusual in the other causes of renal failure in pregnancy. Renal cortical necrosis is not unique to pregnancy. However, pregnancy-related cases account for up to 70% of all cases. This entity is diagnosed based upon the clinical presentation and can usually be established with ultrasonography or CT scanning of the kidneys. The characteristic findings are hypoechoic or hypodense areas in the renal cortex. There is no specific therapy that has been shown to be effective for patients with renal cortical necrosis with many women requiring chronic hemodialysis. Approximately 30%-40% of patients experience at least partial recovery and have markedly compromised creatinine clearances.

Other clinical entities more commonly associated with pregnancy and acute renal failure with varying degrees of proteinuria are seen in patients with hemolysis, elevated liver function tests and low platelets (HELLP syndrome), acute fatty liver of pregnancy, post partum renal failure due to adult hemolytic uremic syndrome (HUS), and thrombotic thrombocytopenic purpura (TTP). Some investigators group these disease processes and preeclampsia under the same rubric of microangiopathic hemolytic processes of pregnancy, because they share a common histologic feature of anemia with evidence of red cell destruction on peripheral smears. The clinical manifestation and the nomenclature of the disease reflect the primary target organ. However, it is believed that there may be a unifying pathophysiologic process of profound vasoconstriction of arterioles resulting from an, as yet, unidentified "toxin" or mechanism likely involving the vascular endothelium. Consequently, in acute fatty liver of pregnancy, although this rare complication of pregnancy is associated with ARF in up to 60% of cases, the target organ is primarily the liver, with accompanying alterations of normal laboratory values such as transaminases, bilirubin, glucose metabolism, and various clotting factors (eg, antithrombin III, fibrinogen). Similarly, in postpartum renal failure resulting from HUS, the kidneys appear to be the target organs with resultant alterations in normal renal functions assays and, in comparison to renal dysfunction associated with HELLP syndrome or acute fatty liver of pregnancy, protracted acute renal failure may result. While HUS is generally a postpartum disease and HELLP syndrome is a form of severe preeclampsia usually confined to the late second or third trimesters, TTP almost always occurs antepartum and, although it may occur in the third trimester, many cases appear before 24 weeks of gestation. TTP is characterized by the pentad of microangiopathic hemolytic

anemia, thrombocytopenia, renal insufficiency, fever, and neurologic abnormalities. The severity of renal dysfunction is usually mild particularly in comparison with the more striking neurological involvement, fever, and thrombocytopenia.

■ DIAGNOSIS OF ARF

Regardless of the underlying cause of ARF, the diagnosis usually hinges on serial analysis of BUN, creatinine, urinalysis, and urinary sediment analysis. It must be emphasized, however, that measurements of BUN and creatinine are relatively insensitive indices of glomerular function. For instance, the GFR may fall by 50% before the serum creatinine values rise. Conversely a relatively large increment in the serum creatinine value reflects relatively small decrement in GFR in patients with preexisting chronic renal disease. (Tables 13-3, 13-4, 13-5)

The clinical approach to the diagnosis of acute renal failure involves a detailed history and physical, urinalysis, flow charts of serial blood pressures, daily weights, urine output, and intake, routine laboratory assessments, and special diagnostic procedures (Table 13-2).

The clinical course of ATN can be divided into three phases, irrespective of the underlying disease process: the initiation phase, the maintenance phase, and the recovery

> **■ TABLE 13-3. Clinical Approach to the Diagnosis of ARF (RF-41)**
>
> History and physical : including drug history, previous records, and detailed review of the hospital chart
> Urinalysis : specific gravity, microscopic, dipstick, and staining for eosinophils
> Flow charts: daily weights, serial blood pressures, serial BUN and creatinine, major clinical events and interventions
> Routine blood chemistry, and hematology tests : BUN, creatinine, electrolytes, red and white cell counts
> Selected special investigations: Urine chemistry, eosinophils, and/or immunoelectrophoresis
> Serologic tests : anti-glomerular basement membrane antibodies, ANA, cryoglobulins, anti–streptolysin O antibodies, and anti-DNase titers
> Radiologic evaluations : plain abdominal films, renal ultrasonography, intravenous pyelography, renal angiography
> Renal biopsy: (rarely used)

■ TABLE 13-4. Urine Indices Used in the Differential Diagnosis of Prerenal and Ischemic Intrinsic Renal Azotemia

Diagnostic index	Prerenal azotemia	Ischemic intrinsic azotemia
Fractional excretion of Na^+ (%) $$\frac{U_{Na} \times P_{cr} \times 100}{P_{Na} \times U_{Na}}$$	<1	>1
Urinary Na^+ concentration (mEq/L)	<10	>10
Urinary creatinine/plasma creatinine ratio	>40	<20
Urinary urea nitrogen/plasma urea nitrogen ratio	>8	<3
Urine specific gravity	>1.018	<1. 012
Urine osmolality (mOsm/kg H_2O)	>500	<250
Plasma BUN/creatinine ratio	>20	<10-15
Renal failure index $U_{Na}/U_{cr}/P_{cr}$	<1	>1
Urine sediment	Hyaline casts	Muddy brown granular casts

phase. In the initiation phase, patients have been exposed to the "insult," either ischemia or toxins, and while the picture is evolving, renal parenchymal injury is not yet established. The initiation phase is followed by the maintenance phase in which the renal parenchymal injury is established and GFR stabilizes at a value of 5 to 10 mL/min. Urine output is usually lowest during this period. This phase typically lasts 1 to 2 weeks, but may be prolonged for 1 to 11 months depending upon the etiology before recovery, if any, is seen. Uremic complications usually arise during this phase. The recovery phase is heralded by a gradual restoration of the urine output and a decline in the serum BUN and creatinine. The recovery phase is frequently accompanied by a marked diuresis which will result in profound electrolyte disturbances unless closely monitored and corrected.

■ MANAGEMENT OF ACUTE RENAL FAILURE

The initial therapy for acute renal failure should be focused on correction of the specific etiology of the renal dysfunction, reestablishing normal fluid and electrolyte abnormalities, being cognizant of potential complications, and maintaining appropriate nutritional and medical requirements. (Tables 13-6, 13-7, and 13-8) Prerenal azotemia is rapidly reversible upon restoration of renal perfusion. The source of the loss of fluid determines the composition of the replacement fluid. Hypovolemia caused by hemorrhage is ideally corrected with packed red blood cells. Isotonic saline is usually an appropriate replacement for plasma losses. Urinary or gastrointestinal fluids are generally hypotonic. Accordingly, initial replacement can be achieved with hypotonic solutions (eg, 0.45% saline) and subsequent replacement should be based on laboratory values. Serum potassium and acid base status should be monitored in all patients. In certain instances, use of insulin and glucose replacement may be necessary to lower the plasma potassium levels. Alternative therapies include sodium polystyrene sulfonate (Kayexalate) orally or as an enema or consideration of dialysis.

Fluid management is particularly difficult in patients with ARF resulting from underlying severe preeclampsia since they are not necessarily volume depleted and are at increased risk for developing pulmonary edema. Liberal use of invasive monitoring with a pulmonary artery catheter has been recommended. In patients with ARF due to severe preeclampsia there may be a poor correlation between the central venous pressure (CVP) value and the pulmonary capillary wedge pressure (PCWP). Therefore, it is preferable to use a pulmonary artery catheter which can measure the PCWP in order to be able to correctly determine the optimal fluid and pharmacological management of such patients. Similarly, measurements of urinary indices may not accurately reflect the volume status of the patient and allow the clinician to differentiate

■ TABLE 13-5. Urine Sediment in the Differential Diagnosis of Acute Renal Failure

Normal or few red blood cells or white blood cells
Prerenal azotemia
Arterial thrombosis or embolism
Preglomerular vasculitis
HUS or TTP
Scleroderma crisis
  Post renal azotemia

Granular casts
ATN (muddy brown)
Glomerulonephritis or vasculitis
  Interstitial nephritis

Red blood cell casts
Glomerulonephritis or vasculitis
Malignant hypertension
Rarely interstitial nephritis

White blood cell casts
Acute interstitial nephritis or exudative
  glomerulonephritis
    Severe pyelonephritis
    Marked leukemic or lymphomatous infiltration
Eosinophiluria (>5%)
    Allergic interstitial nephritis (antibiotics, NSAIDs)
    Atheroembolic disease
Crsytalluria
    Acute urate nephropathy
    Calcium oxalate (ethylene glycol toxicity)
    Acyclovir
    Sulfonamides
    Radiocontrast agents

■ TABLE 13-6. Common Complications of ARF

Metabolic	Neurologic
Hyperkalemia	Neuromuscular irritability
Metabolic acidocis	Asterixis
Hyponatremia	Seizures
Hypocalcemia	Mental status changes
Hyperphosphotemia	Somnolence
Hypermagnesemia	Coma
Hyperurecemia	
Cardiovascular	**Infectious**
Pulmonary edema	Pneumonia
Arrhythmias	Wound infections
Pericarditis	Intravenous line infections
Pericardial effusion	Septicemia
Hypertension	Urinary tract infection
Myocardial infarction	
Pulmonary embolus	
Pneumonitis	
Gastrointestinal	**Other**
Nausea	Hiccups
Vomiting	Decreased insulin catabolism
Malnutrition	Mild insulin resistance
Gastritis	Elevated parathyroid hormone
Gastrointestinal ulcers	Reduced 1,25-dihdroxy and 25-vitamin D
Gastrointestinal bleeding	hydroxyvitamin
Stomatitis or gingivitis	Low total T_3 and T_4
Parotitis or pancreatitis	Normal free T_4
Hematologic	
Anemia	
Bleeding	

between prerenal azotemia and intrinsic renal disease. Patients who do not respond to initial fluid boluses of 500 to 1000 cc should have a pulmonary artery catheter inserted to assist with further management decisions. If the pulmonary capillary wedge pressures indicate euvolemia or hypervolemia and the cause of the renal failure is not prerenal, then efforts should be directed toward medical therapy with diuretics and to selectively dilate the renal vascular bed, such as with the use of renal doses of dopamine. Furosemide (Lasix) administration intravenously is the initial treatment for volume-overloaded patients with ARF. If the initial response is inadequate, the administered dosage is doubled or a continuous furosemide drip is initiated until adequate urine output results (0.5 U/kg/h). As an additional point, all medications should be carefully reviewed and dosages adjusted to maintain appropriate serum levels.

The single most important factor in the appropriate management of intrinsic renal azotemia is the optimization of both cardiovascular function and intravascular volume. The clinician must have an appreciation of the potential complications seen in patients with intrinsic renal azotemia and adopt an aggressive preventative management protocol in order to attempt prevention of significant worsening of acute renal failure. Pregnancy represents a unique challenge in such patients as there are both maternal and fetal concerns.

■ TABLE 13-7. Supportive Management of Intrinsic ARF (RF-41)

Intravascular volume overload	Restriction of salt (1-2 g/d) and water (usually <1 L/d)
	Diuretics (usually loop blockers (± thiazides)
	Ultrafiltration or dialysis
Hyponatremia	Restriction of free water intake (oral and dextrose-containing solutions)
Hyperkalemia	Restriction of dietary potassium intake
	Eliminate K^+ supplements and K^+-sparing diuretics
	K^+-binding ion exchamge resins
	Glucose (50 mL of 50% dextrose) and insulin (10 units regular)
	Sodium bicarbonate (usually 50-100 mEq)
	Dialysis
Metabolic acidosis	Restriction of dietary protein
	Sodium bicarbonate (maintain serum HCO_3^- >15 mEq/L)
	Dialysis

Regardless of the underlying etiology of ARF, there are general guidelines and principles governing its management in pregnancy. As discussed, most cases of ARF complicating pregnancy develop in the postpartum period, thus obviating concerns about fetal well-being. However, in cases of severe preeclampsia/eclampsia or any of the microangiopathic thrombotic processes complicated by ARF, expeditious delivery of the fetus should be carefully considered with appropiate and judicious use of blood product replacement. Oliguria in the pregnant patient is frequently mismanaged. Fluid replacement must be carefully monitored. Indeed, worsening of the medical condition resulting from efforts to reestablish urine production is a common complication of ARF in pregnancy. As with aggressive but inappropriate fluid replacement, the use of potent diuretics, such as furosemide, may increase urine output transiently without correcting the underlying pathology and, in certain instances, such therapy may exacerbate the disease and worsen the clinical condition. One example of this is the oliguric phase of severe preeclampsia which is managed most appropriately with support and minimal fluid replacement rather than aggressively giving fluid and/or diuretics with the intent to simply establish a greater amount of urine production.

The available data support an early and aggressive use of hemodialysis in ARF which is not responding to fluid replacement and diuretics. This is also applicable to the pregnant patient although the use of acute hemodialysis during pregnancy is quite rare. However, following delivery it may indeed be necessary to employ this important clinical modality, particularly for patients experiencing protracted renal failure such as may be seen with hemolytic uremic syndrome or acute cortical necrosis complicating pregnancy. Dialysis has been shown to decrease maternal mortality and accelerate recovery of renal function. Typically, initiation of dialysis should be considered when the BUN reaches 50 to 70 mg/dL or when the serum creatinine

■ TABLE 13-8. Supportive Management of Intrinsic ARF (RF-41)

Hyperphosphotemia	Restriction of dietary phosphate intake. Use PO_4^{3-}-binding agents (calcium carbonate, aluminum hydroxide)
Hypocalcemia	Calcium carbonate (if symptomatic or if sodium bicarbonate is to be administered)
	Calcium gluconate (10-20 mL of 10% solution)
Hypermagnesemia	Discontinue Mg++-containing antacids
Hyperuricemia	Treatment usually not necessary (if <15 mg/dL)
Nutrition	Restriction of dietary protein (~0.5 g/kg/d)
	Carbohydrate (~100 g/d)
	Enteral or parenteral nutrition (if recovery is prolonged)
Drug dosage	Adjust dosage for degree of renal impairment

■ TABLE 13-9. Indications for Dialysis in Pregnancy(RF-41)
Clinical evidence of uremia
Intractable intravascular volume overload
Hyperkalemia or severe acidosis resistant to conservative measures
Prophylactic dialysis when BUN >50-70 mg/dL, or creatinine >6-7 mg/dL

is greater than 6 to 7 mg/dL. These are lower levels than for the nonpregnant patient (Table 13-9).

For women requiring dialysis for renal failure, the reported pregnancy outcomes have been generally poor. In 1980, the European Dialysis and Transplant Association (EDTA) reported a 23% successful pregnancy outcome in women conceiving after starting dialysis. Subsequently, there has been reported a possible improvement with peritoneal dialysis in pregnant women requiring dialysis when compared with the EDTA report. The question of continuing a pregnancy in patients either already dialysis-dependent or who have moderate renal insufficiency at conception but experience a rapid deterioration of renal function during pregnancy leading to chronic dialysis is critically important in counseling women with end-stage renal disease. Pregnancy termination with the hopes of improving renal function does not appear to be a good option. In a recent series of 82 pregnancies in women with chronic renal insufficiency, Hayslett reported that only 15% of women had a return to baseline renal function at 6 months postpartum. More recently, in a review of 2300 dialysis units in the United States, Okundaye and colleagues report that over a 4-year period, 2% of the female dialysis patients of childbearing age became pregnant. Of the hemodialysis women, 2.4% conceived while 1.1% of the peritoneal dialysis women conceived. Of 184 pregnancies occurring in women who conceived after starting dialysis, the infant survival rate was 40.2%. Comparatively, the infant survival rate for the 57 pregnancies in women starting dialysis after conception was 73.6%. There was no difference in outcome between women receiving hemodialysis versus peritoneal dialysis and these investigators do not recommend switching from one modality to another during pregnancy. However, they do report a possible association between improved outcome and increased time and frequency of dialysis. The major complication remains premature birth resulting in both significant mortality as well as morbidity in the surviving infants.

The role of renal biopsy in pregnancies complicated with ARF is not without controversy. Although such a procedure is valuable in many nonpregnant patients and plays a critical role in establishing the specific renal pathology, renal biopsy has potentially significant complications which may be of more concern in the pregnant patient. Consequently, renal biopsy should rarely, if ever, be performed in a patient with ARF while pregnant.

SUGGESTED READINGS

Baylis C, Reckelhoff JF. Renal hemodynamics in normal and hypertensive pregnancy: Lessons from micropuncture. *Am J Kidney Dis.* 17:98;1991.

Brady HR, Brenner BM, Lieberthal W. Acute renal failure. In: Brenner BM, ed. *The Kidney.* 5th ed. Philadelphia, PA: WB Saunders Co;1996:1200-1252.

Christensen T, Klebe JG, Bertelsen V, et al. Changes in renal volume during normal pregnancy. *Acta Obstet Gynecol Scand.* 68:541;1989.

Davidson J. Changes in renal function and other aspects of homeostasis in early pregnancy. *J Obstet Gynaecol Br Commonw.* 1974:81;1003.

Davison J. Renal disease. In: deSwiet M, ed. *Medical Disorders in Obstetric Practice.* Oxford: Blackwell;1984;236.

Davison JM, Dunlop W. Renal hemodynamics and tubular function in normal human pregnancy. *Kidney Int.* 1980;18:152.

DeAlvarez RR. Renal glomerulotubular mechanisms during normal pregnancy: I. Glomerular filtration rate, renal plasma flow and creatinine clearance. *Am J Obstet Gynecol.* 1958;75:931.

Donohoe JF. Acute bilateral cortical necrosis. In: Brenner BM, Lazarus J, eds. *Acute Renal Failure.* Philadelphia, PA: WB Saunders; 1983:252-269.

Dunlop W. Renal physiology in pregnancy. *Postgrad med J.* 1979;55:329.

Dunlop W, Davison JM. The effect of normal pregnancy upon the renal handling of uric acid. *Br J Obstet Gynaecol.* 1977;84:13.

Grunfeld JP, Ganeval D, Bournerias F. Acute renal failure in pregnancy. *Kidney Int.* 1980;18:179-191.

Grunfeld JP, Pertuiset N. Acute renal failure in pregnancy. *Am J Kidney Dis.* 1987;9:359-362.

Hankins GDV, Cunningham FG. Severe preeclampsia and eclampsia: Controversies in management. *Willimas Obstetrics*. 18th ed. (Suppl 12). Norwalk, CT: Appleton & Lange; 1991.

Hankins GDV, Wendel GW JR, Cunningham FG, Leveno KJ. Longitudinal evaluation of hemodynamic changes in eclampsia. *Am J Obstet Gynecol*. 1984;150:506.

Hayslett JP. Postpartum renal failure. *N Engl J Med*. 1985;312:1556-1559.

Krane NK. Acute renal failure in pregnancy. *Arch Intern Med*. 1988;148:2347-2357.

Lee W, Gonik B, Cotton DB. Urinary diagnostic indices in preeclampsia-associated oliguria: Correlation with invasive hemodynamic monitoring. *Am J Obstet Gynecol*. 1987;156:100.

Lindheimer M, Grunfeld JP, Davison JM. Renal disorders. In: Barron WM, Lindheimer M, eds. *Medical Disorders During Pregnancy*. St. Louis, MO: CV Mosby; 2000:39.

Lindheimer MD, Barron WM, Davison JM. Osmotic and volume control of vasopressin release in pregnancy. *Am J Kidney Dis*. 1991;17:105.

Lindheimer MD, Katz AI, Ganeval D, et al. Acute renal failure in pregnancy. In: Brenner BN, Lazarus JM, eds. *Acute Renal Failure*. New York, NY: Churchill Livingstone; 1988:597-620.

Lindheimer MD, Richardson DA, Ehrlich EN, et al. Potassium homeostasis in pregnancy. *J Reprod Med*. 32:517;1987.

Lindheimer MD, Weston PV. Effect of hypotonic expansion on sodium, water and urea excretion in late pregnancy: The influence of posture on these results. *J Clin Invest*. 1969;48:947.

Martin JN, Blake PG, Perry KG, et al. The natural history of HELLP syndrome: patterns of disease progression and regression. *Am J Obstet Gyencol*. 1991;164:1500-1513.

Pertuiser N, Grunfeld JP. Acute renal failure in prepgancy. *Baillieres Clin Obstet Gynaecol*. 1987;1:873.

Pertuiset N, Ganeval D, Grunfeld JP. Acute renal failure in pregnancy: an update. *Semin Nephrol*. 1984;3:232-239.

Stratta P, Canavese C, Colla L, et al. Acute renal failure in preeclampsia-eclampsia. *Gynecol Obstet Invest*. 1987;27:225.

Stratta P, Canavese C, Dogliani M, et al. Pregnancy related acute renal filure. *Clin nephrol*. 1989;32:14.

Usta IM, Barton JR, Amon EA, et al. Acute fatty liver of pregnancy: an experience in the diagnosis and management of fourteen cases. *Am J Obstet Gynecol*. 1994;171:142-147.

Weiner CP. Thrombotic microangiopathy in pregnancy and the postpartum period. *Semin Hematol*. 1987;24:119-129.

Whalley PJ, Cunningham FG, Martin FG. Transient renal dysfunction associated with acute pyelonephritis of pregnancy. *Obstet Gynecol*. 1975;46:174-177.

CHAPTER 14

Amniotic Fluid Embolism

• Gary A. Dildy III and Irene P. Stafford

Amniotic fluid embolism is a catastrophic syndrome occurring during labor and delivery or immediately postpartum. Although presenting symptoms may vary, common clinical features include shortness of breath, altered mental status followed by sudden cardiovascular collapse, disseminated intravascular coagulation (DIC), and maternal death. It was first recognized as a syndrome in 1941, when two investigators described fetal mucin and squamous cells during postmortem examination of the pulmonary vasculature in women who had unexplained obstetric deaths.[1] Since then, many studies, case reports, and series have been published in an attempt to elucidate the etiology, risk factors, and pathogenesis of this mysterious obstetric complication.

The incidence of amniotic fluid embolism (AFE) which includes both fatal and nonfatal cases, ranges between 1 in 12,953 deliveries in the United States, to 1 in 56,500 in the United Kingdom. Incidence data is limited in other parts of the world.[2-4] The true incidence is unclear because this syndrome is difficult to identify and the diagnosis remains one of exclusion, with possible underreporting of nonfatal cases. Diagnostic criteria for AFE as proposed in the national registry are summarized in Table 14-1. There have also been discrepancies in the published maternal mortality rates associated with AFE. In a well-defined US national registry examining 46 cases of AFE, maternal mortality rates were reported as 61%, with a neurologically intact maternal survival rate of 15%[5] for the period 1988 to 1994. Investigators from the United Kingdom report a maternal mortality rate of 37% in their registry of AFE, with 93% of survivors remaining neurologically intact. More recent population-based studies have demonstrated a decreased case fatality rate from AFE (21.6% for

the United States). However, AFE still remains the second leading cause of maternal death in America and the United Kingdom.[6] Fetal outcome is poor when AFE occurs before delivery. The fetal survival rate approaches 40%, though with up to half of surviving neonates developing neurologic abnormalities.[5,6]

Although the United States national registry did not find any maternal demographic risk factors for AFE, they found that 70% of cases occurred during labor, 19% were recorded during cesarean section, and 11% of cases occurred immediately following vaginal delivery.[5] Other studies have also found an increased frequency of AFE in women who underwent cesarean delivery, with rates between 20% and 60%.[4,7] Approximately 50% of these cases were associated with fetal distress, suggesting that amniotic fluid embolus and associated hypoxia preceded cesarean delivery. This interpretation is supported by observations from the United Kingdom in which only one of the five cesarean deliveries in the registry was performed before the diagnosis of AFE.[6] Rupture of membranes was a consistent finding among 78% of women in the US registry, with onset of symptoms occurring within 3 minutes of amniotomy in 11% of cases.[5] Another study found maternal age (mean age, 33 years) and multiparity (mean parity, 2.6) to be associated with AFE.[4] Conflicting data have been reported on multiple gestations. The frequency of twin gestation in the national AFE registry was not increased from baseline population estimates, but was found to be approximately threefold higher in one retrospective analysis.[4]

In one large cohort study examining the association between AFE and induction of labor, AFE was found in twice as many induced women. This association was even stronger for fatal cases (odds ratio, 3.5). In a more

■ **TABLE 14-1. Diagnostic Criteria of AFE**

1. Acute hypotension or cardiac arrest
2. Acute hypoxia, defined as dyspnea, cyanosis, or respiratory arrest
3. Coagulopathy, defined as laboratory evidence of intravascular consumption, fibrinolysis or severe clinical hemorrhage in the absence of other explanations
4. Onset of the above during labor, cesarean section, dilatation and evacuation, or within 30 min postpartum
5. Absence of any other significant confounding condition or potential explanation for the signs and symptoms observed

Source: As suggested by Clark SL, Hankins GD, Dudley DA, et al. Amniotic fluid embolism: analysis of the National Registry. *Am J Obstet Gynecol.* 1995;172:1158-1169.

recent study, no significant association was found between induction of labor and AFE.[3] Increased rates of AFE were also found in women who had placenta previa, polyhydramnios, placental abruption, cervical lacerations, or uterine rupture and in women who underwent operative vaginal delivery.[3,7] Although eclampsia was also strongly associated with AFE in this study, no risk factor has been consistently substantiated in the literature.

■ **ETIOLOGY AND PATHOGENESIS**

The pathogenesis of AFE is poorly understood. Early studies describe the histologic presence of amniotic fluid components in lung tissue during postmortem examination in obstetric patients who had unexplained death.[1] This finding was followed by reports of amniotic fluid debris found in maternal circulation in fatal and nonfatal cases of AFE.[8,9] Conventional wisdom describes the efflux of amniotic fluid components into the maternal vasculature, driven by pressure or electrochemical gradients via lacerations in the lower uterine segment, endocervical vessels, and placental site.[9] Plugging of the cervical vasculature by amniotic fluid elements has been described, although the mechanism by which this leads to AFE is unclear. In addition, elements of amniotic fluid have been isolated in blood and sputum of pregnant women who did not have clinical evidence of AFE.[10,11]

Amniotic fluid contains various concentrations of fetal squamous epithelial cells, lanugo hair, vernix, mucin, zinc coproporphyrin, prostaglandins, and platelet-activating factor. One possible mechanism of disease includes the effect of direct procoagulants found in amniotic fluid on maternal systems. The presence of vasoactive substances, such as platelet-activating factor, in the placenta and amniotic fluid has been shown to cause increased vascular permeability; bronchoconstriction; platelet aggregation; recruitment of leukotrienes, cytokines, and thromboxanes; and the cascade of prostaglandin production.[12] In one small study examining the effect of autologous fetal membranes on the coagulation profile in pigs, findings were significant for decreased platelets, fibrinogen, and antithrombin III. Although these laboratory abnormalities are consistent with AFE, the syndrome of AFE could not be elicited in this study.[13] Similar studies involving primates also failed to model the syndrome despite procoagulant effects of autologous amniotic fluid.[14-16] Currently, there is no suitable animal model for amniotic fluid embolus secondary to the limitations of autologous amniotic fluid.

Laboratory testing for the fetal antigen sialystransferase (sialyl Tn) has shown some diagnostic value with AFE.[17-19] Sialyl Tn is a fetal antigen present in meconium and amniotic fluid detected most accurately with the TKH-2 monoclonal antibody.[19,20] In a small Japanese case series, seven of nine women who were diagnosed with AFE had elevated serum levels of fetal antigen compared with control subjects. In addition, special immunohistochemical stains for the presence of fetal antigen in lung tissue were positive in women who had a history of AFE.[18] An anaphylactic or complement activation reaction to sialyl Tn may explain the mechanism of disease. In one small series, complement activation was found along with high levels of sialyl Tn. Levels of complement C3 and C4 were twofold to threefold lower than normal.[17] When these markers were used for evaluation of anesthesia-induced allergic anaphylaxis; however, similar results were found.[17,21] An alternative immunologic mechanism for AFE involves the possibility of anaphylaxis with massive mast cell degranulation, independent of antigen-antibody–mediated classic anaphylaxis. In early studies, immunohistochemical staining in postmortem cases of AFE revealed elevated numbers of mast cells in the pulmonary vasculature.[22] Tryptase has been examined as a factor involved in anaphylaxis because it is specific to mast cells and has a longer half-life than histamine. In one study using serum tryptase and urinary histamine concentrations as markers for mast cell degranulation, no difference was found between women who had a history of AFE compared with control subjects.[17] Other investigators, however, found elevated tryptase levels in women who had AFE, but these values were compared with nonpregnant control subjects.[23,24] Of note, in some cases when complement is involved in classic antibody-antigen anyphylaxis, mast cell degranulation can occur.[25] The studies evaluating serum tryptase levels in AFE cases did not simultaneously measure complement levels.[23,24]

■ CLINICAL PRESENTATION

Although AFE typically occurs during labor and delivery or immediately postpartum, rare cases of AFE have been reported after midtrimester termination, transabdominal amniocentesis, trauma, and saline amnioinfusion.[26-30] Classic presenting signs and symptoms of AFE include respiratory distress, altered mental status, profound hypotension, coagulopathy, and death.[2] Historical studies have described the presenting symptom as primarily respiratory distress, whereas other studies describe the most common presenting symptom before delivery to be altered mental status. Seizure or seizure-like activity was reported as the intial symptom of 30% of patients involved in the US national registry, followed by dyspnea (27%), fetal bradycardia (17%), and hypotension (13%).[5] Classic signs and symptoms are listed in Table 14-2. The interval between the onset of symptoms and collapse varies between almost immediately to over 4 hours later. Other signs and symptoms include nausea, vomiting, fever, chills, and headache. Diagnostic criteria used for the United States and the UK registry for AFE are listed in Box 14-1.

These symptoms typically occur during labor, cesarean delivery, or dilation and evacuation or within 30 min of delivery with no other explanation for the findings .

Due to the vast overlap of the symptomatology of AFE with other disease states, consideration for the differential diagnosis of AFE is warranted. A differential diagnosis for possible AFE is shown in Box 14-2.

Clinical features of AFE include profound cardiovascular changes. According to the US national registry, all patients who had AFE experienced hypotension. Most women (93%) had some level of pulmonary edema or adult respiratory distress syndrome along with hypoxia.[5] One explanation for these findings includes the possibility of severe bronchospasm related to the presence of fetal elements in the pulmonary vasculature; however, only 15% of patients were found to have bronchospasm.[5]

■ **TABLE 14-2. Signs and Symptoms Noted in Patients with Amniotic Fluid Embolism**

Sign or symptom	Number	%
Hypotension	43	100
Fetal distress	30	100
Pulmonary edema or ARDS	28	93
Cardiopulmonary arrest	40	87
Cyanosis	38	83
Coagulopathy	38	83
Dyspnea	22	49
Seizure	22	48
Atony	11	23
Bronchospasm	7	15
Transient hypertension	5	11
Cough	3	7
Headache	3	7
Chest pain	1	2

Source: Reproduced by permission from Clark SL, Hankins GD, Dudley DA, et al. Amniotic fluid embolism: analysis of a national registry. *Am J Obstet Gynecol.* 1995;172:1158-1169.

Transesophageal echocardiography and pulmonary artery catheterization studies have demonstrated transiently elevated pulmonary artery pressures in cases of AFE along with left ventricular dysfunction, supporting the notion that these pulmonary findings are consistent with cardiogenic shock. There have also been reports of isolated right ventricular dysfunction with high right-sided pressures and tricuspid regurgitation.[14,31-37] In several cases where transesophageal echocardiography was performed during the early course of AFE, left ventricular failure was secondary

■ **BOX-14-1. Diagnostic Criteria for Amniotic Fluid Embolism**

Acute hypotension and/or cardiac arrest

Acute hypoxia diagnosed by dyspnea, cyanosis, and/or respiratory arrest

Coagulopathy or severe clinical hemorrhage in the absence of other explanations

Coma and/or seizures in the absence of other medical conditions or potential explanation for the symptoms/signs observed

■ **BOX-14-2. Differential Diagnosis for Women Presenting with Possible Amniotic Fluid Embolism**

Pulmonary thromboembolism
Transfusion reaction
Hemorrhage
Air embolism
Anaphylaxis
High spinal anesthesia
Placental abruption
Peripartum cardiomyopathy
Eclampsia
Myocardial infarction
Septic shock
Uterine rupture

to impaired left ventricular filling caused by dilation of the right ventricle with deviation of the interventricular septum. Available evidence suggests that the hemodynamic response to AFE initially presents with increased pulmonary vascular resistance and right ventricular failure followed by left ventricular dysfunction (Table 14-3).[14] Myocardial hypoxic injury may be related to decreased cardiac output and impaired filling, resulting in decreased coronary artery perfusion. Although the etiology of these changes is unclear, small studies have reported vasoconstrictive effects of amniotic fluid in animal models.[33,38] This vasoconstriction is often followed by profound

hypotension and shock, most likely resulting from cardiogenic or obstructive causes as described earlier.

After initial survival, hypoxia relates more to noncardiogenic shock, whereby severe alveolar-capillary membrane leak leads to an increase in pulmonary edema and a decrease in oxygenation.[14] In the presence of DIC, hemorrhagic shock may further complicate the management of the patient who has AFE.

DIC is a common feature of AFE. According to the US registry for AFE, 83% of patients demonstrated laboratory abnormalities or clinical findings consistent with DIC, regardless of mode of delivery. Onset was variable, with 50% of cases occurring within 4 hours of presentation, often within 20 to 30 minutes of symptom onset.[5] The presence of clotting factors in amniotic fluid has been linked with the possible activation of the clotting cascade in the pulmonary vasculature of affected women.[39,40] Additional data report that increased levels of plasminogen activator inhibitor—one antigen in amniotic fluid may become active in maternal circulation, leading to consumptive coagulopathy.[41] Within the national registry, 75% of patients who presented with hemorrhage and isolated coagulopathy died despite appropriate resuscitative efforts.

■ MANAGEMENT

Currently, there are no proven laboratory tests that confirm the diagnosis of AFE. Most events occur in an unpredictable manner and often have variable presentation. Initial laboratory data should include: a complete blood count, arterial blood gas, electrolytes, a 12-lead

■ **TABLE 14-3. Hemodynamic Indices (mean ± SD) in Nonpregnant Women, Normal Women in the Third Trimester, and Women with Amniotic Fluid Embolism**

	MPAP (mm Hg)	PCWP (mm Hg)	PVR (dynes/s/cm^{-5})	LVSWI (gm/m/M^{-2})
Nonpregnant (n = 10)	11.9 ± 2.0[a]	6.3 ± 2.1[b]	119 ± 47[b]	41 ± 8[b]
Normal third trimester (n = 10)	12.5 ± 2.0[a]	7.5 ± 1.8[b]	78 ± 22[b]	48 ± 6[b]
AFE (n = 15)	26.2 ± 15.7[c]	18.9 ± 9.2[c]	176 ± 72[c]	26 ± 19[c]

MPAP, mean pulmonary artery pressure; PCWP, pulmonary capillary wedge pressure; PVR, pulmonary vascular resistance; LVSWI, left ventricular stroke work index.

[a]Steven L. Clark (unpublished data).
[b]Clark et al. Central hemodynamic assessment of normal term pregnancy. Am J Obstet Gynecol. 1989;161:1439-1442.
[c]Clark et al. Central hemodynamic alterations in amniotic fluid ambolism. Am J Obstet Gynecol. 1988;158:1124-1126; and unpublished data from the National AFE Registry.

ECG, cardiac enzymes, and a coagulation profile. With the presence of DIC and associated hemorrhage, hemoglobin levels will be decreased and prothrombin and partial thromboplastin times will be increased. Fibrinogen levels will decrease as well. Cardiac enzymes may be elevated and arterial blood gas levels will demonstrate hypoxemia. Electrocardiogram may demonstrate tachycardia with possible right ventricular strain. Chest radiography may demonstrate nonspecific increased opacities and transesophageal echocardiography can reveal severe pulmonary hypertension, acute right ventricular failure, and deviation of the interventricular septum. Ancillary studies, unproven in regard to diagnosing AFE, may be readily available (serum tryptase level), whereas others may not be available (serum TKH-2 antibody to fetal antigen sialyl Tn) or require autopsy (pulmonary mast cell antitryptase, pulmonary TKH-2 antibody to fetal antigen sialyl Tn). The detection of fetal squamous cells in the maternal pulmonary circulation is not pathognomonic for AFE since they have been found in 21% to 100% of pregnant women without AFE; however it is supportive when the clinical condition is suspected and fetal squamous cells are found in large quantities and are surrounded by white blood cells.[11,42]

With or without evidence of hemorrhage as a presenting symptom, blood products should be ordered expeditiously in anticipation of profound bleeding and DIC. Cryoprecipitate may be particularly useful in cases where clotting factors should be replaced in volume-restricted patients. Uterine artery embolism and recombinant factor VII have been used in cases of severe coagulopathy resistant to conventional blood and product replacement.[42-44] In cases with refractory postpartum vaginal bleeding, hysterectomy may be necessary.

Other case reports have described the use of continuous hemodiafiltration, extracorporeal membrane oxygenation, and intra-aortic balloon counterpulsation in cases of AFE.[45-47] In one report, early transesophageal echocardiogram demonstrating severe pulmonary vasoconstriction and cor pulmonale lead to successful rescue using cardiopulmonary bypass.[46]

The primary management goal includes rapid maternal cardiopulmonary stabilization with prevention of hypoxia and maintenance of vascular perfusion. This may require endotracheal intubation to keep oxygen saturation at 90% or greater. Treatment of hypotension should include optimization of preload with infusion of crystalloid solutions. In cases of refractory hypotension, vasopressors such as dopamine or norepinephrine may be necessary. Table 14-4 lists pharmacologic agents that may be used in the management of AFE. Central monitoring for cardiovascular status may assist in these endeavors. In antepartum cases of AFE, careful attention must be paid to the fetal condition. In a mother who is hemodynamically unstable but has not yet undergone cardiac arrest, maternal considerations must be weighed carefully against those of the fetus. The decision to subject such an unstable mother to a major abdominal operation (cesarean section) is a difficult one, and each case must be individualized. However, it is axiomatic in these situations that where a choice must be made, maternal well-being must take precedence over that of the fetus.

According to the national registry, 70% of patients were in labor when AFE occurred. When fetuses were undelivered, the fetal mortality rate approached 20%.[48] Of the surviving fetuses recorded in the registries, 30% were severely acidotic, with a 12% prenatal mortality rate.[5,6] There is a clear relationship between neonatal outcome and event-to-delivery interval in those women suffering cardiac arrest (Table 14-5). Eighty-seven percent of patients in the national AFE registry suffered cardiac arrest. Of these, 40% occurred within 5 minutes of symptom onset. The most common dysrhythmia was found to be electromechanical dissociation, followed by bradycardia and ventricular tachycardia or fibrillation.[5] Inotropic agents may need to be administered to improve myocardial function.

In these cases, administration of all conventional cardiac support measures, including medications used in resuscitation, should be used without delay. The patient should be placed in the left lateral position before chest compressions to avoid compression of the inferior vena cava by the gravid uterus. In cases in which asystole or malignant arrhythmia is present for greater than 4 minutes, perimortum cesarean delivery should be considered. In such women, it is unlikely that the performance of cesarean section would significantly alter the maternal outcome. Even properly performed cardiopulmonary resuscitation, difficult at best in a pregnant woman, provides only a maximum of 30% of normal cardiac output. Under these circumstances, it is fair to assume that the proportion of blood directed to the uterus and other splanchnic beds is minimal. Thus, the fetus will be profoundly hypoxic at all times following maternal cardiac arrest. For the pregnant patient, the standard ABCs of cardiopulmonary resuscitation should be modified to include a fourth category, D: delivery.

Intact fetal survival has been shown to be highest when delivery is accomplished within 5 minutes of maternal

■ TABLE 14-4. Pharmocologic Agents Used to Treat Amniotic Fluid Embolism

Agent	Mechanism of action	Dosage	Comments
Dopamine	Dopaminergic (0.5-5.0 µg/kg/min) vasodilation of renal and mesenteric vasculature β_1-adrenergic (5.0-10.0 µg/kg/min) increased myocardial contractility, SV, CO α-adrenergic (15-20 µg/kg/min) increased general vasoconstriction	2-5 µg/kg/min and titrate to BP and CO	Protect from light. Do not use if injection is discolored.
Norepinephrine	α-adrenergic-peripheral vasoconstriction β-adrenergic-inotropic stimulator of the heart and dilator of coronary arteries	Initial dose 8-12 µg/min and titrate to blood pressure	Contraindicated in hypovolemic hypotension.
Ephedrine	α and β sympathomimetic effects increase blood pressure.	25-50 mg SQ or IM 5-25 mg slow IVP, repeat in 5-10 min if necessary	Peripheral actions partly secondary to release of norepinephrine.
Digoxin	Improved contractility of myocardium	0.5 mg IV push and 0.25 mg q4h x 2, then 0.25-0.37 mg/d	Narrow toxic-to-therapeutic ratio, especially with potassium depletion.
Hydrocortisone sodium succinate	Naturally occurring glucocorticoid, modifies immune system response to diverse stimuli.	500 mg IV every 6 h until condition stabilizes	Sodium retention and hypernatremia may occur if administered beyond 48-72 h.

■ TABLE 14-5. Cardiac Arrest-to-Delivery Interval and Neonatal Outcome

Interval (min)	Survival	Intact survival
<5	3/3	2/3 (67%)
5-15	3/3	2/3 (67%)
16-25	2/5	2/5 (40%)
26-35	3/4	1/4 (25%)
36-54	0/1	0/1 (0%)

Source: Reproduced by permission from Clark SL, Hankins GD, Dudley DA, et al. Amniotic fluid embolism: analysis of the national registry. *Am J Obstet Gynecol.* 1995;172: 1158-1169.

cardiac arrest; however, the decision to deliver should not be abandoned if determined beyond the 5 minute mark.[49,50] There have been reported cases of successful pregnancies following AFE. Although data is limited, there is no evidence to suggest that there is a recurrence risk for AFE in future pregnancies.[37]

Significant maternal morbidity is associated with AFE. Over 75% of patients in the UK registry required intensive care management, with an average length of stay of 5 days among survivors and an average of 34 units of blood products was required in these patients.[6] In the US AFE registry, only 15% of patients who had cardiac arrest survived neurologically intact.[5] Other sequelae include liver hematoma, renal and multisystem failure, and ischemic encephalopathy.

Overall morbidity and mortality of AFE has improved with early recognition of the syndrome and improved resuscitative efforts involving multiple disciplines of medicine. In cases recorded within the UK registry, women who survived AFE had a shorter time frame between symptom onset and treatment (41.5 minutes vs 108 minutes).[6,51,52]

Although there are many new research developments in this field, the etiology and the pathogenesis of AFE remain unclear, and thus, currently, there is no "gold standard" diagnostic test for AFE. AFE remains a diagnosis of exclusion, dependent on bedside evaluation and judgment. Ideal management includes prompt evaluation and intervention for each of the pathologic features found in this complex obstetric condition.

REFERENCES

1. Steiner PE, Lushbaugh C. Maternal pulmonary embolism by amniotic fluid as a cause of obstetric shock and unexplained death in obstetrics. *JAMA.* 1941;117:1245-1254.

2. Morgan M. Amniotic fluid embolism. *Anaesthesia.* 1979;34:20-32.

3. Abenhaim HA, Azoulay L, Kramer MS, Leduc L. Incidence and risk factors of amniotic fluid embolisms: a population based study on 3 million births in the United States. *Am J Obstet Gynecol.* 2008;199:49.e1-49.e8.

4. Knight M, UKOSS. Amniotic fluid embolism: active surveillance versus retrospective data-base review. *Am J Obstet Gynecol.* 2008;199:e9.

5. Clark SL, Hankins GD, Dudley DA, et al. Amniotic fluid embolism: analysis of the national registry. *Am J Obstet Gynecol.* 1995;172:1158-1169.

6. Lewis G. The confidential enquiry into maternal and child health. Saving mothers' lives: reviewing maternal deaths to make motherhood safer—2002-2005. London CEMACH 2007.

7. Kramer MS, Rouleau J, Baskett TF, Joseph KS; Maternal Health Study Group of the Canadian Perinatal Surveillance System. Amniotic fluid embolism and medical induction of labour: a retrospective, population–based cohort study. *Lancet.* 2006;368:1444-1448.

8. Gross PBE. Pulmonary embolism by amniotic fluid: report of three cases with a new diagnostic procedure. *Surg Gynecol Obstet.* 1947;85:315-320.

9. Resnik R, Swartz WH, Plummer MH, et al. Amniotic fluid embolism with survival. *Obstet Gynecol.* 1976;47:295-298.

10. Clark SL, Pavlova Z, Greenspoon J, et al. Squamous cells in the maternal pulmonary circulation. *Am J Obstet Gynecol.* 1986;154:104-106.

11. Lee W, Ginsburg KA, Cotton DB, et al. Squamous and trophoblastic cells in the maternal pulmonary circulation identified by invasive hemodynamic monitoring during the peripartum period. *Am J Obstet Gynecol.* 1986;155:999-1001.

12. Koretsky M, Ramirez M. Acute respiratory failure in pregnancy. An analysis of 19 cases. *Medicine.* 1998;77:41-49.

13. Petroianu GA, Toomes LM, Maleck WM, et al. Administration of autologous fetal membranes: effects on the coagulation in pregnant mini-pigs. *Pediatric Crit Care Med.* 2000;1:65-71.

14. Clark SL. New concepts of amniotic fluid embolism: a review. *Obstet Gynecol Surv.* 1990;45:360-368.

15. el Maradny E, Kanayama N, Halim M, et al. Endothelin has a role in early pathogenesis of amniotic fluid embolism. *Gynecol Obstet Invest.* 1995;40:14-18.

16. Stolte L, van Kessel H, Seelen J, et al. Failure to produce the syndrome of amniotic fluid embolism by infusion of amniotic fluid and meconium into monkeys. *Am J Obstet Gynecol.* 1967;98:694-697.

17. Benson MD, Kobayashi H, Silver RK, et al. Immunologic studies in presumed amniotic fluid embolism. *Obstet Gynecol.* 2001;97(4):510-514.

18. Oi H, Koboayashi H, Hirashima Y, et al. Serological and immunohistochemical diagnosis of amniotic fluid embolism. *Semin Thromb Hemost.* 1998;24(5):479-484.

19. Hiroshi K, Hidekazu, OOI, Hiroshi H, et al. Histological diagnosis of amniotic fluid embolism by monoclonal antibody TKH-2 that recognizes NeuAc alpha 2-6GaINAc epitope. *Hum Pathal.* 1997;28(4):428-433.

20. Kobayashi H, Ohi H, Terao T. A simple, noninvasive, sensitive method for the diagnosis of amniotic fluid embolism by monoclonal antibody TKH-2 that recognizes NeuAc alpha 2-6 Ga1NAc. *Am J Obstet Gynecol.* 1993;168(3):848-853.

21. Harboe T, Benson MD, Oi H, et al. Cardiopulmonary distress during obstetrical anaesthesia: attempts to diagnose amniotic fluid embolism in a case series of suspected allergic anaphylaxis. *Acta Anaesthesiol Scand.* 2006;50(3):324-330.

22. Fineschi V, Gambassi R, Gherardi M, et al. The diagnosis of amniotic fluid embolism: an immunohistochemical study for the quantification of pulmonary mast cell tryptase. *Int J Legal Med.* 1998;111:238-243.

23. Nishio H, Matsui K, Miyazaki T, et al. A fatal case of amniotic fluid embolism with elevation of serum mast cell tryptase. *Forensic Sci Int.* 2002;126(1):53-56.

24. Farrar SC, Gherman RB. Serum tryptase analysis in a woman with amniotic fluid embolism. A case report. *J Reprod Med.* 2001;46(10):926-928.

25. Benson MD. A hypothesis regarding complement activation and amniotic fluid embolism. *Med Hypothesis.* 2007;68(5):1019-1025.

26. Ray Bk, Vallejo MC, Creinin MD, et al. Amniotic fluid embolism with second trimester pregnancy termination: a case report. *Can J Anesth.* 2004;51:139-144.

27. Hassart TH, Essed GG. Amniotic fluid embolism after transabdominal amniocentesis. *Eur J Obstet Gynecol Reprod Biol.* 1983:16:25-30.

28. Maher JE, Wenstrom KD, Hauth JC, et al. Amniotic fluid embolism after saline amnioinfusion: 2 cases and a review of the literature. *Obstet Gynecol.* 1994;83:851-854.

29. Judich A, Kuriansky J, Engelberg I, et al. Amniotic fluid embolism following blunt abdominal trauma in pregnancy. *Injury.* 1998;29(6);475-477.

30. Rainio J, Penttila A. Amniotic fluid embolism as cause of death in a car accident—a case report. *Forensic Sci Int.* 2003;137(2-3):231-234.

31. McDougall RJ, Duke GJ. Amniotic fluid embolism syndrome: case report and review. *Anaesth Intensive Care.* 1995;23:735-740.

32. Clark SL. Hemodynamic alterations associated with amniotic fluid embolism: a reappraisal. *Am J Obstet Gynecol.* 1985;151:617-621.

33. Goetz KL, Wang BC, Madweb JB, et al. Cardiovascular, renal and endocrine responses to intravenous endothelin in conscious dogs. *Am J Physiol.* 1988;255:1064-1068.

34. Koegler A, Sauder P, Marof A, et al. Amniotic fluid embolism: a case with noncardiogenic pulmonary edema. *Intensive Care Med.* 1994;20:45-46.

35. Girard P, Mal H, Laie JJF, et al. Left heart failure in amniotic fluid embolism. *Anesthesiology.* 1986;64:262-265.

36. Shechtman M, Ziser A, Markoits R, et al. Amniotic fluid embolism: early findings of transesophageal echocardiography. *Anesth Analg.* 1999;89:1456-1458.

37. Moore J, Baldisseri MR. Amniotic fluid embolism. *Crit Care Med.* 2005;33(10):279-285.

38. Hankins GD, Snyder RR, Clark SL, et al. Acute hemodynamic and respiratory effects of amniotic fluid embolism in the pregnant goat model. *Am J Obstet Gynecol.* 1993;168:1113-1130.

39. Lockwood CJ, Bach R, Guha A, et al. Amniotic fluid contains tissue factor, a potent initiator of coagulation. *Am J Obstet Gynecol.* 1991;165:1335-1341.

40. Porter TF, Clark SL, Dildy GA, et al. Isolated disseminated intravascular coagulation and amniotic fluid embolism. *Am J Obstet Gynecol.* 1997;174:486.

41. Estelles A, Gilabert J, Andres C, et al. Plasminogen activator inhibitor type 1 and type 2 and plasminogen activators in amniotic fluid during pregnancy. *Thromb Haemost.* 1990;64:281-285.

42. Goldszmidt E, Davies S. Two cases of hemorrhage secondary to amniotic fluid embolus managed with uterine artery embolization. *Can J Anaesth.* 2003;50:917-921.

43. Lim Y, Loo CC, CHia V, et al. Recombinant factor VIIa after amniotic fluid embolism and disseminated intravascular coagulopathy. *Int J Obstet Gynecol.* 2004;87:178-179.

44. Prosper SC, Goudge CS, Lupo VR. Recombinant factor VIIa to successfully manage disseminated intravascular coagulation from amniotic fluid embolism. *Obstet Gynecol.* 2007;109:524-525.

45. Kaneko Y, Ogihara T, Tajima H, et al. Continuous hemodiafiltration for disseminated intravascular coagulation and shock due to amniotic fluid embolism: report of a dramatic response. *Intern Med.* 2001;40:945-947.

46. Stanten RD, Iverson LI, Daugharty TM, et al. Amniotic fluid embolism causing catastrophic pulmonary vasoconstriction: diagnosis by transesophageal echocardiogram and treatment by cardiopulmonary bypass. *Obstet Gynecol.* 2003;102(3):496-498.

47. Hsieh YY, Chang CC, Li PC, et al. Successful application of extracorporeal membrane oxygenation and intraaortic balloon counterpulsation as lifesaving therapy for a patient with amniotic fluid embolism. *Am J Obstet Gynecol.* 2000;183:496-497.

48. Johnson TR, Abbasi IA, Urso PJ. Fetal heart rate patterns associated with amniotic fluid embolus. *Am J Pernatol.* 1987;4:187-190.

49. Morris JA, Rosenbower TJ, Jurkovich GJ, et al. Infant survival after cesarean section for trauma. *Ann Surg.* 1996;223:481-488.

50. Moise KJ, Belfort MA. Damage control for the obstetric patient. *Surg Clin North Am.* 1997;77:835-852.

51. Tuffnell DJ. Amniotic fluid embolism. *Curr Opin Obstet Gynecol.* 2003;15(2):119-122.

52. Conde-Agudelo A, Romero, R. Amniotic fluid embolism: an evidence-based review. *Am J Obstet Gynecol.* 2009;201:445.e1-445.e13.

Acute Fatty Liver of Pregnancy

• *Jennifer McNulty*

Acute fatty liver of pregnancy (AFLP) is an uncommon but potentially fatal complication of pregnancy, which results in microvesicular fat deposition in the liver, resulting in severe liver dysfunction. Hallmarks of the disease include jaundice, coagulopathy, and encephalopathy. Although most commonly a disorder of the late third trimester, rare cases have been reported as early as 23 and 26 weeks. The incidence of AFLP appears to have increased over the past 30 years (from 1:15,900 to 1:6692 deliveries), possibly as more widespread recognition of the disease and identification of milder cases occurs. Prior to the 1970s, maternal and fetal mortality rates were reported to be as high as 75% and 85%, respectively. However, recent reports suggest markedly improved maternal mortality, ranging from 0% to 10% and fetal mortality from 8% to 25%. Deaths have been attributed to bleeding complications, aspiration, renal failure, and sepsis. Survivors of AFLP generally recover without sequelae.

■ PATHOPHYSIOLOGY

The precise etiology of AFLP remains unknown. However, in some cases, an autosomal recessive fetal enzyme deficiency involved in the mitochondrial fatty acid oxidation pathway has been linked to the development of maternal AFLP. The largest study to date of 27 women affected by AFLP found that 19% of the offspring of these pregnancies had long-chain 3-hydroxyacyl coenzyme dehydrogenase (LCHAD) deficiency. In contrast, no newborns had LCHAD deficiency when 81 maternal HELLP syndrome cases were evaluated. It is postulated that toxic metabolites, such as free fatty acids from an impaired fetoplacental unit, result in maternal illness in these cases of AFLP. Importantly, LCHAD deficient infants are at subsequent risk for hepatic steatosis, hypoglycemia, coagulopathy, coma, and death, all of which can be prevented with the use of a special diet and frequent regular feeding. It has been recommended that newborns of all women with AFLP should undergo molecular analysis for LCHAD gene mutations. Nationally, all states have now implemented LCHAD and other fatty acid enzyme disorder testing as part of routine newborn screening via tandem mass spectrometry. Abnormal LCHAD function may represent only one of a variety of fatty acid metabolic disorders resulting in the clinical phenotype of AFLP.

The pathway of impaired mitochondrial oxidation has been implicated in other microvesicular liver disorders in nonpregnant individuals that are remarkably similar to AFLP. Exogenous impairment of mitochondrial oxidation can occur with ingestion of aspirin, valproic acid, and tetracycline, and would, in susceptible individuals with latent oxidative enzyme deficiencies, result in liver dysfunction, such as is seen in Reyes disease, tetracycline toxicity, and valproic acid injury. Common histopathologic findings include the presence of fine fat droplets in swollen hepatocytes, due to the accumulation of triglycerides and particularly in AFLP, free fatty acids. Fat deposits are most prominent in pericentral and mid zones and spare the periportal cells. The microvesicular fat deposition can be missed if the tissue is fixed before examination, and Oil Red O or Sudan stains should be used on frozen tissue sections. Electron microscopy of the liver shows mitochondrial abnormalities. Intrahepatic cholestasis is usual and unlike in preeclampsia, cellular infiltration with lymphocytes is minimal. Although the diagnosis of AFLP can be made by liver biopsy, today the diagnosis is usually made clinically (Tables 15-1 and 15-2).

■ **TABLE 15-1. Clinical Presenting Symptoms of Acute Fatty Liver of Pregnancy**

Always
  Late second/early third trimester onset
Usual
  Jaundice
  Malaise
  Nausea and emesis
Common
  Abdomen pain (epigastric or right upper quadrant)
  Anorexia
  Clinical coagulopathy (GI bleeding, IV site bleeding, pelvic and post surgical bleeding)
  CNS abnormalities (altered sensorium, lethargy, confusion, psychosis, restlessness, coma)
  Edema
  Hypertension with headache

■ **TABLE 15-2. Physical Findings by System in Acute Fatty Liver of Pregnancy**

Central nervous system
  Asterixis
  Fever, low grade
  Mental status changes
Cardiovascular
  Hypertensions
  Tachycardia
Abdomen/gastrointestinal
  Fluid wave or distension
  Guaiac positive stool or emesis
  Pain (right upper quadrant or epigastric)
  Small liver
Genitourinary
  Hematuria
  Oliguria
  Polyuria (occasionally, due to diabetes insipidus)
Dermatologic
  Edema
  Icteric sclera, mucus membranes
  Jaundiced skin
  Mucus membrane(oropharynx, vagina)/IV site bleeding
  Petechiae
  Absent pruritus

■ DIAGNOSTIC TESTS

Noninvasive radiologic techniques have been used in order to avoid liver biopsy and support a clinical diagnosis. Unfortunately, the reported sensitivities are low. Abnormalities in the imaging studies of 19 patients with AFLP were reported in 25% of ultrasounds, 50% of CT scans, and none of the MRI studies. A larger series of ultrasounds from 45 women with AFLP reported abnormalities in just 27%. Imaging studies can be used to exclude biliary obstruction as a cause of jaundice, however.

Table 15-4 reviews the results of common liver assays in normal pregnancy and Table 15-5 presents the laboratory abnormalities encountered in AFLP. The laboratory hallmark of AFLP is hyperbilirubinemia, with values typically elevated to 3 to 10 mg/dL, with a reported range of 3 to 40 mg/dL. Alkaline phosphatase, normally elevated up to twofold in pregnancy, is commonly elevated up to tenfold in AFLP. Due to decreased ammonia utilization by the urea cycle enzymes of the hepatocytes, serum ammonia is elevated, and associated with hepatic encephalopathy. Transaminase elevation is mild to moderate, usually less than 250 to 500 U/mL, but can be greater than 1000 U/mL. Transaminase elevation is less than typically seen in acute hepatitis. Typically SGOT levels (aspartate) are greater than SGPT levels (alanine). Severe liver dysfunction also leads to coagulopathy. Production of vitamin K–dependent clotting factors by the liver is depressed, resulting in another hallmark of AFLP, an elevated prothrombin time. With worsening

■ **TABLE 15-3. Complications of Acute Fatty Liver of Pregnancy**

"PICKLE"
Pancreatitis
Infection (iatrogenic)
Coagulopathy
  Anemia, GI bleeding, intraoperative hemorrhage, vaginal bleeding
Kidney Failure
  Oliguria, uremia, or diabetes insipidus occasionally
Liver Failure
  Acidosis, ascites, hepatic encephalopathy, hypoglycemia, hypovolemia
Edema
  Pulmonary, hypoxia

■ **TABLE 15-4. Liver Assays in Normal Pregnancy**

Bilirubin	No change
Enzymes	
Alkaline phosphatase	Increased twofold
Aminotransferases	No change
γ-glutamyl transpeptidase	No change
LDH	No change
Hemostatic factors	
Clotting factors II, VII, VIII, X	Elevated
Clotting times (PT/PTT)	No change
Fibrinogen	Elevated (by 50%)
Lipids	
Triglycerides	Elevated
Cholesterol	Increased twofold
Proteins	
Albumin	Decreased (by 30% at term)
Globulin	Slightly increased
Hormone-binding proteins	Increased
Transferrin	Increased

■ **TABLE 15-5. Laboratory Abnormalities in Acute Fatty Liver of Pregnancy by Affected System**

Liver
  Elevated
    Alkaline phosphatase
    Ammonia
    Bilirubin (usually 3-15 mg/dL)
    Transaminases (usually <500 U/mL, unless cardiovascular collapse and liver hypoperfusion)
  Decreased
    Antithrombin III activity (usually <20%)
    Fibrinogen
    Clotting factors
    Glucose
Renal
  Elevated
    BUN
    Creatinine
    Proteinuria
    Sodium (if diabetes insipidus)
    Uric acid
    Urobilinogen
  Decreased
    Creatinine clearance
    Urine sodium
Hematologic
  Elevated
    Smear morphology (schistocytes, normoblasts, giant platelets)
    Fibrin split products
    Prothrombin time, partial thromboplastin time
    WBCs (usually >15,000)
  Decreased
    Antithrombin III activity
    Clotting factors
    Fibrinogen
    Hemoglobin/hematocrit
Pancreas
  Elevated
    Amylase
    Lipase

liver failure, the partial thromboplastin time becomes elevated. Decreased fibrinogen production results from further liver dysfunction. A profound depression of antithrombin III (ATIII) activity is also reported in AFLP, to a far greater degree than in preeclampsia or HELLP syndrome. ATIII activity is not significantly affected by normal pregnancy, or pregnancy with chronic hypertension alone. The low levels in AFLP are probably due to derangement in liver production, but may also be associated with accelerated consumption and DIC. Despite the marked decrease in ATIII, which is a natural inhibitor of coagulation, clinical large vessel thrombosis does not occur, perhaps due to the proportional impairment of clotting activators.

Hypoglycemia is often present and is presumed to be due to impairment of glycogenolysis within the liver, resulting from depression of glucose-6-phosphatase activity. Approximately 15% of patients with AFLP will have severe hypoglycemia and over half will require glucose supplementation with 10% dextrose to maintain adequate blood glucose.

Laboratory evaluation also reveals dysfunction of other organ systems. Renal insufficiency appears to be universal in AFLP, but infrequently requires dialysis. An elevated serum creatinine has been documented in some patients before the development of liver failure, and renal insufficiency may not be due to hepatorenal syndrome as has been postulated. Instead, it may be due to inhibition of beta oxidation of fat in the kidneys, as in the liver, and thus might be a direct effect of the underlying mitochondrial dysfunction on the kidneys. Autopsy findings in patients with AFLP have shown microvesicular deposition of fat in the renal tubules. In addition, diabetes insipidus has been noted in up to 10% of patients with AFLP, resulting in polyuria and hypernatremia. The etiology is not yet clear. Pancreatitis, associated with microvesicular fat deposition in the pancreas, results in elevated amylase and lipase in some patients. Although hypoglycemia due to liver impairment is common in AFLP, hyperglycemia may be present if there is pancreatitis.

■ DIFFERENTIAL DIAGNOSIS

Table 15-6 outlines a comparison of liver diseases in pregnancy which must be distinguished from AFLP, a task which is sometimes difficult. Atypical preeclampsia and HELLP syndrome (*h*emolytic anemia, *e*levated *l*iver function test, and *l*ow *p*latelets) are probably the most common conditions the obstetrician will consider as alternate diagnoses to AFLP. Features in common to these entities include elevated transaminases, thrombocytopenia, and frequently an elevated serum creatinine. In addition, proteinuria and even hypertension are frequent in patients with AFLP, as is always seen in preeclampsia, and usually in HELLP syndrome. Importantly, in both AFLP and preeclampsia/HELLP, delivery is ultimately curative. Clinical jaundice, apparent when the bilirubin rises above 2 to 3 mg/dL, is a hallmark in AFLP, but uncommon in preeclampsia/HELLP syndrome. While an elevated prothrombin time is a hallmark of AFLP, the prothrombin time and fibrinogen levels are usually normal in preeclampsia/HELLP, unless placental abruption or fetal death has occurred with associated DIC. Hypoglycemia, common in AFLP, is not expected in preeclampsia/HELLP. Cholestasis of pregnancy is the most common liver disease in pregnant women. This entity can be associated with elevated transaminases and bilirubin, but usually to a lesser degree than in AFLP. Importantly, unlike in AFLP, cholestasis is associated with pruritus.

The clinical presentation may be similar in both AFLP and viral hepatitis, including malaise, nausea, emesis, and a tender right upper quadrant. Fulminant acute viral hepatitis is typically associated with much higher transaminase values than AFLP, usually >1000 U/L. In addition, unlike many patients with AFLP, hypertension and proteinuria are not present. Risk factors may be identified for hepatitis, including drug exposure or known hepatitis exposure. Finally, hepatitis does not have a predilection for the third trimester.

Both hemolytic uremic syndrome (HUS) and thrombotic thrombocytopenic purpura (TTP) share some features with AFLP, including thrombocytopenia, renal insufficiency, microangiopathic anemia, and alterations in mental status. However, the coagulopathy which is a hallmark of AFLP is not found in TTP or HUS cases, in which the prothrombin time and fibrinogen levels will be normal. In addition, antithrombin III activity is normal in TTP and HUS.

■ MANAGEMENT

The most critical component of caring for a woman with AFLP is delivery of her fetus. There is no clear benefit to immediate cesarean delivery versus induction of labor and vaginal delivery with meticulous supportive care. In fact, in one report of 28 patients with AFLP, almost all of the maternal hemorrhagic complications occurred in association with surgical trauma. However, factors such as known fetal growth restriction and uteroplacental insufficiency, non-reassuring fetal status by fetal heart rate monitoring, and early gestational age with a markedly unfavorable cervix may appropriately influence a decision to choose cesarean section over vaginal delivery. Coagulation parameters should be corrected prior to surgical delivery, and consideration given to a vertical midline incision, avoiding the dissection associated with a Pfannenstiel incision. The use of an intraperitoneal, closed suction drain, as well as a similar subcutaneous drain (or delayed secondary closure) can also be considered. If vaginal delivery can be accomplished, avoidance of episiotomy in the presence of a coagulopathy is suggested. Anesthesia should be carefully planned, and regional anesthesia considered if coagulation abnormalities can be corrected. If not, and general anesthesia is chosen, inhalation agents with the potential for hepatotoxicity (such as halothane) should be avoided. The use of isoflurane has been described. In addition, the dose of narcotics, which are metabolized by the liver, should be adjusted.

Additional supportive care for AFLP includes monitoring for hypoglycemia, treatment of coagulopathy with transfusion when clinically indicated, optimizing nutrition, and surveillance for infection. Although

■ TABLE 15-6. Differential Diagnosis of Acute Fatty Liver in Pregnancy

	Fatty liver of pregnancy	Acute viral hepatitis	HELLP syndrome/preeclampsia/eclampsia
Onset (I/II/III trimester)	II/III, most >35 wk, rare reports <30 wk	Any	II/III (after 20 wk)
Clinical findings	Malaise, nausea/emesis, jaundice, mental status changes, abdomen pain, +/− hemorrhage, +/− preeclampsia	Malaise, nausea/emesis, jaundice, abdomen pain	Malaise, hypertension, proteinuria, nausea, abdomen pain, rare jaundice, +/− seizures, +/− oliguria, +/− coagulopathy
Laboratory			
Transaminases (U/mL)	↑ usually <500	↑ commonly >1000	Normal to ↑ 50× (> if liver hematoma)
Bilirubin (mg/dL)	↑ usually 3-10	↑	↑ occasionally (usually <2-3×)
Prothrombin time	↑	+/− ↑	Normal unless DIC/IUFD/abruption
Alkaline phosphatase	↑	+/− ↑	↑ occasionally
Other	↑ ammonia, very ↓ antithrombin III, ↓ platelets, ↓ fibrinogen, ↑ WBC, ↑ creatinine, proteinuria, ↓ glucose	+ hepatitis serology, ↓ antithrombin III	Moderately ↓ antithrombin III, proteinuria, ↓ platelets, ↑ creatinine, ↑ uric acid
Liver histopathology	Centrilobular microvesicular fat, cholestasis	Marked inflammation and necrosis	Periportal fibrin deposits, hemorrhagic hepatocellular necrosis, inflammation
Treatment	Immediate delivery, supportive	Supportive	$MgSO_4$ seizure prophylaxis, delivery (delayed in very selected preterm cases), antihypertensive treatment

	Cholestasis of pregnancy	Hemolytic uremic syndrome	Thrombotic thrombocytopenia purpura
Onset (I/II/III trimester)	III, rare reports II	Any	Any, 60% <24 wk
Clinical findings	Pruritus, (worst in PM, palms and soles), +/− jaundice	Hypertension, acute renal failure, nausea/emesis, may have fever and neurologic findings, hallmarks are microangiopathic anemia and severe thrombocytopenia.	Often neurologic findings, fever and renal dysfunction, hallmarks are microangiopathic anemia and severe thrombocytopenia.
Laboratory			
Transaminases (U/mL)	↑ (usually <300)	Usually normal	Usually normal
Bilirubin (mg/dL)	Often ↑ (usually <5)	↑ (unconjugated)	↑ (unconjugated)
Prothrombin time	Usually normal, may be ↑	Usually normal	Usually normal
Alkaline phosphatase	↑ (up to 4 × normal)	Usually normal	Usually normal

(Continued)

■ TABLE 15-6. Differential Diagnosis of Acute Fatty Liver in Pregnancy (*Continued*)

	Cholestasis of pregnancy	Hemolytic uremic syndrome	Thrombotic thrombocytopenia purpura
Other	↑ serum bile acids	Normal antithrombin III, usually normal fibrinogen, ↓ WBC, ↓ platelets (often <20,000), significantly ↑ creatinine , ↑ uric acid, ↑ LDH, +/− proteinuria	Normal antithrombin III, usually normal fibrinogen, ↑ WBC, ↓ platelets (often <20,000), normal – slightly ↑ creatinine, ↑ LDH, +/− proteinuria, ↓ ADAMTS13 activity, + antiADAMTS13 antibodies
Liver histopathology	Centrolobular cholestasis, no inflammation	Unknown	Unknown
Treatment	Ursodeoxycholic acid, corticosteroids of reported benefit, vitamin K	For nondiarrheal associated HUS probably plasma exchange, FFP infusion, hemodialysis, ?corticosteroids/immunosuppressive agents	Plasma exchange, FFP infusion pending initiation of plasma exchange, ?corticosteroids/immunosuppressive agents

transfusion with antithrombin III has been suggested in light of its severe depression in patients with AFLP, this approach is not known to be of clinical benefit. Worsening of liver and renal function can be seen for up to 2 to 3 days after delivery. Additional therapies which have been reported empirically in very small numbers of patients with uncertain benefit have included plasma exchange and albumin dialysis. Plasma exchange was used for six patients in one small series who continued to worsen from 2 to 9 days after delivery. Albumin dialysis (molecular adsorbent recirculating system or MARS) has been utilized in nonpregnant patients with hepatic encephalopathy and reported in two AFLP patients on days 3 and 9 after delivery. Although there are several reported cases of liver transplantation for patients with ongoing liver failure in the immediate postpartum period, it has been argued that with ongoing supportive care, all patients with AFLP will ultimately experience complete resolution of the liver failure. Importantly, AFLP has been recognized to recur in subsequent pregnancy, in a small number of cases. At least one such case was associated with LCHAD heterozygosity in the patient. Table 15-7 presents the cornerstones of supportive care for patients with AFLP.

■ **TABLE 15-7. Management Cornerstones for Acute Fatty Liver of Pregnancy by Affected System**

General
  Admit to ICU
  Consultation as needed with gastroenterology/hepatology, critical care specialist, nephrology
Respiratory
  Secure airway if encephalopathy or comatose and ventilate, supplemental oxygen—otherwise as needed
  Evaluate for pulmonary edema
Central nervous system
  Minimize encephalopathy
    Decrease endogenous ammonia
      Protein-restrict diet, although of uncertain benefit for encephalopathy
  Neomycin orally 6-12 g/d to decrease ammonia producing intestinal bacteria
      Lactulose by mouth or NG tube, 45 mL q6-8h to evaluate colon and acidify the gut lumen
    Avoid hepatic metabolized medication (certain inhalation anesthetics, narcotics)
Bleeding/coagulopathy
  Transfuse
    FFP, cryoprecipitate, packed red cells, platelets
  GI protection
    H2 blockers (ranitidine 50 mg IV q8h, famotidine 20 mg IV q12h)
    Or sucralfate 1 g po q6h or 1 h before meals when eating
Renal/electrolytes
  Avoid hypovolemia
  Correct electrolyte abnormalities
  Surveillance for hypoglycemia
    Maintain glucose >60 mg%
    Dextrose 20% solution, at 125 cc/h provides about 2000 cal/d
  Synthetic dDAVP if diabetes insipidus
Infection surveillance
  Culture/treat if evidence of pneumonia (ventilator/aspiration), urosepsis (bladder catheter), bacteremia (IV lines), wound (if post operative)

SUGGESTED READINGS

Bacq Y, Riely CA. Acute fatty liver of pregnancy: the hepatologist's view. *The Gastroenterologist.* 1993;1:257-264.

Castro MA, Fassett MJ, Reynolds TB, et al. Reversible peripartum liver failure: a new perspective on the diagnosis, treatment, and cause of acute fatty liver of pregnancy, based on 28 consecutive cases. *Am J Obstet Gynecol.* 1999;181:389-395.

Ibdah JA. Acute fatty liver of pregnancy: an update on pathogenesis and clinical implications. *World J Gastroenterol.* 2006;12:7397-7404.

Knight M, Nelson-Piercy C, Kurinczuk J. A prospective national study of acute fatty liver of pregnancy in the UK. *Hepatology.* 2008;57:951-956.

Pereira SP, O'Donohue J, Wendon J, et al. Maternal and perinatal outcome in severe pregnancy-related liver disease. *Hepatology.* 1997;26:1258-1262.

Porter TF. Acute fatty liver of pregnancy. In: Dildy GA, Belfort MA, Saade GR, et al, eds. *Critical Care Obstetrics.* 4th ed. Boston, MA: Blackwell Science; 2004.

Usta IM, Barton JR, Amon EA, et al. Acute fatty liver of pregnancy: an experience in the diagnosis and management of fourteen cases. *Am J Obstet Gynecol.* 1994;171:1342-1347.

Yang Z, Yamada J, Zhao Y, et al. Prospective screening for pediatric mitochondrial trifunctional protein defects in pregnancies complicated by liver disease. *JAMA.* 2002;288: 2163-2166.

Neurologic Emergencies during Pregnancy

• William H. Clewell

A patient with a neurological emergency does not present with a diagnosis but rather with one or several clinical manifestations. The nature of the presentation, sequence of events, and constellation of signs and symptoms suggests a differential diagnosis. Starting from the presentation, the physician must select diagnostic tests and procedures and then, once a diagnosis is made, initiate treatment. The differential diagnosis may be altered by pregnancy and diagnostic procedures employed may be different from those one would use for nonpregnant patients. We will consider the following presentations: headache, seizures, altered state of consciousness, and motor or sensory changes. This signs and symptoms approach was chosen because patients do not usually come to the physician with a diagnosis but with a change in their condition, appearance of symptoms, and the need for care.

■ HEADACHE

Headache is a common complaint in pregnancy. Patients who report having had the same problem for some time prior to pregnancy do not usually have a neurological emergency. Chronic and recurrent headaches may be due to tension, migraine, sinusitis, pseudotumor cerebri or in many cases be unexplained. Migraine headaches are relatively common during reproductive age of women and often become less frequent and severe in pregnancy. In a minority of migraine sufferers, however, they may present for the first time or become more severe in pregnancy. They must be distinguished from other more immediately dangerous conditions. Many patients who think they have migraines do not have the classical pattern of aura, headache, and nausea. Headaches which, aside from frequency, are similar to those the patient has experienced in the past can

generally be considered to not represent a neurological emergency and can be managed symptomatically. Medications used for the treatment of migraine headache are listed in Table 16-1. If headaches become more frequent and severe or have accompanying neurologic manifestations, then they require further evaluation.

Onset of a new headache or the occurrence of a headache with a different location, quality, or accompanying neurologic symptoms demands further evaluation. Figure 16-1 and Table 16-2 outline an approach to the evaluation of headache in pregnancy. The sudden onset of headache requires immediate evaluation and perhaps admission to the hospital. Headache is a common feature of preeclampsia which must be considered in any patient in the second half of pregnancy. Since preeclampsia consists of a constellation of clinical and laboratory abnormalities, appropriate clinical and laboratory evaluation should be able to determine if it is a likely diagnosis in a specific patient (see Chap 5).

The differential diagnosis of sudden, severe headache in pregnancy is the same as that for the nonpregnant patient with the addition of preeclampsia. It includes subarachnoid hemorrhage, intracerebral hemorrhage, cortical vein thrombosis, meningitis, and mass lesions (tumors or abscesses). Subarachnoid hemorrhage can be due to ruptured cerebral aneurysms, arteriovenous malformations (AVM) or, rarely, preeclampsia or eclampsia.

Cerebral aneurysms usually occur on the vessels of the circle of Willis or the proximal portions of the vessels arising from it. These saccular or berry aneurysms can be found in any patient but are more common in patients with Marfan syndrome or familial polycystic kidneys. Bleeds from aneurysms are more common in older patients (generally over age 30) and tend to occur in late

TABLE 16-1. Medications for Migraine

Medication	Class	Dosage	Route of administration	Safety in pregnancy
Acetaminophen	Pain reliever	4 g/d max	po or pr	Yes
Codeine	Narcotic	30-90 mg q 3-4 h	po	Yes
Meperidine (Demerol)	Narcotic	25-100 mg q 3-6 h	po, IM, or IV	Yes
Ibuprofen	Nonsteroidal	Up to 3200 mg/d (divided doses)	po	Avoid in late pregnancy (beyond 32 wk)
Fioricet[a]	Sedative, pain reliever, vasoconstrictor	2 tabs q 4 h, 6/d max	po	Yes
Midrin[b]	Vasoconstrictor, sedative, pain reliever	2 caps, then 1 q h, no more than 5 in 12 h	po	Yes
Caffeine	Vasoconstrictor	500 mg in 50 mL IV, may repeat	po or IV	Yes
Imitrex[c]	Vasoconstrictor	po 300 mg/d SC 6 mg (max, 12 mg/d)	po, SC, nasal spray	Yes
Ergotamine and caffeine	Vasoconstrictor	2 mg + 200 mg, then 1 mg + 100 mg 2 caps; 30 min	po or pr	No
Nortriptyline	TCA (prophylaxis)	25-100 mg qhs	po	Yes
Amitriptyline	TCA (prophylaxis)	50-100 mg qhs	po	Yes
Sertraline	SSRI (prophylaxis)	50-100 mg qhs	po	Probably yes
Fluoxetine	SSRI (prophylaxis)	20-40 mg qhs	po	Probably yes
Propranolol	β-blocker (prophylaxis)	80-120 mg qd	po	Low risk of IUGR
Nadolol	β-blocker (prophylaxis)	20-80 mg qd	po	Risk of IUGR
Atenolol	β-blocker (prophylaxis)	25-100 mg qd	po	Risk of IUGR
Carbamazepine	Anticonvulsant (prophylaxis)	Up to 1200 mg/d	po	Risk of malformations (first trimester)

TCA, tricyclic antidepressant; SSRI, selective serotonin reuptake inhibitor.
[a]Butalbital (50 mg), acetaminophen (325 mg), caffeine (40 mg).
[b]Isometheptene mucate (40 mg), dicloralphenazone (100 mg), acetaminophen (325 mg).
[c]Sumatriptan.

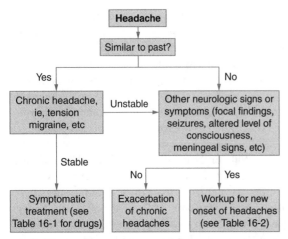

FIGURE 16-1. Workup of headache.

TABLE 16-2. Workup for New Headaches

Rule out preeclampsia
    Clinical evaluation BP, edema, proteinuria)
    Laboratory
Rule out mass lesions
    MRI, CT, or MRA
Rule out infection
    LP
    Clinical evaluation
Rule out AVM or aneurysm
    MRI, CT, or MRA

■ TABLE 16-3. CNS Hemorrhage: Condition at Presentation (Hunt and Botterell Scale)

Grade	Hemorrhage condition
I	Alert, with/without nuchal rigidity
II	Drowsy/severe headache, no CNS deficit except cranial nerves
III	Focal CNS deficits (mild hemiparesis)
IV	Stupor with severe CNS deficit
V	Moribund

pregnancy. In contrast, hemorrhage from an AVM tends to occur in younger patients (peak between 15 and 20 years) and is equally likely at all gestational ages. There is no way to clinically distinguish between bleeding from an AVM, a berry aneurysm, or preeclampsia. These patients all present with sudden onset of severe headache, nausea and vomiting, and meningeal signs. They may have focal neurological deficits, altered state of consciousness, seizures, and hypertension. The condition of the patient at presentation is the most important prognostic feature (see Table 16-3).

The diagnosis of possible subarachnoid hemorrhage in pregnancy starts with a high index of suspicion raised by the presentation. Clinical and laboratory evaluation for possible preeclampsia/eclampsia must be accomplished, since it is the more common diagnosis and if confirmed requires specific therapy and possible delivery as the definitive treatment. If preeclampsia and eclampsia are ruled out, the cornerstone of evaluation is CNS imaging with CT, MRI, or MRA. A head or cervical spine CT exposes the uterus to less than 1 mrad of radiation. Magnetic resonance imaging is more sensitive than CT and entirely avoids the issue of radiation exposure. There is very limited data on the safety of Gadolinium compounds used for MRI imaging in pregnancy. The American College of Radiology recommends against their use "unless absolutely necessary." Cerebral angiography may also be used to pinpoint the site of bleeding. Contrast dyes used in x-ray angiography pose no significant risk to the fetus beyond the radiation exposure. Spinal tap will serve to confirm the presence of subarachnoid blood and rule out meningitis as the cause of the headache. Simultaneously, with the initiation of the diagnostic workup, neurological and neurosurgical consultation should be obtained.

Surgical management of both AVM and berry aneurysms can be accomplished in pregnancy but if the patient is near term, consideration of delivery prior to or simultaneously with the surgical repair should be considered. Surgery under hypotensive anesthesia or hypothermia can be well tolerated by the fetus. Continuous fetal heart rate monitoring is needed during and after surgery. Anesthetic medications generally suppress fetal heart rate variability and can make monitor interpretations more difficult. If fetal bradycardia occurs, it is desirable to raise the maternal blood pressure to improve utero-placental perfusion. Careful attention to maternal oxygenation will improve fetal condition. Almost all women known to have an AVM or berry aneurysm deliver by cesarean section. If the lesion has been surgically treated by excision in the case of AVM or clipping in the case of aneurysm, then vaginal delivery can be safely conducted.

■ SEIZURE

When a pregnant woman presents with a seizure, the first question to ask is whether she has a seizure disorder. The second question to ask oneself is whether this represents eclampsia (Fig 16-2). Seizure disorders occur in approximately 0.5% of the population and are the most common neurologic complications of pregnancy. There appears to be an increase in seizure frequency in pregnancy, but it is unclear how much of this increase is due to increased susceptibility to seizures and how much is due to declining blood drug levels. Both the volume of distribution and hepatic clearance of anticonvulsant drugs are increased in pregnancy. This can be especially dramatic in the case of phenytoin. The renal clearance of phenobarbital also increases in pregnancy. These physiologic changes result in falling anticonvulsant levels while the patient is maintained on a constant dose.

A woman who, when not pregnant, experienced at least one convulsion per month can expect an increase in seizure frequency during pregnancy. When a pregnant woman, whose seizures have been well controlled prior to conception, presents with a recurrence of seizures, one must confirm adequate blood levels of her anticonvulsant medication. Infants of epileptic women have a higher incidence of birth defects than the general population. This risk is present for women not on medication as well as those on anticonvulsants. The magnitude of the risk increases with the severity of the maternal condition and the number of drugs required to control the seizures.

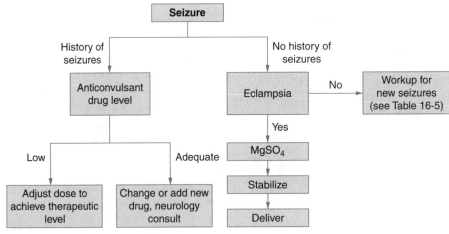

FIGURE 16-2. Workup for seizures.

A variety of malformations have been associated with maternal anticonvulsant use. Dysmorphic facial features are seen with a variety of agents. Distal digital hypoplasia occurs in 15% to 30% of infants exposed to phenytoin and carbamazepine. Neural tube defects appear in 1% to 2% of infants exposed to valproic acid in the first trimester. It is unclear whether the anomalies seen with anticonvulsant therapy are due to the direct embryotoxic effect of drugs or relative folate deficiency or antagonism. Dietary supplementation with folic acid in doses of 0.5 to 1 mg/d, starting prior to conception, seems reasonable but direct proof of efficacy in patients on anticonvulsants is lacking.

Use of anticonvulsants in the third trimester may contribute to bleeding problems in the fetus and newborn. While the mother's clotting system appears to be unaffected by anticonvulsants, about one-half of exposed newborns have a deficiency of vitamin K–dependent clotting factors. Maternal vitamin K supplementation of 20 mg/d, for 2 weeks prior to delivery, results in normal clotting parameters in the newborn. In case of preterm labor, a single 10 mg intramuscular dose to the mother should be adequate. Since most infants receive 1 mg of vitamin K intramuscularly at birth, clinical hemorrhagic disease of the newborn is quite rare even in patients on anticonvulsants.

The new onset of seizures, especially in the third trimester or postpartum, should be considered due to eclampsia until proven otherwise. The initial treatment should be magnesium sulfate as outlined in Chap 5.

Earlier in pregnancy or with eclampsia ruled out, the initial therapy can be with phenytoin. If the patient is in status epilepticus, this can be accomplished with an intravenous loading dose of 18 to 20 mg/kg with a maximum rate of 50 mg/min. Transient hypotension and heart block can occur with rapid intravenous infusion of phenytoin. The patient should be on a cardiac monitor during this therapy. For patients not in status epilepticus, oral treatment is appropriate and safer.

Status epilepticus is a life-threatening emergency and treatment must be initiated immediately to preserve both maternal and fetal well-being. Prolonged seizure activity can lead to lactic acidosis, cardiovascular instability, and irreversible brain injury. Initial steps in therapy are to establish an airway and venous access. The Epilepsy Foundation of America has published a timetable for the treatment of status epilepticus (Table 16-4).

Once the acute seizure is controlled, the patient must be evaluated for etiology. Potential causes include trauma, infection, metabolic disorders, space-occupying lesions, central nervous system bleeding, and drug use. Neurological consultation should be obtained as soon as the workup is started (see Fig 16-2 and Table 16-5).

A pregnant woman with a seizure disorder may be on one or several of the commonly used anticonvulsants. While none have been shown to be completely safe for the fetus, uncontrolled seizures are unequivocally dangerous to both the mother and the fetus. Table 16-6 lists the doses, therapeutic blood levels, and side effects of the commonly used drugs.

■ TABLE 16-4. Suggested Timetable for the Treatment of Status Epilepticus

Time (min)	Action
0-5	Diagnose status epilepticus by observing continued seizure activity or one additional seizure.
	Give oxygen by nasal cannula or mask: position patient's head for optimal airway patency, consider intubation if respiratory assistance is needed.
	Obtain and record vital signs at onset and periodically thereafter; control any abnormalities as necessary; initiate EEG monitoring.
	Establish IV line; draw venous blood samples for glucose level, serum chemistries, hematologic studies, toxicology screens, and determination of antiepileptic drug levels.
6-9	If hypoglycemia is established or a blood glucose determination is not available, administer glucose. In adults, give 100 mg of thiamine followed by 50 mL of 50% glucose by direct push into the IV.
10-20	Administer either 0.1 mg/kg of diazepam at 5 mg/min by IV. If diazepam is given, it can be repeated if seizures do not stop after 5 min. If diazepam is used to stop the status, phenytoin should be administered next to prevent recurrent status.
21-60	If status persists, administer 15-20 mg/kg of phenytoin no faster than 50 mg/min in adults and 1 mg/kg/min in children by IV; monitor ECG and blood pressure during infusion. Phenytoin is incompatible with glucose-containing solutions. The IV should be purged with normal saline before the phenytoin infusion.
>60	If status does not stop after 20 mg/kg of phenytoin, give additional doses of 5 mg/kg to a maximum dose of 30 mg/kg. If status persists, give 20 mg/kg of phenobarbital by IV at 100 mg/min. When phenobarbital is given after benzodiazepine, the risk of apnea is great and assisted ventilation is usually required. If status persists, give anesthetic dose of drugs such as phenobarbital or pentobarbital; ventilatory assistance and vasopressors are virtually always necessary.

Source: From Epilepsy Foundation of America. Treatment of status epilepticus. *JAMA.* 1993;270:854-859.

■ TABLE 16-5. Workup of New Onset Seizures

Rule out CNS bleeding
  MRI, CT, or MRA
  LP
  Neurologic and/or neurosurgical consultation
Rule out CNS infection
  LP
Rule out metabolic disorder
  Electrolytes
  BUN/creatinine
  Calcium
  Glucose
Rule out drug exposure
  Urine drug screen (cocaine, methamphetamine, etc)
Neurologic examination for focal signs
EEG

■ ALTERED STATE OF CONSCIOUSNESS AND FOCAL NEUROLOGIC SIGNS

When a patient presents with altered state of consciousness, it is often accompanied or preceded by seizure, headache, or focal neurologic signs. When it occurs without these other features, one must consider drug exposure or a catastrophic intracerebral event such as massive hemorrhage or stroke. In these latter conditions, the onset of the event may not have been witnessed and only the fully developed situation is observed. The evaluation of patients with altered consciousness is similar to that of new onset of seizures. Often the patient has had a seizure which was not witnessed and she is found in the postictal state. Because of its serious consequences and relatively high prevalence, eclampsia must be considered in any patient with altered consciousness. Once eclampsia is eliminated

■ **TABLE 16-6. Anticonvulsants Commonly Used in Pregnancy**

Drug (µg/mL)	Maternal effects	Fetal effects	Usual dosage	Therapeutic levels
Carbamazepine (Tegretol)	Drowsiness, leucopenia ataxia hepatotoxicity	Possible craniofacial and neural tube defects	400-1200 mg in divided doses	4-10
Ethosuximide (Zarontin)	Nausea, hepatotoxicity, leucopenia, thrombocytopenia	Possible teratogenesis	500 mg/d	40-100
Gabapentin (Neurontin)	Leukopenia, drowsiness, ataxia	Too little data to report	900-1800 mg/d in divided doses	Not followed
Phenobarbital	Drowsiness, ataxia	Possible teratogenesis, coagulopathy, neonatal depression, withdrawal	60-240 mg/d as single dose	10-35
Phenytoin (Dilantin)	Nystagmus, ataxia, gingival hyperplasia, megaloblastic anemia	Possible teratogenesis, coagulopathy, hypocalcemia	300-600 mg/d as single dose	10-20 (free phenytoin, 1-2)
Primidone (Mysoline)	Drowsiness, ataxia, nausea	Possible teratogenesis, coagulopathy, neonatal depression	750-2000 mg/d, divided	5-12
Valproic acid	Ataxia, drowsiness, alopecia, hepatotoxicity, thrombocytopenia	Neural tube defects, possible craniofacial and skeletal defects	12-15 mg/kg/d, divided doses	50-100

and a thorough neurologic examination is completed, the cornerstone of evaluation is brain imaging by MRI or CT. Figure 16-3 outlines the initial steps in evaluation and management of this emergency.

Thrombotic Stroke

Thrombotic stroke is relatively rare in the reproductive age group. The overall incidence is one per 20,000 live births. About half of the pregnancy-associated events occur in the immediate postpartum period. The other half occurs predominantly in the late second and third trimesters. Certain conditions predispose to it including hypertension, diabetes, hyperlipidemias, smoking, collagen vascular disease, and some thrombophilias. During the first 24 hours, attention should be paid to maintaining normal blood sugar and adequate arterial pressure to ensure cerebral perfusion. Bed rest assists in cerebral perfusion by avoiding orthostatic changes in blood pressure. Heparin appears to play a minor role in the acute phase but in certain circumstances it is useful in preventing recurrence. Intracranial hypertension may develop and must be controlled

with dexamethasone and osmotic diuresis with mannitol. In the absence of vascular instability, maternal stroke poses little threat to the fetus. If associated with thrombophilia, this condition may pose an independent threat to fetal well-being.

Embolic Stroke

Embolic stroke usually occurs in the settings of valvular heart disease, atrial septal defect, cardiomyopathy, or arrhythmia. Such underlying etiologies are especially more common in nonhemorrhagic strokes in younger patients. For these reasons, cardiac evaluation is essential to the evaluation of maternal stroke. Once the diagnosis of embolic stroke is confirmed, the management is similar to thrombotic stroke with the exception of anticoagulation. As with thrombosis, heparin does little to improve the acute condition but is useful to prevent recurrence. In many cases anticoagulation should be delayed for 7 to 10 days to avoid converting an infarct into a hemorrhagic infarct.

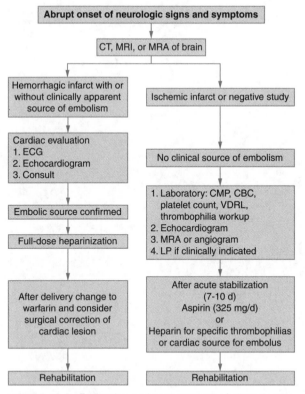

FIGURE 16-3. Evaluation and management of altered state of consciousness.

SUGGESTED READINGS

American College of Obstetricians and Gynecologists. *Seizure Disorders in Pregnancy.* Washington, DC: ACOG Educational Bulletin 231; 1996.

Hiilesmaa VK. Pregnancy and birth in women with epilepsy. *Neurology.* 1992;42(suppl 5):8.

Walker SP, Permezel M, Berkovic SF. The management of epilepsy in pregnancy. *BJOG.* 2009;116:758.

Silberstein SD. Headaches in pregnancy. *Neurol Clin.* 2004; 22:727.

Silberstein SD. Evaluation and emergency treatment of headache. *Headache.* 1992;32:396.

CHAPTER 17

Advanced Cardiac Life Support of the Pregnant Patient

• *Robert A. Raschke*

Cardiopulmonary arrest in pregnancy is very uncommon—occurring only once in every 30,000 pregnancies. Even at the busiest medical centers, this will only total a few cases per year. Because it is uncommon, it is difficult to study. Most of what we know regarding cardiopulmonary resuscitation (CPR) in pregnancy is based on animal experiments or observational studies in humans. There are no published randomized controlled clinical trials of CPR during pregnancy, and few clinicians have had the experience of running many obstetrical codes.

Advanced cardiac life support (ACLS) guidelines have been developed principally for sudden death from ischemic heart disease, a relative rarity during pregnancy. During pregnancy, arrest most often occurs in previously healthy woman related to acute events such as pulmonary embolism or hemorrhage. The unpredictability and rarity of sudden death during pregnancy makes preparation difficult. The single most important factor for improving the survival of mother and baby is a well-prepared, time-conscious, team approach.

The focus of this chapter will be to help you plan this approach. We will review pertinent pathophysiology, causes of cardiopulmonary arrest, preparation for ACLS response, and how to run a code from the aspect of the bedside clinician. It should be noted that the ACLS guidelines published by American College of Cardiologists are considered the gold standard in the United States. Nothing in this chapter should be interpreted as to conflict with these guidelines, but I have taken the liberty of offering simplification in a few areas, and expounding in a few others. Review of the ACLS guidelines reveal three major modifications for the pregnant patient that we will explain in detail: (1) focus on early endotracheal intubation, (2) leftward displacement of

the uterus during chest compressions, and (3) consideration of perimortem caesarean delivery within 4 minutes of onset of arrest. These few basics are easy to remember, and are the most important contents of this chapter.

■ CLINICAL PATHOPHYSIOLOGY OF CARDIAC ARREST IN PREGNANCY

Maternal cardiopulmonary adaptation to pregnancy allows a balanced delivery of oxygen to the mother's tissues and the uterus. The fetal cardiovascular system delivers oxygen to fetal tissues and returns blood to the placenta. The resulting circulatory interaction drives gas exchange from mother to fetus and maintains adequate oxygen delivery to the tissues. Protective mechanisms in normal pregnancy include increased maternal plasma volume, red blood cell mass, and cardiac output. The fetus develops an increased hemoglobin concentration with enhanced oxygen affinity. Clinical experience and animal experimentation indicate that during normal pregnancy, maternal systemic and uterine oxygen delivery far exceed the minimal level necessary to sustain maternal and fetal life—demonstrating a remarkable reserve to compensate for threatening conditions. During cardiopulmonary arrest, however, oxygen delivery to maternal tissue and the uterus is dramatically reduced or eliminated completely. Maternal or fetal adaptations to such severe insult are insufficient to sustain tissue viability. Death begins in minutes.

Pathophysiological Rationale for CPR Recommendations in Pregnancy

Some normal physiological changes of late pregnancy have deleterious effects on oxygen delivery. By approximately

TABLE 17-1. Interval from Death of Mother until Perimortem Caesarean Delivery of Surviving Infants: 1900 to 2004			
Interval (min)	All surviving infants	% of total healthy infants	% surviving with neurological injury
0-5	54 (1 with CNS injury)	71%	2%
6-10	12 (3 with CNS injury)	12%	25%
11-15	9 (2 with CNS injury)	9%	22%
>15	11 (5 with CNS injury)	8%	45%
Total	86	100%	

20 weeks' gestation, the gravid uterus begins to compress abdominal and pelvic blood vessels, particularly the inferior vena cava and aorta. This diminishes preload to the heart, decreases maternal stroke volume, and may decrease uteroplacental oxygen delivery. In about 10% of women, these effects are so profound that the patient will become hypotensive in a supine position, even in the absence of illness. Uterine aortocaval compression has two important clinical consequences during maternal arrest: (1) it must be temporarily relieved to optimize the effectiveness of CPR, and (2) it provides an opportunity to definitively improve maternal survival, since perimortem delivery can have a profound benefit on maternal hemodynamics.

In nonpregnant patients, chest compression is estimated to produce cardiac output approximately 30% of normal. Although the effectiveness of chest compressions in pregnancy is unknown, it is likely diminished by aortocaval compression. In healthy late term pregnancy, the gravid uterus can be shifted off the inferior vena cava if the patient is positioned in 15° left lateral decubitus position. This has been shown to result in a 25% increase in cardiac output. Therefore, when performing CPR on the patient with a gestational age >20 weeks, manual displacement of the uterus to the left and upward, or rotating the patient so that their left hip is down (blanket roll under the right hip), is recommended. Alternately, a Cardiff resuscitation wedge, specially designed to maintain the patient in 27° left lateral decubitus position, can be used. Lateral decubitus positioning greater than 30% have been shown to be associated with significantly reduced force generation during chest compressions.

Pathophysiological Rationale for Perimortem Caesarean Delivery—the 4-Minute Rule

Although the maneuvers discussed above may partially relieve vascular compression, perimortem delivery should theoretically be more effective. It has been shown that caesarean delivery immediately increases the cardiac output in healthy women by 30%. Delivery should drastically reduce the cardiac output demand of the uterus and placenta, which consume approximately 30% of maternal cardiac output near term, and also provide approximately a 500-mL autotransfusion. Additionally, delivery allows resuscitative access to the infant.

Katz and colleagues have reviewed all published data on perimortem caesarean deliveries from 1900 through 2004. Their combined analyses show that 71% of babies that survived maternal arrest with a good neurological outcome were delivered in 5 minutes or less (see Table 17-1) and that the rate of neurological injury among survivors increases dramatically as time to delivery increases. Maternal benefit of perimortem caesarean delivery is less well documented. Many case reports illustrate maternal recovery from refractory shock upon perimortem caesarean delivery, but publication bias should be considered when interpreting these reports.

The 4-Minute Rule

If the mother remains pulseless, and the baby is viable, caesarean delivery should be started by 4 minutes and completed by 5 minutes into the code.

Note that there is no rule that says delivery cannot be initiated *before* 4 minutes. If CPR is ineffective, or the cause of the arrest is unlikely to be reversed within 4 minutes (for instance, abruption) it is prudent to proceed directly to caesarean.

As an individual pregnancy progresses, increasing potential for maternal hemodynamic compromise by the enlarging uterus, and rapidly improving potential viability of the fetus lead to three clinically important pathophysiological states:

1. *Less than 20 weeks' gestation.* Insignificant hemodynamic compromise from uterus; baby nonviable. No benefit in perimortem caesarean delivery.

2. *Twenty to twenty-three weeks' gestation.* Possible hemodynamic compromise from uterus; baby unlikely to be viable. Perimortem caesarean delivery may be considered to save mother.

3. *Twenty-four weeks' or greater gestation.* Probable hemodynamic compromise from uterus; baby viable. Perform perimortem caesarean as indicated during arrest to benefit mother and baby.

If the patient's obstetrical dates are unknown, they can be estimated by bedside examination. The uterine fundus is usually palpable at the level of the umbilicus at approximately 20 weeks' gestation, and grows cephalad at a rate of about a centimeter per week. Therefore, potential fetal viability can be determined at the bedside if the uterine fundus is palpable at least 4 cm above the umbilicus in the supine position. Portable ultrasound can be useful for determining gestational age, but should not interfere with resuscitation.

Keep in mind that a great deal of preparation, both before and during the code is necessary to successfully perform a perimortem caesarean within 5 minutes.

Pathophysiological Rationale for Early Endotracheal Intubation

Note in the section above that in order to do a perimortem caesarean delivery, the patient will generally need to have been intubated. Physiological changes of late pregnancy increase the risk of life-threatening complications of endotracheal intubation about tenfold. Increased maternal oxygen consumption and a 20% reduction in the functional residual capacity of the lung due to compression by the gravid uterus, result in rapid oxygen desaturation if gas exchange is interrupted. Edema and hyperemia of the upper airway make airway bleeding more common and visualization of the vocal cords more difficult. Airway edema is further exacerbated in the presence of fluid overload due to preeclampsia. Decreased gastric motility and relaxation of esophageal sphincter tone increase the risk for aspiration.

Because of these factors, the decision to forego bag mask ventilation, and proceed directly to endotracheal intubation is generally made more rapidly in the pregnant patient. Intubation should be performed by the most experienced person available with difficult airway equipment available at the bedside. Efforts to prevent aspiration should be undertaken including avoidance of unnecessarily prolonged bag-masking (that will cause

gastric distention), and application of cricoid pressure during intubation to help diminish the risk of passive aspiration. Use of neuromuscular blocking agents and rapid sequence intubation can help prevent active vomiting leading to aspiration. Airway edema may necessitate the use of slightly smaller endotracheal tubes.

When pregnant patients are intubated in non-arrest situation, placement of a nasogastric tube and preoxygenation with 100% FiO_2 should be considered prior to intubation. We also routinely notify the obstetrical team of any elective intubation beforehand, and arrange for a second physician experienced in airway management to provide backup in case a difficult airway is encountered.

Code Pharmacology and Cardioversion

Little information is available regarding the use of code medications in pregnancy. Vasopressor agents commonly used in ACLS protocols, such as norepinephrine and vasopressin, are known to decrease uterine blood flow. However, the infant's best chance of survival is maternal survival. Therefore in full arrest, ACLS protocol pharmacology is not altered by pregnancy. Standard defibrillation/cardioversion energies are not altered by pregnancy. The electrical impedence of the chest wall is not significantly altered by pregnancy, and deleterious effects of maternal defibrillation/cardioversion have not been reported in infants.

■ THE CAUSES OF CARDIOPULMONARY ARREST IN PREGNANCY

The approach to ACLS in nonpregnant patients has a strong focus on managing the complications of ischemic heart disease, particularly shockable ventricular arrhythmias. By contrast, obstetrical arrest usually has a non-arrhythmogenic cause. In the standard ACLS terminology, this equates with "pulseless electrical activity" (PEA). The term "PEA/asystole" basically includes all causes of pulselessness not caused by ventricular tachycardia or ventricular fibrillation—in other words all causes of full arrest that an electric shock won't fix. Typically, the cause of PEA/asystole during pregnancy is difficult to initially determine. Yet, survival is usually dependent upon making a specific diagnosis and treating it.

The American College of Cardiology has offered the memory aid "**Hs** and **Ts**" to help clinicians remember the causes of PEA/asystole. Pregnancy entails some causes of cardiac arrest never (or rarely) seen in non-pregnant patients, such as amniotic fluid embolism, and

■ **TABLE 17-2. Differential of PEA/asystole in Pregnant Patients: the Hs and Ts**

Hs	Ts
Hypovolemia	**T**hrombosis/embolism
• Abruptio placentae	• Pulmonary embolism
• Placenta previa/	• Myocardial infarction
accreta/increta	• Amniotic fluid embolism
• Subcapsular hepatic	• Venous air embolism
hematoma	**T**ension pneumothorax
• Ectopic pregnancy	**T**amponade
• Uterine rupture	**T**oxins/tablets: epidural
Hypoxia	anes-**T**-hesia
Hyperkalemia/	
hypermagnesemia	
[**H**⁺] ↑ (acidosis)	
Hypoglycemia	
Hypertension-related	
complications of	
eclampsia/pre	
eclampsia	

hypermagnesemia. Therefore I have taken the liberty of altering the Hs and Ts slightly to apply them to the pregnant patient (Table 17-2). It is beyond the scope of this chapter to deal with each of these exhaustively; however, brief mention of a few is worth making because they require rapid clinical diagnosis and emergent therapy.

Hypovolemia

In an arrest, this refers to acute hemorrhage. A memory aide is not necessary if the bleeding is overt—it is the *occult* massive hemorrhage that requires some diagnostic effort. Because of hypervolemia of pregnancy, a pregnant patient can sustain massive blood loss before manifesting significant changes in vital signs. Most occult bleeds causing maternal arrest are of uteroplacental origin, such as abruption. Vaginal bleeding is often observable, but up to 2.5 L of blood can be concealed between the myometrium and placenta, so the hemodynamic effect may be much more severe than the apparent amount of blood loss. Consider hepatic subcapsular hematoma in the patient with preeclampsia who had complained of right-upper-quadrant pain.

Hypermagnesemia

Consider this diagnosis in any patient receiving intravenous magnesium for preterm labor or preeclampsia,

particularly those with renal insufficiency. Hyporeflexia is a physical finding compatible with severe hypermagnesemia. Electrocardiographic findings are similar to those seen in hyperkalemia, including peaked T-waves, and broadening of the QRS. Ultimately the ECG will demonstrate a sine-wave morphology as the QRS and T merge.

Thrombosis/Embolism: Pulmonary Embolism

Pregnancy is a thrombophilic state with a five- to tenfold increased risk for venous thromboembolism. Pulmonary embolism is the commonest cause of death in pregnancy accounting for approximately 20% of maternal mortality. Some patients with pulmonary embolism present with syncope or sudden death without prominent preceding dyspnea, or severe hypoxemia. Although bedside echocardiogram is not useful for the diagnosis of pulmonary embolism in general, it is sensitive during arrest because a patient in severe shock from a pulmonary embolism will have a dilated and hypocontractile right ventricle.

Thrombosis/Embolism: Amniotic Fluid Embolism

This catastrophic event usually occurs immediately following delivery, although it can occur at any time during pregnancy. It is uncommon, but has a mortality rate in excess of 50%. Pathophysiologically, it is most like anaphylaxis. It often presents with fulminant hypotension, hypoxemia, neurological deterioration, and bleeding secondary to disseminated intravascular coagulation (DIC). Echocardiography in patients with amniotic fluid embolism can show acute right heart failure secondary to pulmonary arteriospasm. It can be very difficult to tell amniotic fluid embolism and pulmonary embolism apart in a perimortem situation.

A few other causes of maternal death do not easily fit into this memory aid, but should not be forgotten—these include septic shock, congenital or acquired heart disease, and aortic dissection.

■ INSTITUTIONAL AND PERSONAL PREPARATION

Much of the work involved in successfully conducting ACLS in a pregnant patient occurs well before the arrest. The institution needs to have a plan in place to provide the required personnel and equipment to the patient's bedside with minimal delay around the clock. In obstetrical codes, this is complicated by the potential to require a bedside Caesarean section and neonatal resuscitation. At our institution, oversight of this process is provided by a medical staff committee that meets every month.

The code team needs to be able to immediately provide the following services around the clock:

- Code team leadership
- Airway management
- Drug preparation/administration
- Caesarean delivery
- Record keeping
- Chest compressions
- Vascular access
- Rhythm monitoring/defibrillator
- Neonatal resuscitation

Each individual in the team should be an expert at his or her particular assignment, but studies have shown significant deficiencies in the knowledge of caregivers in regards to obstetrical arrest. ACLS certification and recertification are helpful. Our institution and others have the advantage of utilizing a simulation center to practice code responses.

Personnel not assigned a specific task on the code team should steer clear of the patient's room. In general, onlookers increase the noise and stress level of the code, detracting from the code team's performance. One exception to consider occurs in teaching institutions. We incorporate residents into our code team, but only doing tasks that they are well trained in, such as providing chest compressions and vascular access.

Although many experienced clinicians are likely to be present at the code, and any code member might have a good suggestion, codes run best when there is one established leader giving all the orders. Establishing authority for code leadership requires some forethought and discussion between specialties.

People who assume responsibility for running codes are familiar with a few prerequisites of the job. It is the responsibility of the code leader to make sure each other member of the team is doing their job. The code leader should also anticipate the needs of the patient during the code. For instance, with the knowledge that perimortem caesarean delivery might required, it's incumbent upon the person running the code to be sure that the patient is intubated, and all equipment and personnel necessary to deliver and resuscitate the baby is available within the first 4 minutes of the code. This will not be possible in the unprepared institution or unprepared code leader.

■ A STEPWISE APPROACH FOR MANAGEMENT OF A PREGNANT WOMAN IN CARDIOPULMONARY ARREST

Disclaimer: The American College of Cardiology algorithms are the gold standard for running codes in the United States. Nothing contained in our chapter is intended to conflict with those algorithms, but we have sought to simplify them a bit, and focus them on the care of the pregnant patient. The reader should refer to the ACLS 2005 guidelines for full details (see App A through C).

Consider the following scenario: you are designated as the code leader and you have just entered the room of a pregnant patient with a viable fetus who is pulseless and apneic. Basic life support has already begun.

1. *Establish leadership.* Note time of arrest and gestational age. Mentally plan to initiate perimortem Caesarean within 4 minutes, if pulse not re-established by then.
2. *Assess the airway and breathing.* (A and B of the "ABC"s). Give 100% oxygen. Instruct airway team to proceed with intubation.
3. *Assess CPR.* Ensure manual displacement of uterus to the left or place patient left side down. Chest compressions should be hard and fast—100 compressions per minute. If no pulse with compressions, consider immediate caesarean. Also consider immediate delivery if the cause of the arrest is unlikely to be reversible within 4 minutes (for instance abruption).
4. *Allocate a team member to establish central venous access.* Large-bore catheters such as 9-French introducer in the internal jugular or subclavian position are preferred in case massive transfusion is required.
5. *Assess team resources.* Be sure that personnel and equipment necessary to perform caesarean delivery and to resuscitate the baby are present.
6a. *Check the rhythm.* Rhythm interpretation in the pulseless patient can be simplified, since only ventricular fibrillation (Fig 17-1) and fast ventricular tachycardia cause pulselessness in the absence of another primary threat to life. Ventricular tachycardia can be monomorphic or polymorphic (Figs 17-2 and 17-3). An overall approach to rhythm interpretation is illustrated in Fig 17-4.
6b. *If the rhythm is ventricular tachycardia or ventricular fibrillation, shock the patient.* Remove the fetal monitor lead prior to shock. Refer to Fig 17-5.

The stark distinction in ACLS algorithms between pulseless ventricular arrhythmias and PEA/asystole is

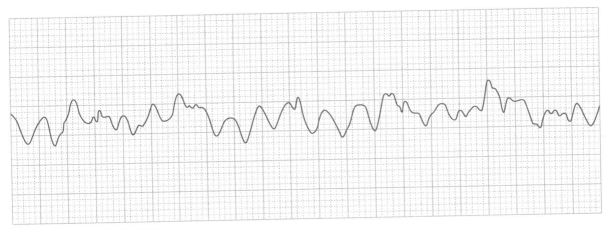

FIGURE 17-1. Ventricular fibrillation.

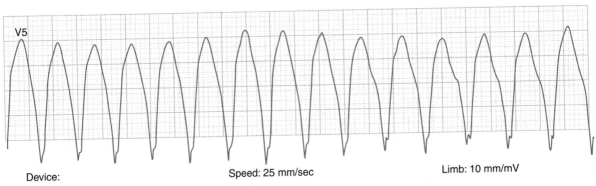

Device: Speed: 25 mm/sec   Limb: 10 mm/mV

FIGURE 17-2. Ventricular tachycardia (monomorphic).

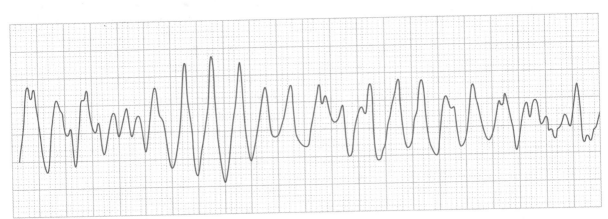

FIGURE 17-3. Ventricular tachycardia (polymorphic).

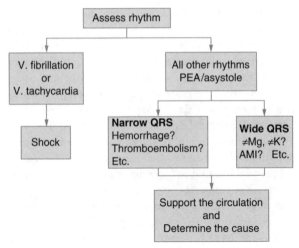

FIGURE 17-4. Simplified approach to rhythm interpretation in pulseless patient.

important to properly guide immediate therapy, but in an arrest situation, the code leader will often jump back and forth between these two algorithms as the patient's clinical condition changes. Pregnant patients often suffer episodes of ventricular fibrillation and ventricular tachycardia in the course of an arrest, even though the underlying threat to life is actually one of the causes of PEA/asystole. These arrhythmias are likely secondary to acute cardiac ischemia secondary to shock, or severe metabolic derangements caused by

---

Ventricular fibrillation (VF) or pulseless ventricular tachycardia (VT)
Shock once at 150 J biphasic*, (360 J monophasic) restart CPR immediately and continue for 2 min

↓

Reassess rhythm, *if still VF or VT:* shock again
Resume CPR immediately, give vasopressin 40 U IV, and continue CPR for 2 min

↓

Reassess rhythm, *if still VF or VT:* shock again
Resume CPR immediately, give amiodarone 300 mg IV, and continue CPR for 2 min

*Recommended shock energy is device-specific. Check your defibrillator for optimal shock energy.

FIGURE 17-5. If pulselessness is caused by a ventricular fibrillation or ventricular tachycardia, proceed stepwise.

---

a noncardiac insult. So even if the initial rhythm is ventricular fibrillation or ventricular tachycardia, the code leader should still consider the differential of PEA/asystole (see below). *Have 4 minutes gone by yet? If so, and no pulse, proceed to perimortem caesarean delivery.*

7. *If the patient is not in VF or VT, look to the PEA/asystole algorithm.*

7a. *Support the circulation.* Give epinephrine 1 mg IV or vasopressin 40 units IV. Some patients with PEA have electrical mechanical dissociation—that is, there is electrical activity in the heart, but no discernable mechanical systole. Others still have a mechanically functioning ventricle, but the blood pressure generated is too low to generate a palpable pulse. Generally, there is no way to tell these apart in a code (and no absolute need to do so). However, patients in the later group have a better prognosis and particularly may benefit from further hemodynamic support with intravenous fluids and additional pressor agents such as norepinephrine.

7b. *Consider the cause.* Survival of patients in PEA/asystole is dependent on rapidly determining and reversing the underlying cause. A list of causes of PEA/asystole in pregnancy was considered earlier in this chapter. It is the responsibility of the code leader to rapidly consider this differential and make a clinical decision on which are likely enough to warrant specific therapy. There is often not enough time in a code to perform laboratory or radiographical studies to confirm specific diagnoses, therefore the code leader has to rely on bedside diagnosis.

A focused history may provide clues to the cause of PEA/asystole—the patient may have been admitted for a deep venous thrombosis and complained of sudden onset dyspnea before collapsing. A targeted bedside examination might reveal conjunctival pallor, and an abnormally firm and hard uterus related to abruption. As the code leader recalls the differential diagnosis of PEA/asystole at the bedside, the appropriate history and physical examination can be elicited. This is the best chance the code leader has for determining the etiology of the arrest.

Review of the cardiac rhythm can also provide some clues. A wide QRS complex (≥ 0.12 s) indicates that the electrical-chemical environment is abnormal (eg, hyperkalemia or hypermagnesemia) or that the conduction system of the heart is dying (eg, myocardial infarction). A wide QRS isn't specific though because any cause of PEA/asystole can ultimately result in a wide complex QRS as the heart becomes ischemic. A narrow complex QRS indicates that the conduction system of the heart is functional. This is typically seen earlier in arrest, for instance, in patients who are hemorrhaging or who have suffered pulmonary embolism.

If available, portable ultrasonography can be very helpful so long as it doesn't interfere with ACLS. It might show a dilated hypocontractile right ventricle consistent with pulmonary embolism, or a hyperdynamic, underfilled left ventricle in hemorrhagic shock. Abdominal/pelvic ultrasound may demonstrate occult hemorrhage in the liver or uterus.

7c. Treat the cause

If You Think the Patient Is Hemorrhaging:
Push IVF rapidly using low resistance IV tubing (blood transfusion tubing) with a manual pump. A liter of fluid can be given in less than 5 minutes with the appropriate equipment. Standard IV Infusion pumps deliver inadequate rates for resuscitation (typically < 1 L/h), but rapid infusion pumps can be very helpful. Patients that are pulseless from bleeding will likely require large volumes of packed red blood cells as well as fresh frozen plasma and platelets—best to get the blood bank working on all needed blood products immediately. Hemostasis may require surgical intervention.

If You Think the Patient Is Hypermagnesemic or Hyperkalemic:
Give CaCl, 5 mEq IV and repeat if warranted. Electrocardiographic abnormalities related to these electrolyte abnormalities generally normalize with 1 to 2 doses. Further treatment of hyperkalemia may include intravenous bicarbonate 50 mEq, nebulized albuterol 10 mg, and intravenous insulin 10 units + intravenous D50 1 ampule.

If You Think the Patient Has a Pulmonary Embolism:
Give intravenous fluids to optimize preload of the right ventricle. Norepinephrine can be used to support the circulation if a pulse is recovered. In some cases, circulatory support will restore a pulse. Despite the high risk of bleeding complications, systemic thrombolytic therapy can be considered in several situations. If a pulse is recovered, and the need for immediate delivery abates, thrombolytic therapy may be considered if in the clinician's judgment the pulmonary embolism remains life-threatening. This will dangerously complicate hemostasis should a caesarean delivery be required within the next 24 hours or so, but in some patients the potential benefit may outweigh the risk. Echocardiography is often helpful in this situation since severe right heart failure is highly predictive of poor prognosis and argues in favor of aggressive therapy. Thrombolytic therapy can also be considered *after* perimortem caesarean if maternal circulation is not restored. This very difficult decision might be appropriately made in situations in which there is no other reasonable hope for maternal survival but to give lytics and risk bleeding. We have observed our obstetricians achieve reasonable surgical hemostasis during caesarean delivery in a patient who had just received 50 mg of tissue plasminogen activator (tPA)—the agent we use to treat arrest from pulmonary embolism. The operative team should take part in the decision to give thrombolytics—as it may subsequently befall them to ligate the uterine arteries or crossclamp the aorta. Catheter-directed thrombolysis and thrombectomy are options in some institutions, but are unlikely to be as rapidly applied.

If You Think the Patient Has Amniotic Fluid Embolism:
Support the circulation as above, consider cardiopulmonary bypass.

Consider the full differential diagnosis of PEA/asystole listed in Table 17-2. Other causes including hypoglycemia, tension pneumothorax, and tamponade require specific therapy not listed in the algorithm above.

By Now, 5 Minutes Have Certainly Passed, and Caesarean Delivery Should Have Been Completed if Pulse Was Not Restored:
We have focused on resuscitation of the pulseless patient in the section above, but the appendices include ACLS algorithms for the treatment of unstable patients *with a pulse* related to tachycardia (App B) and bradycardia (App C)

■ POST-ARREST CARE

In many critically ill obstetrical patients, there is a fine and somewhat artificial line between CPR, and post-code resuscitation. The code "ends" when a pulse is detected, and CPR is stopped. But the reason the patient arrested often persists and requires ongoing therapy. We have separated out continued post-arrest therapy from that likely to be administered during CPR. Remarkable neurologic recovery has been observed in pregnant patients who have survived prolonged cardiopulmonary arrest. We advocate an aggressive approach in the hours and days after a cardiac arrest.

Here are some things to consider in the hour after the code.

- Consider non-closure of the abdominal incision if caesarean was necessary. This will facilitate direct access for ligation maternal vessels if necessary and allow for cross clamping vascular structures, in extreme cases. It will also ameliorate the possibility of abdominal compartment syndrome.
- Resuscitated patients who have suffered massive hemorrhage or amniotic embolism are likely to have developed consumptive and dilutional coagulopathy. They will likely require further transfusion therapy with fresh frozen plasma and platelets. Cryoprecipitate is often required to repair hypofibrinogenemia. Oxytocin and prostaglandins can be administered to correct uterine atony. Rewarming of the hypothermic patient may improve hemostasis. Activated factor VII (45-90 mcg/kg) has occasionally been a useful hemostatic adjunct. Interventional radiology can often provide hemostasis of uterine arterial origin via embolization.
- Massive transfusions may be associated with complications such as hydrostatic pulmonary edema, transfusion-related lung injury, and hypocalcemia from citrate toxicity.
- Intra-abdominal hemorrhage can lead to abdominal-compartment syndrome, wherein elevated intra-abdominal pressure is transmitted to the chest and essentially tamponades the heart. This syndrome is treated by laparotomy.
- In cases of massive pulmonary embolism, surgical thrombectomy can be life-saving. Thrombolytic therapy is not contraindicated in pregnancy and can also be life-saving.
- Many important causes of maternal arrest and death are not included in the Hs and Ts. Sepsis and preeclampsia are examples that don't have specific ACLS interventions, but may require emergent post resuscitative treatment. In particular, patients with severe preeclampsia/eclampsia may suffer from posterior reversible encephalopathy syndrome requiring emergent antihypertensive therapy.

Additional Considerations: Therapeutic Hypothermia

Two randomized controlled trials demonstrate that patients who suffer cardiac arrest secondary to ventricular fibrillation have improved neurological outcomes if they are treated with 24 hours of mild hypothermia (32-34°C). Pregnant patients were excluded from these studies, and few pregnant patients have primary ventricular fibrillation as the cause of their arrest. Nevertheless, there is no compelling logic to argue that hypothermia should benefit cerebral recovery only when the cerebral perfusion insult was caused by ventricular fibrillation. Therefore, some believe that the benefit of hypothermia therapy can be extrapolated to patients with PEA/asystole. We consider hypothermia therapy in pregnant women who do not regain consciousness within an hour of arrest, even if the arrest is not due to ventricular arrhythmia. Therapeutic hypothermia is a potentially dangerous intervention that should only be performed by clinicians experienced in its application.

Somatic Support of the Brain Dead Mother to Achieve Fetal Viability

Rarely, a pregnant woman suffers brain death while carrying a fetus that is not yet viable. This may occur when the cause of the death is an intracranial hemorrhage, brain trauma, or brain tumor. Such patients may demonstrate hemodynamic instability, but may not suffer cardiopulmonary arrest. Multiple reports have described somatic support of the mother's body in order to bring the baby close enough to term for a good chance of survival. In one case at our institution, a 23 week old infant was brought to 30 weeks maturity and successfully delivered. Homeostasis of cardiopulmonary, endocrine, and other somatic systems requires a committed critical care team, but can yield a bright outcome in the midst of tragedy.

■ CONCLUSION

Consider these closing thoughts. An obstetrical code is a situation in which a physician is essentially called upon to save two lives in less than 5 minutes. Although it's lucky that obstetrical arrests are rare, their infrequency degrades our ability to study them and our readiness to deal with them when the sudden need arises. Understanding the pathophysiology, and preparing ahead of time—on an individual and institutional level—are the keys to providing the best chance for the mother and the baby to survive. If you are ever called upon to manage an obstetrical code, use the ACLS algorithms, intubate early, displace the uterus to the left during chest compressions, and remember the 4-minute rule.

SUGGESTED READINGS

American Heart Association: Guidelines 2005 for cardiopulmonary resuscitation and emergency cardiovascular care. Cardiac arrest associated with pregnancy. ACLS 2005. *Circulation.* 2005;112:IV-150-IV-153.

Atta E, Gardner M. Cardiopulmonary resuscitation in pregnancy. *Obstet Gynecol Clin North Am.* 2007;34:585-597.

Campbell TA, Sanson TG. Cardiac arrest and pregnancy. *J Emerg Trauma Shock.* 2009;2:34-42.

Castrén M, Silfvast T, Rubertsson S, et al. Task Force on Scandinavian Therapeutic Hypothermia Guidelines, Clinical Practice Committee Scandinavian Society of Anaesthesiology and Intensive care Medicine. Scandinavian clinical practice guidelines for therapeutic hypothermia and postresuscitation care after cardiac arrest. *Acta Anaesthesiol Scand.* 2009 Mar;53(3):280-288.

Cunningham FG, Leveno KJ, Bloom SL, Hauth JC, Gilstrap L, Wenstrom KD. Maternal physiology. In: Cunningham FG, Leveno KJ, Bloom SL, Hauth JC, Gilstrap L, Wenstrom KD, eds. *Williams Obstetrics.* 22nd ed. New York, NY: McGraw-Hill; 2005.

Katz V, Balderston K, DeFreest M. Perimortem cesarean delivery: Were our assumptions correct? *Am J Obstet Gynecol.* 2005;192:1916-1921.

Katz VL, Dotter DJ, Droegemueller W. Perimortem cesarean delivery. *Obstet Gynecol.* 1986;68(4):571.

Mallampalli A, Guy E. Cardiac arrest in pregnancy and somatic support after brain death. *Crit Care Med.* 2005;33(suppl 10):325S-331S.

Meschia G. Placental respiratory gas exchange and fetal oxygenation. In: Creasy RK, Resnick R, eds. *Maternal-Fetal Medicine: Principles and Practice.* 5th ed. Philadelphia, PA: W.B. Saunders; 2004:199-208.

Munnur U, de Boisblanc B, Suresh MS. Airway problems in pregnancy. *Crit Care Med.* 2005;33(suppl 10):259S-268S.

Soar J, Deakin CD, Nolan JP, et al. European Resuscitation Council Guidelines for Resuscitation 2005: Section 7. Cardiac arrest in special circumstances. *Resuscitation.* 2005;67S1:S135-S170.

Strong TH, Lowe RA. Perimortem cesarean section. *Am J Emerg Med.* 1989;7:489-494.

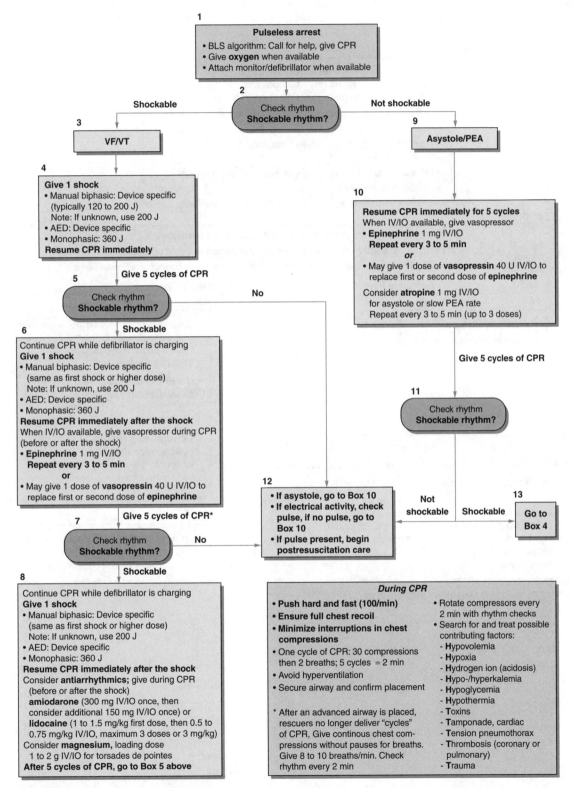

APPENDIX A. ACLS Algorithm for Pulseless Arrest.

1

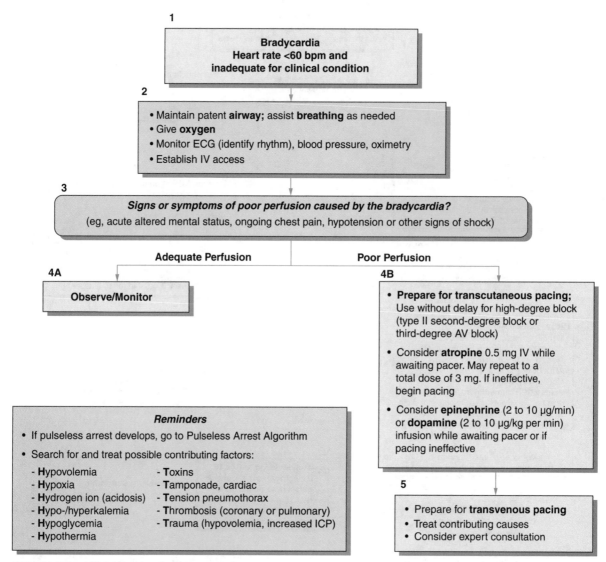

> **Bradycardia**
> **Heart rate <60 bpm and**
> **inadequate for clinical condition**

2

- Maintain patent **airway;** assist **breathing** as needed
- Give **oxygen**
- Monitor ECG (identify rhythm), blood pressure, oximetry
- Establish IV access

3

Signs or symptoms of poor perfusion caused by the bradycardia?
(eg, acute altered mental status, ongoing chest pain, hypotension or other signs of shock)

Adequate Perfusion   **Poor Perfusion**

4A

Observe/Monitor

4B

- **Prepare for transcutaneous pacing;**
  Use without delay for high-degree block
  (type II second-degree block or
  third-degree AV block)

- Consider **atropine** 0.5 mg IV while
  awaiting pacer. May repeat to a
  total dose of 3 mg. If ineffective,
  begin pacing

- Consider **epinephrine** (2 to 10 µg/min)
  or **dopamine** (2 to 10 µg/kg per min)
  infusion while awaiting pacer or if
  pacing ineffective

Reminders
- If pulseless arrest develops, go to Pulseless Arrest Algorithm
- Search for and treat possible contributing factors:

  - **H**ypovolemia   - **T**oxins
  - **H**ypoxia   - **T**amponade, cardiac
  - **H**ydrogen ion (acidosis) - **T**ension pneumothorax
  - **H**ypo-/hyperkalemia   - **T**hrombosis (coronary or pulmonary)
  - **H**ypoglycemia   - **T**rauma (hypovolemia, increased ICP)
  - **H**ypothermia

5

- Prepare for **transvenous pacing**
- Treat contributing causes
- Consider expert consultation

APPENDIX B. ACLS Algorithm for Bradycardia.

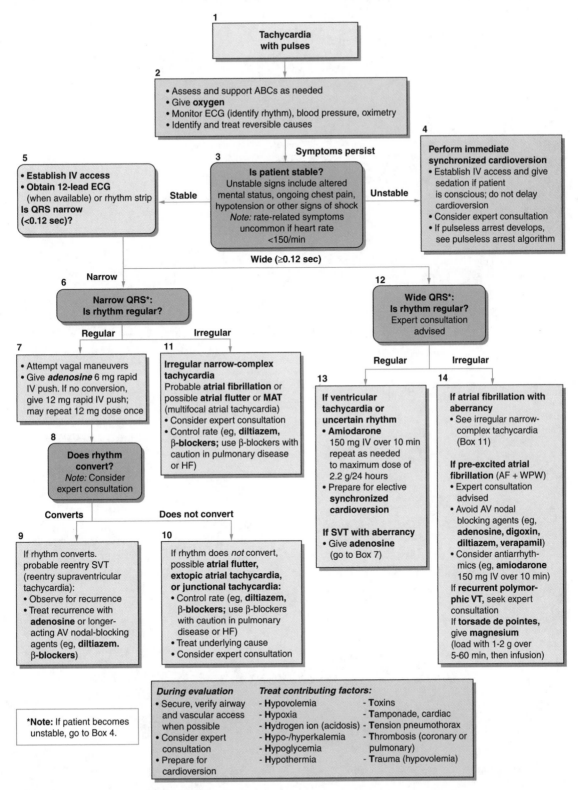

1

Tachycardia
with pulses

2
- Assess and support ABCs as needed
- Give **oxygen**
- Monitor ECG (identify rhythm), blood pressure, oximetry
- Identify and treat reversible causes

Symptoms persist

3
Is patient stable?
Unstable signs include altered mental status, ongoing chest pain, hypotension or other signs of shock
Note: rate-related symptoms uncommon if heart rate <150/min

4
Perform immediate synchronized cardioversion
- Establish IV access and give sedation if patient is conscious; do not delay cardioversion
- Consider expert consultation
- If pulseless arrest develops, see pulseless arrest algorithm

Stable — Unstable

5
- **Establish IV access**
- **Obtain 12-lead ECG** (when available) or rhythm strip
Is QRS narrow (<0.12 sec)?

Wide (≥0.12 sec)

Narrow

6
Narrow QRS*:
Is rhythm regular?

Regular — Irregular

12
Wide QRS*:
Is rhythm regular?
Expert consultation advised

Regular — Irregular

7
- Attempt vagal maneuvers
- Give *adenosine* 6 mg rapid IV push. If no conversion, give 12 mg rapid IV push; may repeat 12 mg dose once

11
Irregular narrow-complex tachycardia
Probable **atrial fibrillation** or possible **atrial flutter** or **MAT** (multifocal atrial tachycardia)
- Consider expert consultation
- Control rate (eg, **diltiazem, β-blockers**; use β-blockers with caution in pulmonary disease or HF)

8
Does rhythm convert?
Note: Consider expert consultation

Converts — Does not convert

13
If ventricular tachycardia or uncertain rhythm
- **Amiodarone** 150 mg IV over 10 min repeat as needed to maximum dose of 2.2 g/24 hours
- Prepare for elective **synchronized cardioversion**

If SVT with aberrancy
- Give **adenosine** (go to Box 7)

14
If atrial fibrillation with aberrancy
- See irregular narrow-complex tachycardia (Box 11)

If pre-excited atrial fibrillation (AF + WPW)
- Expert consultation advised
- Avoid AV nodal blocking agents (eg, **adenosine, digoxin, diltiazem, verapamil**)
- Consider antiarrhythmics (eg, **amiodarone** 150 mg IV over 10 min)
If recurrent polymorphic VT, seek expert consultation
If torsade de pointes, give **magnesium** (load with 1-2 g over 5-60 min, then infusion)

9
If rhythm converts. probable reentry SVT (reentry supraventricular tachycardia):
- Observe for recurrence
- Treat recurrence with **adenosine** or longer-acting AV nodal-blocking agents (eg, **diltiazem. β-blockers**)

10
If rhythm does *not* convert, possible **atrial flutter, extopic atrial tachycardia, or junctional tachycardia:**
- Control rate (eg, **diltiazem, β-blockers**; use β-blockers with caution in pulmonary disease or HF)
- Treat underlying cause
- Consider expert consultation

*Note: If patient becomes unstable, go to Box 4.

During evaluation
- Secure, verify airway and vascular access when possible
- Consider expert consultation
- Prepare for cardioversion

Treat contributing factors:
- Hypovolemia
- Hypoxia
- Hydrogen ion (acidosis)
- Hypo-/hyperkalemia
- Hypoglycemia
- Hypothermia

- Toxins
- Tamponade, cardiac
- Tension pneumothorax
- Thrombosis (coronary or pulmonary)
- Trauma (hypovolemia)

APPENDIX C. ACLS Algorithm for Tachycardia.

CHAPTER 18

Trauma and Pregnancy

• *Cathleen M. Harris*

■ SCOPE OF THE PROBLEM

Trauma complicates up to 6%-7% of pregnancies, and trauma registries indicate that 4%-8% of trauma cases involve pregnant women. The rate of fetal mortality after trauma is significant (3%-38% after blunt abdominal trauma), and fetal loss can occur without significant maternal injury. Thus, all pregnant women should be evaluated after trauma, even in the setting of a minor incident.

Pregnant women are hospitalized for injuries more commonly than many physicians realize. In 2002, there were 4.1 injury hospitalizations per 1000 deliveries in the United States (16,982 cases). When compared to nonpregnant trauma patients, pregnant women are younger, less severely injured, and more likely to be African American or Hispanic. Twenty percent of pregnant trauma patients tested positive for drugs or alcohol in one study. In one series, 19%-24% of trauma patients delivered when they required hospitalization for an injury.

■ TRAUMA-RELATED MATERNAL ADAPTATIONS TO PREGNANCY

Physiological changes of pregnancy directly affect how pregnant women respond to trauma, and how providers should interpret examination findings and laboratory values. Table 18-1 provides a summary of pertinent changes.

■ MECHANISM OF TRAUMA

According to a study of cases reported to the NTDB between 1994 and 2001, the mechanisms for injuries were as follows: motor vehicle crash (55%), fall (13%), interpersonal violence (10%), bicycle/recreation (4%), pedestrian struck (4%), and other (11%).

Motor vehicle crashes account for two-thirds of trauma during pregnancy overall, a fact that is not surprising when one reviews trends in automobile use. The average number of miles driven annually by women of reproductive age increased from 3721 to 8258 during 1975 to 2001. Pregnant women have similar rates of using seat belts (14%) and seat position (70% driver) as nonpregnant women. Nonetheless, it is estimated that the rate of fetal death due to motor vehicle crashes now exceeds infant death by a factor of 7.

Partner violence is an important contributor to maternal trauma. In 1999, homicide was the third leading cause of injury-related death for women aged 15 to 44 years, after motor vehicle crashes and suicide, and it was the second leading cause among women <24 years and black women (3× higher than whites). The pregnancy-associated homicide ratio was 1.7 per 100,000 live births, with firearms being the leading mechanism of homicide (57%).

Patterns of Injury

Blunt abdominal trauma accounts for two-thirds of cases. Blunt trauma most often results from motor vehicle crashes, falls, pedestrian injuries, and assaults are other sources of blunt trauma. The uterus is protected within the pelvis until 12 weeks, so chances of injury are limited. At 20 weeks, the uterus is at the level of the umbilicus. After 20 weeks, the fundal height (in centimeters) corresponds to weeks of gestation. The bladder is displaced upward as the uterus grows, making it an intra-abdominal organ vulnerable to injury. The uterine wall becomes thinner and the relative amount of amniotic fluid decreases with advancing gestation; these changes contribute to the possibility of adverse placental or fetal effects.

■ TABLE 18-1. Trauma-Related Maternal Adaptations to Pregnancy

Category	Adaptation	Clinical consequences
Cardiovascular system	Cardiac output increases 30%-50% Pulse increase (10-15 bpm) Blood pressure declines	Adaption to tolerate blood loss
Hematological system	Plasma volume increases 40%-50% RBC mass increases 30%	Dilutional anemia Circulating blood volume 6 L
Pulmonary system	Minute ventilation increases 30%-40% FRC decreases 20%	Respiratory alkalosis normal Decreased Pco_2 Rapid desaturation if supine or apneic
Uterus and placenta	20%-30% shunt Marked increase in uterine size Placental flow, high flow and low resistance circuit	Potential rapid blood loss Abdominal organs displaced Supine hypotension
Gastrointestinal system	Slowed stomach emptying Organ displacement	Risk of aspiration Site of injury influences organ damage

Penetrating trauma typically involves gunshot or stab wounds. Gunshot wounds are more common, but the risk of death is decreased in pregnant women compared with nonpregnant women. The gravid uterus provides protection to abdominal organs, so wounds are less likely to cause bowel or vascular injury. However, upper abdominal wounds can be associated with complex bowel injuries in late pregnancy, since the bowel is displaced. Gunshot wounds to the abdomen may enter the uterus and cause fetal injury in up to 70% of cases, with a high fetal mortality rate (40%-65%).

Pelvic fracture represents a serious injury, often with hypovolemic shock due to retroperitoneal or intra-abdominal hemorrhage. Pelvic fracture during pregnancy is associated with a high maternal mortality rate (9%) and fetal mortality (35%), although the fracture type and classification does not appear to affect obstetric (OB) outcomes. Pelvic fracture alone is not a contraindication to vaginal delivery, but severely dislocated or unstable fractures may be a reason to consider cesarean as the route of delivery.

■ MATERNAL AND FETAL OUTCOMES AFTER TRAUMA

Maternal Injury

Fractures, dislocations, sprains, and strains are the most common maternal diagnoses after trauma. However, internal injuries are most highly associated with maternal death. This is likely related to an increased severity of hemorrhage and relative difficulty in diagnosing intra-abdominal pathology. Uncommon types of maternal injuries reported in published literature include thoracic aorta rupture or liver rupture. In rare instances, severe burns, electrical injury, or spinal cord injury can affect pregnancy—the patient should be treated in the same fashion as a nonpregnant individual. Regardless of the type of maternal injury, a variety of adverse sequelae have been reported. Trauma can affect pregnancy outcomes via direct uteroplacental injury, or may be a marker for behavioral risk factors; thus, both short- and long-term complications are possible.

Fetal Death

A 3-year study of fetal death certificates from 16 states identified 240 fetal deaths due to maternal trauma (3.7 per 100,000 live births). Motor vehicle crashes accounted for 82% of cases, with firearms and falls accounting for 6% and 3% of cases, respectively. Fifteen- to nineteen-year olds had the highest rate of fetal deaths, at 9.3 per 100,000. Placental injury was cited in 42% of cases, and maternal death in 11% of cases. The risk of fetal or infant death is strongly influenced by gestational age at delivery. The most common reported risk factors for fetal death include ejection from car, maternal death, maternal tachycardia, abnormal fetal heart rate pattern, lack of restraints, and high injury severity score (>9-15). Other important clinical risk factors include prolonged maternal hypotension or hypoxemia, abruption, uterine rupture, and direct uterine trauma.

Adverse Pregnancy Outcomes: PTL, Abruption, Fetomaternal Hemorrhage, Uterine Rupture

Women hospitalized for trauma during pregnancy due to motor vehicle crashes are well-known to be at increased risk for placental abruption and cesarean delivery, and their infants are at higher risk for respiratory distress syndrome and fetal death. However, uninjured pregnant women experiencing trauma are also at risk for preterm labor and placental abruption (relative risks of 7.9 and 6.6, respectively). The worst outcomes are seen among women who deliver during the initial trauma hospitalization. Complications in such cases include maternal death, fetal death, uterine rupture, or abruption. Women with prenatal injury (but not delivery) also are at risk for adverse outcomes at delivery, including abruption, preterm labor, and maternal death.

Preterm contractions are common among third trimester trauma patients (25%), but these resolve spontaneously in 90%. Even after trauma center discharge, the risk for preterm birth and low birth weight is twice as high for the rest of the pregnancy, and is higher with increasing injury severity or trauma <24 weeks' gestation. Risk factors most predictive of PTL include gestational age >35 weeks, assaults and pedestrian collisions, according to one study. It is important to monitor women carefully during the remainder of their pregnancy even after the initial trauma episode.

Placental abruption is one of the most common complications of blunt abdominal trauma. Typical signs and symptoms include vaginal bleeding, painful contractions, and fetal distress. However, the clinical presentation can be subtle in cases where there is concealed hemorrhage. Historical risk markers include low education level, nonwhite race, lack of seat belt use, and high-speed collision. Clinical risk factors include maternal tachycardia, abdominal pain, vaginal bleeding, PROM, uterine contractions, and abnormal fetal heart rate pattern. The risk of abruption is 1% to 5% after minor trauma, but up to 40% to 50% after severe injury.

Fetomaternal hemorrhage (FMH) involves fetal bleeding into the maternal bloodstream. FMH is seen in up to 30% of severe trauma. The clinical consequences can be severe, such as fetal death due to acute hemorrhage, fetal hydrops, and maternal sensitization to RhD or other minor antigens. Fortunately, the mean fetal blood loss is typically low, with 98% of cases less than 30 mL. FMH is usually detected via Kleihauer-Betke (KB) testing, but can be evaluated using flow cytometry or other methods.

Uterine rupture is estimated to occur in 0.6% of all maternal traumas. Uterine rupture is the result of direct abdominal impact with high force. The extent of injury and clinical presentation are highly variable. Seventy five percent of cases involve the fundal region of the uterus, and fetal death is common. Among cases of uterine rupture after trauma, maternal death was seen in 10%—much higher than for cases of uterine rupture due to other causes. Clinical features include uterine pain or tenderness, non-reassuring fetal heart rate pattern, abdominal distension, peritoneal signs, and vital sign changes from minimal tachycardia to hypovolemic shock.

Direct fetal trauma complicates <1% of all pregnancies following trauma. Most cases result from serious maternal injury or from penetrating trauma. Unusual fetal consequences of trauma include limb-body wall complex, fetal subdural hemorrhage, and fetal CNS damage, such as hydrocephalus or cerebral palsy. Cases of uterine rupture with fetal death and fetal spinal fracture have been reported, even with seat belts.

■ APPROACH TO THE PATIENT

Initial Management

Pregnant trauma victims are typically evaluated in a level I trauma unit. The trauma team is composed of emergency room (ER) or trauma physicians and nurses, as well as anesthesia personnel. An OB physician and nurse should be on standby for secondary assessment, once the patient is stabilized and the initial evaluation is complete. Persons able to perform neonatal resuscitation, as well as delivery and neonatal equipment, should be immediately available.

Physical examination for the pregnant trauma patient should include all elements as in nonpregnant women, with additional attention to items pertaining to pregnancy. Pregnancy can be confirmed by examination of the uterus, ultrasound, and/or serum HCG testing.

Primary Survey

The initial assessment should take only a few minutes. The ABCDE framework allows for a complete yet efficient exam, and is no different from any other nonpregnant patient. *It is important to stabilize the mother first, and then turn attention to the pregnancy and fetus.*

A—Airway	Immobilize the cervical spine. Clear obstruction or secretions. Maintain neutral head position. Use laryngeal mask airway or endotracheal tube if needed.
B—Breathing	Check respiratory rate and effort. Supply supplemental oxygen in most cases. Use continuous pulse oximetry.
C—Circulation	Assess pulse and BP, including orthostatics if needed. Establish two large-bore IV lines. Replete blood loss with isotonic crystalloid in a 3:1 ratio.
D—Disability	Assign injury severity score (ISS)[a] or Glasgow Coma Scale (GCS) score Report alertness (alert, respond to voice or pain, unresponsive).
E—Expose the patient	Remove all clothing; inspect the entire body for wounds or ecchymoses.

[a]ISS scores have a similar predictive value for pregnant women vs nonpregnant individuals.

Secondary Assessment

After initial stabilization, evaluate for specific maternal injuries and assess fetal well-being. Adjunctive laboratory tests focus on injury patterns related to the mechanism of injury, patient complaints, or suspicious findings on exam. A secondary survey includes an early vaginal and rectal examination, with attention to dilation and effacement of the cervix. If vaginal bleeding is present in the second or third trimester, cervical examination should be deferred until sonography excludes placenta previa. Gestational age can be initially estimated by fundal height, and is confirmed by bedside ultrasound. External fetal monitoring should be performed on patients at viability or greater, typically 23 weeks and beyond.

■ ANCILLARY TESTING

Cardiotocography

External fetal monitoring (EFM) is one of the most sensitive clinical tools for detecting placental abruption after trauma. Continuous EFM is more sensitive in detecting placental abruption than ultrasonography, KB testing, or physical examination. Among women with contractions every 10 minutes or more, the risk of abruption is 20%.

EFM should be a routine part of a trauma evaluation when the fetus is viable (>23 weeks' gestation). The duration of monitoring should be at least 4 hours. If abnormal findings are seen, such as contractions >6 to 8 times per hour, or a Class II FHR pattern (fetal tachycardia, fetal heart rate (FHR) decelerations, or decreased FHR variability), the risk of adverse OB outcomes increases. In this case, continuous EFM should be extended to 24 to 48 hours. Cesarean delivery should be considered if a Class III FHR pattern is identified.

Blood tests

Standard laboratory tests to order for female trauma patients include: CBC, BMP (electrolytes and glucose), Type and Cross, PT/PTT, fibrinogen, Kleihauer-Betke (KB), toxicology screen, urinalysis (and HCG if needed). If indicated, arterial blood gas testing should be done if respiratory function is compromised.

Be aware that "normal ranges" for laboratory results are based on nonpregnant persons. Notable pregnancy-related changes to common tests are as follows: mildly elevated WBC and physiologic anemia. The arterial pH is increased along with decreased serum bicarbonate level and arterial Pco_2. Maternal fibrinogen levels are increased. In fact, the most sensitive laboratory indicator of abruption is a decreased fibrinogen content.

The Kleihauer-Betke (KB) test detects fetal hemoglobin in the maternal circulation. Although some recent studies question its use, a positive KB test (>0.01 mL of fetal RBC) has been associated with significant fetomaternal hemorrhage and preterm labor. One study reported that women with a positive KB test had a likelihood ratio of 20.8 for PTL. However, another study found that the rate of positive KB tests in low-risk women was not different than in maternal trauma patients. Thus, an isolated positive KB test does not necessarily indicate fetomaternal hemorrhage; other causes such as hemoglobinopathy should be considered and clinical correlation is advised (see Table 18-2).

Imaging Studies

It is important to obtain quick, reliable imaging in the setting of maternal trauma. **Do not avoid or delay necessary exams due to concerns about fetal radiation exposure.** Ultrasound (US) is the method of choice for evaluating pregnant trauma patients. US can be used to detect abnormal fluid or air collections in the abdomen. US is mainly used to determine basic pregnancy information, such as fetal heart rate, fetal size and position, amniotic fluid

■ TABLE 18-2. Common Laboratory Studies for Pregnant Trauma Patients

- Complete blood count
- Comprehensive metabolic panel
- Urinalysis
- Urine drug screen
- Type and screen
- Kleihauer-Betke
- Fibrinogen and PT/PTT
- Basic OB ultrasound: number of fetuses, FHR, fetal position, amniotic fluid volume, placental location and appearance, gestational age assignment, basic anatomy (if possible)
- Additional imaging studies as clinically indicated

volume, location and appearance of the placenta. Ultrasonic features of placental abruption can be variable, and it plays a limited role in making a diagnosis. Acute hemorrhage is difficult to confirm, since blood has an echotexture similar to myometrium, but retroplacental lucencies may be seen days after abruption. Actually, ultrasound has a sensitivity of only 50% to detect abruption.

FAST (focused assessment with sonography in trauma) US reduces the need for x-ray or CT scan, shortens the time to surgery, and is associated with shorter hospital stays and fewer complications. After initial sonogram, 96% of gravid trauma patients required no tests using ionizing radiation,

in one study. Overall, the sensitivity of FAST US to detect intra-abdominal injury in pregnancy is 61% to 83%, and the specificity is 94% to 100%. Abdominal CT may be more sensitive to detect small amounts of fluid, retroperitoneal hemorrhage, and solid organ injury, but efforts should be made to decrease radiation exposure to the extent possible. Although MRI may be an alternative, its long study time and the limited accessibility of MRI units render this approach suboptimal in an emergency setting.

Theoretical fetal risks of ionizing radiation to the fetus include excess cases of childhood cancer (mainly leukemia), with an estimated risk of 1 in 2000. The potential for congenital anomalies, growth restriction, or mental retardation requires at least 200 mGy of exposure during organogenesis or the fetal period. Most patients can be reassured that the potential fetal risk after a typical trauma evaluation is negligible. A suggested algorithm for imaging pregnant patients is depicted below (Fig 18-1).

■ OTHER CONSIDERATIONS

Rh Immune Globulin

All Rh-negative patients should receive Rh immune globulin (RhIG) 300 μg IM within 72 hours of an episode of trauma, in order to prevent maternal sensitization. For women with a positive KB test, additional RhIG can be administered, with an additional 300 μg for each 30 mL of fetal RBCs in the maternal circulation.

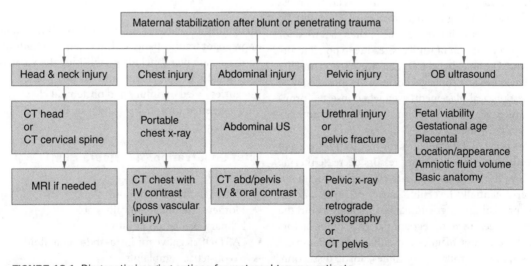

FIGURE 18-1. Diagnostic imaging options for maternal trauma patients.

MCA Doppler Testing

Consideration may be given to fetal MCA Doppler testing in cases where large fetomaternal hemorrhage is suspected. This test reliably detects severe fetal anemia, which can cause fetal hydrops or death. Sonographic features of hydrops include placentomegaly, subcutaneous edema, fetal ascites, and pleural or pericardial effusion.

Tetanus Prophylaxis

Tetanus is a rare, potentially fatal disease caused by the anaerobe *Clostridium tetani*. Wounds that are crushed, devitalized, or contaminated with dirt or rust are considered to be tetanus-prone. Open fractures, punctures, and abscesses are also associated, but severity of the wound does not determine the risk. All wounds should be cleaned and debrided if necessary. Tetanus toxoid should be given if the last booster was more than 10 years prior. If a vaccination history is unknown, tetanus toxoid can be considered when convenient. If the last immunization was >10 years ago, then tetanus immune globulin (TIG) should be given. The tetanus toxoid (TT) dose is 5 IU IM, while TIG prophylaxis dosing is 250 to 500 units IM (in opposite extremity to TT).

■ CPR AND PERIMORTEM CESAREAN DELIVERY

In rare cases, pregnant women may have life-threatening injuries that require CPR and ACLS procedures. There are several modifications for pregnant patients, which may improve the effectiveness of resuscitation. It is important to secure the airway early, using continuous cricoid pressure before and during intubation attempts. Use an ETT 0.5 to 1 cm smaller in internal diameter than that used for a nonpregnant woman of similar size, due to possible airway edema. Use an exhaled CO_2 detector to confirm ETT placement, since an esophageal detector is more likely to suggest esophageal placement, even when inserted properly. Reduce ventilation volumes, since the mother's diaphragm is elevated.

Follow usual ACLS guidelines for medications used in ACLS protocols. Although vasopressors decrease uterine blood flow, there are no alternative agents or regimens. Consider potentially reversible causes of cardiac arrest when approaching the gravid patient. In addition to the same causes seen in nonpregnant patients, other factors may include excess magnesium sulfate, preeclampsia/eclampsia, acute coronary syndromes, aortic dissection, pulmonary embolism, stroke, amniotic fluid embolism, trauma, and drug overdose.

To improve circulation, the woman should be on her left side with her back angled 15° to 30° back from the left lateral position. At this point, one may start chest compressions. Alternatively, a wedge can be placed under the woman's right side, or one rescuer can kneel next to the woman's left side and pull the gravid uterus laterally. With respect to defibrillations, there are no modifications in dose or pad position. It is important to remove any fetal or uterine monitors prior to delivering a shock.

Cesarean delivery has been shown to be life-saving for fetuses at viability or beyond. Gestational age and the interval from cardiac arrest to delivery determine the chance of survival and the risk for neurological impairment. A retrospective review of 61 cases indicated 93% of surviving infants were born within 15 minutes of death, with most survivors (70%) delivered by 5 minutes.

Cesarean delivery not only plays a role in saving the life of the fetus, but may improve resuscitation efforts for the mother. Mechanisms for improving maternal outcome after emergency cesarean include relieving vena cava compression and improving thoracic compliance. In one series of 38 perimortem cesareans (with 34 surviving infants), 20 cases were due to "resuscitatable" causes. Fully 13 mothers were revived and discharged from the hospital in good condition. In cases where hemodynamic status was reported, 12 of 18 showed a return of pulse and BP after cesarean.

■ APPROACH TO THE PATIENT— SUMMARY

Many hospitals have established protocols for evaluation of pregnant trauma patients. Important elements of standardized care plans include establishing the viability and gestational age of pregnancy, and triaging women into risk categories based on injury and obstetrical characteristics. One suggested protocol is shown in Fig. 18-2 (adapted from Muench et al).

Brief Observation (4-6 Hours EFM) Sufficient if

- Maternal trauma is minor
- Mother is hemodynamically stable
- Primary evaluation negative
- FAST-US negative for intra-abdominal fluid
- No obstetric complaints

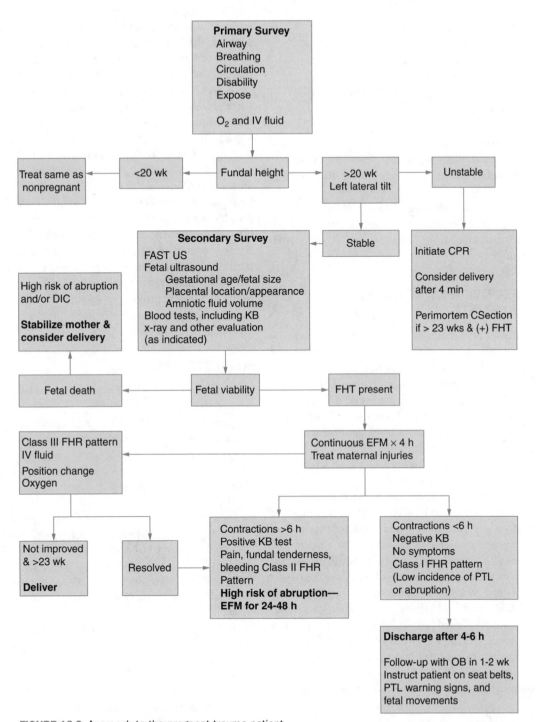

FIGURE 18-2. Approach to the pregnant trauma patient.

- Less than six contractions per hour
- Class I FHR pattern
- Normal examination and laboratory data

Prolonged Observation (24-48 Hours EFM) Required if

- Multiple or severe maternal injuries
- Mother hemodynamically unstable
- Obstetric symptoms are present (bleeding, ROM)
- Contractions more than six per hour during first 4 to 6 hours
- Abnormal FHR pattern on CTG
- Abnormal examination (eg, fundal tenderness)
- Abnormal laboratory data (eg, +KB, abnormal fibrinogen).

■ EFFECTIVENESS OF MATERNAL RESTRAINTS

Fetal outcome after motor vehicle crashes is most strongly associated with crash severity, injury of the mother, and proper maternal restraints (whether or not an airbag deploys). It is estimated that about 50% of fetal losses in motor vehicle crashes could be prevented if all pregnant women used their seat belts properly. Only 48.7% of women reported receiving counseling about seat belt use during prenatal care in one multistate survey.

Women >30 years, with more than a high school education, were most likely to wear seat belts in the last trimester, while women under age 20, black, and less educated women were the most likely to report being hurt in a crash during pregnancy. One study reported that women using seat belts are not at increased risk for adverse fetal outcomes after a crash, compared with pregnant women not in a crash. However, those who did not wear seat belts during a crash were 1.3 times more likely to have a low birth weight infant, and 2 times more likely to have excessive bleeding than belted women in a crash. Although there is little data regarding the effects of airbag deployment, case series seem to indicate no increased risk of abruption or fetal compromise. NHSTA recommends that the chest and uterine fundus be at least 10 in from the airbag cover.

■ MATERNAL INJURY PREVENTION

Studies indicate that women who experience physical violence are at higher risk for pregnancy loss and low birth weight infants. Universal screening for domestic violence is recommended by professional organizations, such as the American Medical Association (AMA), American College of Obstetricians and Gynecologists (ACOG), and the American Academy of Family Physicians (AAFP). Should a patient indicate that intimate partner violence is a concern, assistance is available from the National Domestic Violence Hotline (1-800-799-SAFE). This 24-hour, toll-free hotline provides information and referrals from anywhere in the United States.

Evidence to date suggests that correct use of seat belts and airbags does reduce the likelihood of maternal injury and fetal loss after a motor vehicle crash. Women should be advised to place their lap belt low across the hips and under the maternal abdomen. The shoulder harness should like between the breasts and over the midline of the clavicle. Airbags should not be disabled due to pregnancy. Prenatal care visits and emergency room encounters provide an opportunity for providers to give health messages to their pregnant patients regarding the importance of proper seat belt use.

SUGGESTED READINGS

ACEP Board of Directors. Emergency ultrasound guidelines. *Ann Emerg Med.* 2009;53:550-570.

American Heart Association. Part 10.8: cardiac arrest associated with pregnancy. *Circulation.* 2005;112:IV150-IV153.

Bochicchio GV, Haan J, Scalea TM. Surgeon-performed focused assessment with sonography for trauma as an early screening tool for pregnancy after trauma. *J Trauma.* 2002;52:1125-1128.

Brown MA, Sirlin CB, Farahmand N, Hoyt DB, Casola G. Screening sonography in pregnant patients with blunt abdominal trauma. *J Ultrasound Med.* 2005;24:175-181.

Cahill AG, Bastek JA, Stamilio DM, Odibo AO, Stevens E, Macones GA. Minor trauma in pregnancy—is the evaluation unwarranted? *Am J Obstet Gynecol.* 2008;198:208e.1-208e.5.

Chang J, Berg CJ, Saltzman LE, Herndon J. Homicide: a leading cause of injury deaths among pregnant and postpartum women in the United States, 1991-1999. *Am J Pub Health.* 2005;95:471-477.

Chang J, Elam-Evans LD, Berg CJ, et al. Pregnancy-related mortality surveillance—United States, 1991-1999. *MMWR Surveillance Summaries.* 2003;52(SS02):1-8.

Curet MJ, Schermer DR, Demarest GB, Bieneik EJ, Curet LB. Predictors of outcome in trauma during pregnancy: identification of patient who can be monitored for less than 6 hours. *J Trauma.* 2000;49:18-25.

Cusick SS, Tibbles CD. Trauma in pregnancy. *Emerg Med Clin N Am.* 2007;25:861-872.

DeSantis-Klinich K, Flannagan CAC, Rupp JD, Sochor M, Schneider LW, Pearlman MD. Fetal outcome in motor-vehicle crashes: effects of crash characteristics and maternal restraint. *Am J Obstet Gynecol.* 2008;198:450.e1-450.e9.

Dhanraj D, Lambers D. The incidences of positive Kleihauer-Betke test in low-risk pregnancies and maternal trauma patients. *Am J Obstet Gynecol.* 2004;190:1461-1463.

El Kady D, Gilbert WM, Anderson J, Danelsen B, Towner D, Smith LH. Trauma during pregnancy: an analysis of maternal and fetal outcomes in a large population. *Am J Obstet Gynecol.* 2004;190:1661-1668.

Hill CC, Pickinpaugh J. Trauma and surgical emergencies in the obstetric patient. *Surg Clin North Am.* 2008;28:421-440.

Hyde LK, Cook LJ, Olson LM, Weiss HB, Dean JM. Effect of motor vehicle crashes on adverse fetal outcomes. *Obstet Gynecol.* 2003;102:279-286.

Ikossi DG, Lazar AA, Morabito D, Fildes J, Knudson MM. Profile of mothers at risk: an analysis of injury and pregnancy loss in 1,1195 trauma patients. *J Am Coll Surg.* 2005;200:49-56.

Katz V, Balderston K, DeFreest M. Perimortem cesarean delivery: were our assumptions correct? *Am J Obstet Gynecol.* 2005;192:1916-1920.

Katz V, Dotters DJ, Droegmeuller W. Perimortem cesarean delivery. *Obstet Gynecol.* 1986;68:571-576.

Kuo C, Jamieson DJ, McPheeters JL, Meikle SF, Posner SF. Injury hospitalizations of pregnant women in the United States, 2002. *Am J Obstet Gynecol.* 2007;196:161.e1-161.e6.

Leggon RE, Wood GC, Indeck MC. Pelvic fractures in pregnancy: factors influencing maternal and fetal outcomes. *J Trauma.* 2002;53:796-804.

Lu EJ. Chapter 23. Surgical procedures in pregnancy: trauma in pregnancy. In: *Gabbe: Obstetrics: Normal and Problem Pregnancies.* 5th ed. Churchill, Livingstone. An Imprint of Elsevier, Philadelphia, PA; 2007.

Mattox KL, Goetzl L. Trauma in pregnancy. *Crit Care Med.* 2005;33:385S-389S.

Meroz Y, Elchalal U, Ginosar Y. Initial trauma management in advanced pregnancy. *Anesth Clin.* 2007;25:117-129.

Morris S, Stacey M. ABC of resuscitation: resuscitation in pregnancy. *BMJ.* 2003;327:1277-1279.

Muench MV, Baschat AA, Reddy UM, et al. Kleihauer-Betke testing is important in all cases of maternal trauma. *J Trauma.* 2004;57:1094-1098.

Patel SJ, Reede DL, Katz DS, Subramaniam R, Amorosa JK. Imaging the pregnant patient for nonobstetric conditions: algorithms and radiation dose considerations. *Radiographics.* 2007;27:1705-1722.

Rhee P, Nunley MK, Demetriades D, Velmahos G, Doucet JJ. Tetanus and trauma: a review and recommendations. *J Trauma.* 2005;58:1082-1088.

Schiff MA, Holt VL. Pregnancy outcomes following hospitalization for motor vehicle crashes in Washington state from 1989 to 2001. *Am J Epidemiology.* 2005;161:503-510.

Sirin H, Weiss HB, Sauber-Schatz EK, Dunning K. Seat belt use, counseling and motor-vehicle injury during pregnancy: results from a multi-state population-based survey. *Matern Child Health J.* 2007;11:505-510.

Sperry JL, Casey BM, McIntire DD, Minei JP, Gentilello LM, Shafi S. Long-term fetal outcomes in pregnant trauma patients. *Am J Surg.* 2006;192:715-721.

Theodorou DA, Velmahos GC, Souter I, et al. Fetal death after trauma in pregnancy. *Am Surg.* 2000;66:809-812.

Weiss HB. Hidden epidemic of maternal, fetal, and neonatal mortality and injury from crashes: a case of societal neglect? *Transportation Research Record: Journal of the Transportation Research Board. No. 1956.* Washington, DC: Transportation Research Board of the National Academies; 2006:133-140.

Weiss HB, Songer TJ, Fabio T. Fetal deaths related to maternal injury. *JAMA.* 2001;286:1863-1868.

Weiss HB, Strotmeyer S. Characteristics of pregnant women in a motor vehicle crashes. *Injury Prevention.* 2002;8:207-210.

Whitten M, Irvine LM. Postmortem and perimortem caesarean section: what are the indications? *J Royal Soc Med.* 2000; 93:6-9.

CHAPTER 19

Transport of the Critically Ill Obstetric Patient

• *John P. Elliott*

The broad framework of regionalization is based on the notion that sophisticated perinatal care should be available to every patient within a designated region, even if it is not specifically available at each hospital within the region. The level of care provided within individual hospitals is determined by the availability of technology, skilled nursing and medical personnel, and other related support services. Thus, when transport becomes necessary, it is to match a patient to the level of technology and support she and her baby need.

■ INDICATION FOR MATERNAL TRANSPORT

Maternal transport to a tertiary facility should be considered when the facility at which a patient is located does not have the capacity to manage actual or anticipated complications of either mother or child. Low analyzed 463 maternal transports in the United States over a 6-month period, noting prematurity as the primary reason for transport in 330 (71%) cases, hemorrhage in 79 (17%), pregnancy induced hypertension in 41 (9%), and eclampsia in 8 (2%). In a study done by the author, acute maternal medical complications were the indication for transport in 360 of 1541 (23.4%) maternal patients transported in Arizona over an 18-month period. Fifty-two percent had hypertensive crises, 36% had hemorrhage, 6% were trauma victims, and 3% had respiratory compromise.

■ OBSTETRIC INTENSIVE CARE DURING TRANSPORT

In general, critical care obstetric patients should be stabilized at the referring hospital prior to transport.

Hypertensive emergencies such as severe preeclampsia should be treated with magnesium sulphate to stabilize the neuromuscular irritability that can progress to eclamptic seizures. In addition, diastolic hypertension should be lowered to 100 to 105 mm Hg by cautious administration of intravenous hydralazine or labetalol. Third trimester bleeding due to placenta previa or abruptio placentae can cause hypovolemic shock and disseminated intravascular coagulopathy (DIC). The estimated blood loss should be replaced with crystalloid solution such as normal saline or lactated Ringer solution in a 3:1 ratio (3 mL of crystalloid for each milliliter of blood loss). Because maternal intravascular volume increases by about 50% during pregnancy, signs and symptoms of shock may not be apparent until blood loss approaches 2000 to 2500 mL. Magnesium sulfate may also be used as a tocolytic. DIC is treated with blood component therapy (see Chap 2). During transport, left-side recumbent positioning should be utilized to optimize uteroplacental function, as described below. Table 19-1 illustrates an example of typical maternal transport standing orders.

■ MATERNAL TRAUMA

Transport of the pregnant trauma victim requires special knowledge and skills by the transport team. The uterus may be injured without signs of direct physical trauma. Abrupt deceleration with resulting contra-coup forces can be harmful to both the fetus and the placenta. In most cases of maternal trauma, every effort should be made to stabilize serious maternal injuries prior to transport. All pregnant patients beyond 18 weeks' gestation should be transported in left lateral tilt position to prevent hypotension from aorto-caval compression. Supine hypotension

Premature labor and/or rupture of membranes (PROM), multiple pregnancy, abnormal presentations

Prior to transport

1. Assess blood pressure (BP), temperature, pulse, respiratory rate, and fetal heart tones.
2. Assess contractions (frequency, duration, quality), status of membranes; time of PROM (if applicable), color, and how PROM was confirmed. If membranes intact, may perform vaginal exam as needed. If PROM, do not do digital exam.
3. Administer medications as ordered by obstetric transport director.
4. Start IV (if absent) with 18 or 16 g catheter; 1000 mL LR at 50-150 mL/h. Fluid restrict, when necessary.
5. Left/right lateral uterine displacement.
6. Record above data, obtain consent for transport, and obtain copies of the patient's chart.
7. Assess maternal/fetal condition and call maternal-fetal physician, if necessary, for consultation and further orders.
8. Help facility prepare for birth, if imminent; notify dispatch if neonatal transport team is needed.

During transport

1. Vital signs with fetal heart tones q15min.
2. Administer tocolytics and other medicines, prn.
3. Record above information.
4. Explain procedures to patient and family; reassure patient.

Emergency medications

- Terbutaline: 0.25 mg SQ when contraction frequency is more than q10min, providing there are no contraindications such as maternal heart disease, maternal diabetes mellitus, shortness of breath, tachycardia, or heavy maternal bleeding. May repeat every 1/2 to 1 h if pulse <120.
- Meperidine: 25-50 mg IVP for labor pain. May repeat every hour. Observe pulse and BP closely. For other causes of pain, speak with medical director before administering.
- Magnesium sulfate: IVPB 40 g/1000 mL LR. Bolus 6 g over 10-15 min. Follow with 3 g/h via infusion pump to suppress contractions—adjust as needed. Note: 6 g bolus diluted to not greater than 10% solution. May use 100 mL bag of LR or NS for MgSO$_4$ bolus.
- Antidote for magnesium toxicity: Calcium gluconate Ig, slow IV push, over 3 min. Observe BP closely.
- Continually assess urine output, deep tendon reflexes, and respiratory rate/effort.

Preeclampsia/eclampsia

Prior to transport

1. Assess vital signs, fetal heart tones, and deep tendon reflexes.
2. Assess contractions (frequency, duration, quality), status of membranes (see PROM/premature labor orders).
3. Right/left lateral uterine displacement.
4. Start IV. Mainline 1000 mL LR, infuse at 0-100 mL/h as indicated by cardiopulmonary status, etc (hold total fluids at 75 mL/h, if possible).
5. Mix MgSO$_4$ 40 g/1000 mL LR (6 g bolus diluted to not greater than 10% IV solution). May use 100 mL bag of NS or LR for MgSO$_4$ bolus.

6. Administer medicines as indicated by condition:
   MgSO$_4$ 4-6 g IV bolus over 10-15 min, considering patient's weight, urine output, and deep tendon reflexes. MgSO$_4$—continuous infusion of 2-3 g/h via infusion pump
7. Foley catheter if patient cannot void, or is oliguric.
8. Record above information, obtain copy of chart, obtain consent to transport.
9. Assess maternal/fetal condition for transport and call maternal-fetal physician for consultation or further orders.

During transport

1. Take vital signs with fetal heart tones q15 min.
2. Administer medicines, prn.
3. Explain procedures to the patient and the family.
4. Foley catheter, prn.

Emergency medications

- Hydralazine: First choice for hypertension. May require hydration before medicating. Give when diastolic ≥110 mm Hg. Give 2-10 mg IV push every 15-20 min until BP begins to decrease. Stop when diastolic blood pressure is 100-105 mm Hg or a total of 30 mg given. Consult medical director.
- Labetalol: Give when diastolic ≥110 mm Hg. 20 mg (8 mL) over 2 min IV push. If desired effect not reached after 10 min, give 40 mg (16 mL) IV push. Call medical director.
- Oxygen: 12 L by non-rebreathing mask, prn.
- Morphine: 2-5 mg, slow IV push for acute pulmonary edema.
- Furosemide: 20-40 mg, slow IV push over 2-3 min for acute pulmonary edema.

Eclampsia

- Establish airway: Provide supplemental oxygen. Assist with bag/mask or endotracheal intubation, as needed.
- If seizure persists: Rebolus with 2 g MgSO$_4$ (total bolus should not exceed 8 g).
- If seizure persists after second MgSO$_4$ bolus: Sodium amobarbital IV push 250 mg over 3-5 min (discuss with medical director).

Hemorrhage (General)

Prior to transport

1. Assess vital signs and fetal heart tones.
2. Assess contractions, status of membranes, extent of bleeding, number of bleeding episodes, and amount of blood loss (weigh pads, when possible).
3. O$_2$ 12 L/non-rebreathing mask.
4. Start IV with 16 g needle. Infuse 1000 mL LR using blood transfusion tubing at 125 mL/h or as necessary to maintain adequate blood pressure and urine output greater than 30 mL/h.
5. With active bleeding or suspected abruption, place a second IV line. Use 16 g catheter.
6. Check hemoglobin/hematocrit, type and cross (or screen).
7. May travel with blood infusing. Use NS to clear tubing.
8. Administer medications as ordered (IV ritodrine and terbutaline are contraindicated). See Premature Labor, PROM Section for tocolytics.

(Continued)

9. Foley catheter.
10. Assess maternal-fetal condition for transport and call maternal-fetal physician, prn.
11. Record above information, obtain copy of chart, and permit for transport.
12. No vaginal exam unless placenta previa has been ruled out; then, if necessary, perform gentle vaginal examination or sterile speculum examination to document cervical status prior to departure.

During transport

1. Check vital signs and fetal heart tones q15min, or as deemed necessary.
2. Check blood loss, keep pad count.
3. Record above information.
4. Reassess the patient and call maternal-fetal physician for consultation or further orders.

Acute hemorrhage with hypoperfusion

1. O_2 12 L/non-rebreathing mask.
2. Start additional IV lines and increase IV fluids, as needed.
3. Military antishock trousers (MAST) application, as indicated (see Chap 18).
4. Left/right lateral uterine displacement.
5. Elevate feet.
6. If hypotensive, consider ephedrine 5-25 mg slow IV push. Observe BP closely. Call obstetric transport director.

Acute postpartum hemorrhage

1. Oxytocin 20-30 u/L NS, 125-150 mL/h.
2. Methylergonovine 0.2 mg, IM. Contraindicated in the presence of maternal hypertension or sepsis.
3. 15-Methyl $F_{2\alpha}$ 0.25 mg, IM. Contraindicated in the presence of maternal asthma or pulmonary hypertension. Call medical director.

Excessive nausea and vomiting

• Promethazine 25 mg, IV.

Emergency delivery

1. Perform emergency delivery whenever imminent during transport.
2. May perform small midline episiotomy, as necessary, to prevent laceration.
3. Cut and clamp the umbilical cord 1/2 in from stump.
4. Administer oxytocin 10-20 units, IM or added to full IV bag after placenta is delivered.
5. Obtain cord blood when time permits.
6. Resuscitate newborn (see Chap. 26), provide warmth, O_2 by bag and mask, with intubation, prn. If estimated time of arrival is greater than 20 min and situation permits, obtain chem strip for glucose.
7. For neonatal glucose less than 40 mg/dL, give dextrose 10% IV or gavage, if necessary. Give 2-4 mL/kg over 3-5 min.

may significantly compromise the maternal cardiac output and placental perfusion. Should the patient require a backboard for neck or back stabilization, the entire backboard can be tilted to the left by placing rolled sheets or towels under the right side of the board. The fetal heart rate should be auscultated in all traumatic maternal injuries. The absence of fetal heart tones may be associated with placental abruption and/or fetal death. The uterus should also be examined carefully for evidence of tenderness or rigidity. Vaginal bleeding should be ruled out in all gravid trauma patients.

The emergency medical system (EMS) in the United States is efficient at triaging trauma victims to designated trauma centers. However, when considering transport of a pregnant woman from an accident scene, the EMS system often fails to recognize that the fetus/neonate also needs to be treated at an appropriate level facility. Level I trauma patients in the second or third trimester of pregnancy ideally should be transported to a hospital that combines Level I trauma capabilities with Level III obstetric and neonatal facilities.

■ THE OBSTETRICAL TRANSPORT CREW

Transport of the critically ill obstetric patient often requires personnel with skills beyond that of the typical advanced life support/emergency medical ambulance crew. These care providers may be cross-trained adult trauma nurses or dedicated obstetrical nurses. They must have an excellent working knowledge of maternal physiology and the process of labor. Experience with obstetric drugs and fetal monitoring is also essential. The ability to perform advanced cardiac life support, to interpret electrocardiograms, and to perform successful endotracheal intubation are important skills for a perinatal flight nurse to possess (Table 19-2). Table 19-3 lists the recommended equipment for perinatal transport along with a detailed plan for equipment organization/flight-kit planning.

■ TABLE 19-2. Maternal Flight Nurse Skills and Qualifications

Skills
1. Vaginal speculum examination; digital cervical examination
2. Vaginal delivery
3. Advanced cardiac life support—certified
4. Intubation—maternal and/or neonatal

Qualifications/requirements
1. Basic and advanced cardiac life support capable
2. Neonatal resuscitation capable
3. National certification in obstetrics
4. Three years of tertiary obstetric experience
5. Successful completion of maternal flight nurse course/examination

---

■ TABLE 19-3. Equipment for Maternal Transport

Contents of maternal flight nurse delivery bag[a]

Ob delivery kit

- Bulb syringe
- Suction trap
- Self-inflating resuscitation bag
- Infant and newborn mask
- Infant hat
- Pediatric stethoscope
- Infant blanket pack
- Portawarm mattress
- Sterile gloves (latex and nonlatex)

- 1 chux
- Cord clamp (2)
- Scissors (curved/straight) (2)
- Curved Kelly clamp
- Short ring forceps
- Plastic placenta bag
- Cloth towels (2)
- Sterile 4 × 4 in gauze (2)
- Bulb syringe

(Continued)

TABLE 19-3. Equipment for Maternal Transport (*Continued*)

Contents of maternal flight nurse pharmacy bag[a]

$MgSO_4$ 10 g (2)
Furosemide 20 mg (2)
Oxytocin 10 U (3)
$MgSO_4$ 10 g (3)
Normal saline 10 mL (3)

Thermometer
TB syringe (2)
3 mL syringe (2)

Dimenhydrinate (2)
Narcotic sheets

Bretylium 500 mg (2)
Verapamil 5 mg (3)

Epinephrine 1:10,000 (2)
Calcium gluconate 10% (1)
Diphenhydramine (2)

Ephedrine 50 mg (3)
Dextrose 50% 50 mL
Hydralazine 20 mg (2)
$D_{10}W$ vial 5 mL (2)
Hep-lock

Band-aids
Needles
  19 g (3)
  22 g (3)
  Filter (3)
Cord clamp (2)
Aspirin (2)
Tylenol (2)
Epinephrine 1:1000 (3)

Sodium bicarb 50 cc jet (1)
2% lidocaine 100 mg jet (2)
Procainamide 1 g (1)

Methylergonovine 0.2 mg (2)

Labetalol 100 mg (2)
Terbutaline 1 mg (3)
Ammonium salts (2)
Promethazine HCl 25 mg (2)
Albuterol, unit dose 2.5 mg (2)
Alcohol swabs
Labels
Hep-lock cap

Drug labels (4)

Inventory
Atropine 1 mg (2)
Lidocaine 1 g/50mL (1)
Sodium amobarbital 250 mg (1)

Meperidine 100 mg (1)
Diazepam 10 mg (4)
Morphine 10 mg (1)
Naloxone 0.4 mg (2)

Contents of top portion maternal flight nurse medical bag[a]

3-mL syringe (2)
Tuberculin syringe (2)
Insulin syringe (1)
Stopcock
19-gauge needles
Syringes
  10 mL
  20 mL
  30 mL
  60 mL

100 mL normal saline (2)

Bite stick
Drug bag

Alcohol wipes
Virowipes

Contents of base portion maternal flight nurse medical bag[a]

250 mL D_5W
500 mL NS
Cardiac electrodes

1000 mL LR
500 mL LR

Sterile speculum

Orange

Laryngoscope handle and bulb

Blades

Green

In self-seal bags
Chemstrips
Alcohol wipes

Yellow

IV start kit
Nonsterile gloves (latex and nonlatex)

McIntosh (3, 4)
Miller (0, 1, 3)

Spare "C" batteries (2)

Xylocaine gel
Benzoin (2)
1-in adhesive tape
10-mL syringe

Lancets
Cotton balls

KY jelly
Betadine jelly
Nitrazine paper
Tape-measure
Blood tubes
Purple (2)
Red (2)
Vacutainer
Alcohol
Band-aids
Tourniquet
Needles
Small self-seal bag (2)
Urine dipstick
Plastic bags (2)
Flashlight
Peri pads (2)

Mainline tubing
IV Catheters
16 gauge (3)
18 gauge (3)
24 gauge (2)
23-gauge butterfly
T connector
Tourniquet

Sterile gloves (latex and nonlatex)

Contents of outside pockets maternal flight nurse medical bag[a]

Left side

Micro drip extension set

Blood tubing with pump
Salem pump

Top handle pocket

Micro drip extension set

Stopcock
60-mL syringe
needles

Top center

Stethoscope
Doppler and gel
BP cuff (regular and oversized)

Bottom center

Emesis bag
Adult BVM oxygen
Bag
Leg BP cuff
Charts (3)
Self-inflating
Ambu-bag
Red isolation bag (1)

Right side

Stylette
Adult
Pediatric
End-tidal CO_2 detector

Zipper bag

PEEP valve
Magill forceps
Oral airways
Medium adult

Small adult

Infant
ET tubes
2.0
2.5
3.0
3.5
7.0
7.5
8.0
7.0 Endotrol
Beck airways airflow monitor

---

[a]Description of some components of the maternal flight nurse bag by brand name does not necessarily infer endorsement of that brand.

The comprehensive care of the critically ill obstetric patient during transport requires care providers that have a detailed knowledge of maternal physiologic adaptations and a comprehensive understanding of the disease processes unique to obstetrics. The combination of perinatal regionalization and a skilled perinatal transport service may improve outcome for both mother and baby.

SUGGESTED READINGS

Baxt WG, Moody P. The impact of a rotorcraft aeromedical emergency care service on trauma mortality. *JAMA.* 1983; 249:3047-3051.

Elliott JP, Foley MR, Young L, et al. Transport of obstetrical critical care patients to tertiary centers. *J Reprod Med* 1996: 41;171-175.

Elliott JP. Magnesium sulfate as a tocolytic agent. *Am J Obstet Gynecol.* 1983;147:277-284.

Elliott JP, O'Keeffe DF, Freeman RK. Helicopter transportation of patients with obstetric emergencies in an urban area. *Am J Obstet Gynecol.* 1982;143:157-162.

Elliott JP, Sipp TL, Balazs KT. Maternal transport of patients with advanced cervical dilatation—to fly or not to fly? *Obstet Gynecol.* 1992;79:380-382.

Elliott JP, Trujillo R. Fetal monitoring during emergency obstetric transport. *Am J Obstet Gynecol.* 1987;157:245-247.

Kanto WP, Bryant J, Thigpen J, et al. Impact of a maternal transport program on a newborn service. *South Med J.* 1983; 76:834-837.

Katz VL, Hansen AR. Complications in the emergency transport of pregnant women. *South Med J.* 1990;83:7-10.

Knox GE, Schnitker KA. In-utero transport. *Clin Obstet Gynecol.* 1984;27:11-16.

Low RB, Martin D, Brown C. Emergency air transport of pregnant patients: the national experience. *J Emerg Med.* 1988; 6:41-48.

Tsokos N, Newnham JP, Langford SA. Intravenous tocolytic therapy for long distance aeromedical transport of women in preterm labour in Western Australia. *Asia-Oceania J Obstet Gynaecol.* 1988;14:21-25.

CHAPTER 20

Anesthesia for the Complicated Obstetric Patient

• *Lisa A. Dado*

A thorough understanding of the nature of the parturient's pain is the first aspect in providing optimal obstetric anesthetic care. Once the biology and pathophysiology of this special acute pain is discussed, then the benefits of analgesia for this pain will appropriately follow. Pharmacology of local anesthetics and related drugs will be reviewed, with special emphasis on complications associated with their administration. A variety of techniques including epidural, subarachnoid, and other regional techniques will be discussed with benefits and complications reviewed. General anesthesia for cesarean section delivery will be outlined. A variety of special consideration patients will be addressed including: (1) The preeclamptic patient, (2) preterm birth patient on tocolytics, (3) HIV-positive mothers, (4) coagulopathies, (5) cardiac disease, and (6) pulmonary disease.

■ NATURE OF THE PATIENT'S PAIN

The current concept of pain focuses on the peripheral nervous system relaying a stimulus to the central nervous system for interpretive evaluation—the somatosensory system (Fig 20-1). The peripheral system consists of afferent neurons which are embedded in body tissues awaiting nociceptive (painful) stimuli. These afferent neurons are termed Ad (A-delta) and C-fibers. These fibers transverse into the spinal segments and synapse at the dorsal spinal ganglion. Here, substance-P is released causing the painful effect to be initiated. From each spinal segment stimulated, these messages ascend through one of two pathways to the thalamus for further modulation: the lateral spinothalamic tract or the medial lemniscus tract. Once at the thalamus, adjustment and regulation from inherent emotional and psychological factors occurs. The data support the emphasis on the importance of perceptual factors that influence a patient's total pain experience (Table 20-1). The psychodynamics of prior experience, motivation, anxiety, anticipation of pain, attention, personality, and ethnic and cultural factors all influence the modulation of substance-P release, affecting the pain experience. From the thalamus, this information is synthesized in the sensory cortex for relay to the many effector sites which contribute to the pain response. Once pain has been perceived, there is an initiation of the pain response which has neuroendocrine, behavioral and psychological implications.

In humans, there is a 300% to 600% increase in epinephrine and 200% to 400% increase in norepinephrine levels produced during severe pain experienced in active labor. There is a 200% to 300% increase in cortisol levels, as well as, increases in corticosteroid and adrenocortictropic hormone levels reaching their peaks at or after delivery. During labor the cardiac output increase is 40% to 50% with a further 20% to 30% increase during painful contractions. The systolic and diastolic blood pressures also increase by 20 to 30 mm Hg. These increases in cardiac output (CO) and systolic blood pressure (SBP) lead to a significant increase in left ventricular stroke work that may be harmful to patients with preeclampsia, hypertension, cardiac valvular disease, pulmonary hypertension, or severe anemia.

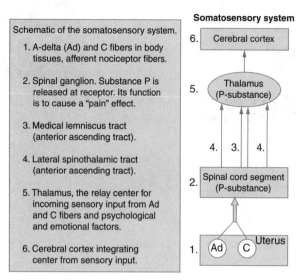

Schematic of the somatosensory system.

1. A-delta (Ad) and C fibers in body tissues, afferent nociceptor fibers.

2. Spinal ganglion. Substance P is released at receptor. Its function is to cause a "pain" effect.

3. Medical lemniscus tract (anterior ascending tract).

4. Lateral spinothalamic tract (anterior ascending tract).

5. Thalamus, the relay center for incoming sensory input from Ad and C fibers and psychological and emotional factors.

6. Cerebral cortex integrating center from sensory input.

FIGURE 20-1. Schematic of the somatosensory system.

With the sympathetic-induced lipolytic metabolism, increases in free fatty acids and lactate produce relative maternal acidosis. Increased sympathetic activity increases metabolism and oxygen consumption, and decreases gastrointestinal and urinary bladder motility. Respiratory rate is increased with resultant respiratory alkalosis. The kidney compensates by excreting HCO_3^-. Diminished $PaCO_2$ levels below 25 to 27 mm Hg may result in increased uteroplacental resistance and reduced oxygen delivery to the fetus.

During peak contractions, there is a reduction of intervillous blood flow leading to a significant decrease in placental gas exchange. This exaggerates the already dramatic reduction in uterine blood flow, secondary to the increases in norepinephrine and cortisol (Table 20-1).

■ EFFECTS OF ANALGESIA

By blocking nociceptive input, there is a reduction in the release of catecholamines, adrenal corticotropic hormone, and cortisol in the parturient (Table 20-2). Effective analgesia significantly reduces pain-related hemodynamic changes. Maternal cardiac output fluctuations are modulated and oxygen consumption is reduced. Gastric and bladder motility is not adversely affected by neuroblockade. Cautious epidural analgesia has been reported to provide a vasomotor blocking effect which increases intervillous blood flow and oxygen delivery to the fetus.

The first stage of labor refers to the beginning of cervical dilation and effacement until its completion. The second stage of labor extends from complete cervical dilation

■ TABLE 20-1. Pain Perception	
Psychological	Anxiety, fear, emotional arousal
Behavioral	Verbalization, motor activity
Neuroendocrine	Hyperventilation—maternal respiratory
	Endocrine (stress) response
	↑ adrenocorticotropic hormone (ACTH), ↑ cortisol
	↑ epinephrine, norepinephrine
	↑ lipolytic metabolism—metabolic acidosis
	Cardiovascular Response
	↑ systemic vascular resistance
	↑ cardiac output
	↑ blood pressure
	↑ oxygen consumption
	↑ left ventricular stroke work
	Gastrointestinal function
	↓ gastric motility
	↑ risk for gastroesophageal reflux/aspiration
	↑ nausea and vomiting
	Urinary function
	↓ emptying—urinary retention oliguria
Fetal effects	↓ uterine blood flow
	↑ fetal heart rate alterations

■ TABLE 20-2. Analgesic Effects	
Psychological	↓ Anxiety, ↓ fear, ↑ emotional stability
Behavioral	↓ Motor activity
Neuroendocrine	↓ Respiratory alkalosis (maternal)
	↓ Catechol release
	↓ Cortisol
	↓ Adrenocorticotropic hormone (ACTH)
	↓ Metabolic acidosis (maternal)
	↓ Cardiac output
	↓ Oxygen consumption
	↓ Left ventricular stroke work
	Normal gastrointestinal function
	Normal urinary function
Fetal effects	↑ Uterine blood flow
	More stability in fetal heart rate tracing

until delivery of the infant. The third stage is the delivery of the placenta. (Table 20-2)

Transmission of pain during the first stage of labor is from spinal segments (pain fibers) T_{10}, T_{11}, T_{12}, and L_1 and the second and third stage of labor is from S_2, S_3, and S_4 (Fig 20-2). It is important for the care provider to understand the differences between the pain conduction (spinal levels) during the first stage of labor, as compared with the second and third stage, in order to provide appropriately directed analgesia. It is also important to consider that pain may also be due to the pathology of the gestation, such as abruptio placenta, infection, adnexal torsion, or appendicitis, and these may be *masked* if total neuroblockade is achieved from T_4 to S_5 at the onset of labor. Only segments necessary for the specific pain of labor should be blocked (Table 20-3). Relatively decreased fetal perfusion has been reported to occur both in the presence and absence of overt maternal hypotension secondary to a sympathectomy-mediated reduction in uterine blood flow.

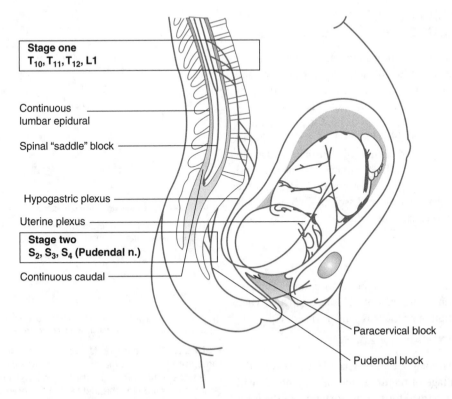

Stage one
T_{10}, T_{11}, T_{12}, L1

Continuous lumbar epidural

Spinal "saddle" block

Hypogastric plexus

Uterine plexus

Stage two
S_2, S_3, S_4 (Pudendal n.)

Continuous caudal

Paracervical block

Pudendal block

FIGURE 20-2. Note the completely separate pain fibers responsible for pain in the first and second stages of labor: T_{10}-L_1 versus S_2-S_4.

■ TABLE 20-3. Innervation of Pelvic Viscera	
Uterus	Motor fibers from parasympathetic pelvic nerves from S_2, S_3, S_4, and sympathetic sensory
Tubes/ovaries	Motor fibers from parasympathetic pelvic nerves from S_2, S_3, S_4, and sympathetic sensory fibers via the ovarian plexus from T_{12}, L_1
Broad ligament	Motor fibers from parasympathetic pelvic nerves from S_2, S_3, S_4, and sympathetic sensory fibers via the hypogastric plexus from T_{12}, L_1
Cervix	Motor fibers from parasympathetic pelvic nerves from S_2, S_3, S_4, and sympathetic sensory fibers via the hypogastric plexus from T_{12}, L_1
Vagina	Motor fibers from parasympathetic pelvic nerves from S_2, S_3, S_4, and sympathetic sensory fibers via the hypogastric plexus from T_{12}, L_1
Vestibule/hymen	Erectile vasodilator fibers from parasympathetic pelvic nerves from S_2, S_3, S_4
Labia	Posterior labial nerve S_2, S_3, and perineal branch of the posterior femoral cutaneous nerve S_1, S_2, S_3
Clitoris	Erectile vasodilator fibers from parasympathetic pelvic nerves from S_2, S_3, S_4
Perineum	Motor and sensory innervation from the pudendal nerve arising from S_2, S_3, S_4
Bladder	Sympathetic fibers from T_{11}, T_{12}, L_1, L_2 via the superior/inferior hypogastric plexuses control the sphincter and parasympathetic fibers from S_2, S_3, S_4 control filling/emptying of the bladder
Anus	Motor and sensory innervation from the pudendal nerve arising from S_2, S_3, S_4

Source: Reproduced with permission from John J Bonica. *Principles and Practice of Obstetric Analgesia and Anesthesia.* 2nd ed. Malvern, PA: Williams & Wilkins; 1995.

■ PHARMACOLOGY OF LOCAL ANESTHETICS AND RELATED DRUGS

The desired action of all local anesthetics is the reversible blockade of nerve conduction and, therefore, the cascade of events producing perception of pain. These drugs prevent the development of an action potential in a nerve by blocking sodium channels responsible for propagating a response in the nerve fiber (Fig 20-3). Local anesthetics exist in both charged and uncharged form. The uncharged state of the drug crosses the lipid nerve membrane and enters the cell. Once in the cell, it reequilibrates into the charged form that is readily dissolved in water. This charged form now reaches the sodium channels and blocks them from inside. (Table 20-3)

Ionization

The capacity for an uncharged species to assume a charged form, is the essential property of all local anesthetics. They are a combination of a weak base and a strong acid.

$$B + H^+ \neq BH^+$$

As a general principle, lowering the pH will increase the ionized percentage of the drug, and raising the pH will increase the uncharged form of the drug. Since the local anesthetics are usually supplied in an acidic medium, the

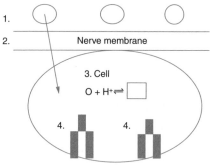

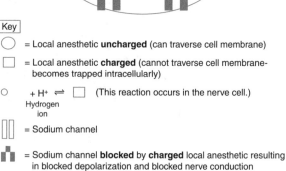

Key

◯ = Local anesthetic **uncharged** (can traverse cell membrane)

☐ = Local anesthetic **charged** (cannot traverse cell membrane-becomes trapped intracellularly)

○ + H⁺ ⇌ ☐   (This reaction occurs in the nerve cell.)
Hydrogen
ion

▯▯ = Sodium channel

▮▮ = Sodium channel **blocked** by **charged** local anesthetic resulting in blocked depolarization and blocked nerve conduction

FIGURE 20-3. Uncharged (**1**) local anesthetic passes through the nerve membrane (**2**) into the *cell* (**3**) where the local anesthetic gains a H⁺ (hydrogen ion) to become charged *blocked* Na⁺-channel (**4**) in the nerve cell by the charged local anesthetic does not allow the nerve to propagate a nerve impulse.

addition of $NaHCO_3$ will increase the relative uncharged portion allowing the drug to cross the nerve membrane more readily resulting in a quicker onset of block.

Usual Doses

0.1 cc $NaHCO_3$/10 cc bupivicaine

1.0 cc $NaHCO_3$/10 cc lidocaine

Precipitation of the local anesthetic will occur if too much $NaHCO_3$ is added. Comparative properties of lidocaine and bupivacaine are outlined in Table 20-4.

Protein Binding

Protein binding is another property important to understand. All local anesthetics bind to albumin and μ-1-acid glycoprotein (AAG). It is the free portion of the drug that is responsible for toxicity. In pregnancy, albumin levels are depressed, so AAG binding becomes most important. AAG is released in response to surgery, trauma, infection, and inflammation. Once AAG sites are saturated with local anesthetics, the free drug levels progressively increase. Protein binding also decreases with decreasing pH. Therefore, in an acidotic environment a high proportion of free drug with the potential for cardiac or neurotoxicity should be anticipated.

Absorption

Absorption of local anesthetics refers to the movement of the drug from the site of injection to the bloodstream. Therefore, the more vascular the area and the larger the total dose of anesthetic used, the higher the resulting serum level of the drug. The addition of a vasoconstrictor (epinephrine) to the local anesthetic can decrease the absorption and, therefore, *toxicity* of the drug used. (Table 20-4)

Toxicity

Local anesthetic toxicity may manifest with central nervous system or cardiac effects. As the doses increase, disinhibition and CNS excitation occurs producing seizures. Local anesthetic bind and inhibit cardiac Na^+, Ca^{2+}, and K^+ channels as concentrations increase causing cardiac arrest. Treatment of adverse reactions depends on the severity of their effects from spontaneous recovery, to supportive care with oxygen and maintaining the airway, to ACLS.

Ropivacaine is a local anesthetic with similar characteristics to bupivicaine. This is produced solely as the S-enantiomer, whereas bupivicaine is a mixture of the S and R forms. This S-form has less ability to bind Na-channels in the myocardial conduction system. Therefore, there is less risk of cardiotoxicity with ropivacaine. As seen in Table 20-4, ropivacaine and bupivicaine have very similar physical properties except for the margin of safety, in ropivacaine, which produces less toxic side effects. There also appears to be *less of a motor block* compared to bupivacaine, which theorhetically should improve patient satisfaction during the laboring process. Caution has been used in administering this agent as it has several side effects that occur in a significantly high occurrence (>10% of patients). These include

■ TABLE 20-4. Properties of Lidocaine, Bupivacaine, and Ropivacaine

Property	Lidocaine	Bupivacaine	Ropivacaine
Molecular weight	234	288	274
pK_a	7.7 (at pH 7.4, more drug in basic form)	8.1	8.0
Lipid solubility (directly related to speed of onset)	↑↑↑↑↑	↑↑	↑↑↑
Protein binding	64%	95%	94%
Elimination $T_{1/2}$ (h)	1.6	2.8	1.9
Maximum dose[a]	5 mg/kg (350 mg in a 70-kg patient) (7 mg/kg with epinephrine)	2-3 mg/kg (175 mg in a 70-kg patient)	>2 mg/kg
Toxicity	Seizures	Cardiac arrest	Seizures with much larger doses

[a]1% = 10 mg/cc; 0.25% bupivacaine = 2.5 mg/cc; 0.2% ropivacaine = 2.0 mg/cc.

cardiovascular: hypotension (dose-related and age-related: 32%-69%), maternal bradycardia (6%-20%), gastrointestinal: nausea (11%-29%), vomiting (7%-14%), and neuromuscular and skeletal: back pain (7%-10%) of patients.

Epidural Analgesia/Anesthesia

Lumbar epidural block is the most common form of analgesia used to provide relief from the nociceptive pathways during the stages of labor. The epidural space is the interval superiorly bounded by the foramen magnum, inferiorly by the lower end of the dural sac, anteriorly by the posterior longitudinal ligament, and posteriorly by the ligamentum flavum. The approach to the epidural space is posteriorly through the skin, subcutaneous fat, supraspinous ligament, interspinous ligament, ligamentum flavum and into the epidural space (Fig 20-4).

The size of the epidural space varies along its course with the largest diameter existing at the L_2 interspace with a range of 4 to 9 mm. A simple maneuver which helps to open up the bony entrance to the epidural space is flexion of the lumbar spine (Fig 20-5).

The contents of the epidural space include fat, vertebral venous plexus, lymphatics, arteries, and dural spinal nerve projections. In pregnancy, with the increase in intra-abdominal pressure, the venous plexus becomes distended. This phenomenon, and the accompanying increase in epidural fat that occurs during pregnancy, functions to substantially reduce epidural volume. Therefore, pregnant patients usually require less volume of local anesthetic, as compared to nonpregnant controls, to produce a similar level of blockade.

Once the epidural catheter is in place, local anesthetic is administered according to the appropriate pain pathway and corresponding stage of labor. In the first stage of labor, T_{10} block is sufficient. In the late first stage and second stage of labor, the nerves to be blocked include the sacral area so the parturient should be dosed in the semi-Fowler position to allow downward spread of the local anesthetic. Finally, for predelivery and the third stage of labor, the parturient may be seated upright (with a vena cava tilt) to secure sacral root spread of the drug (Fig 20-6). This blockade may be achieved by intermittent bolus injections or by continuous infusion of the drug with changes in patient positioning altering the level of blockade.

With the uppermost level of analgesia at T_{10}, the five lowermost vasomotor segments supplying the pelvis, lower trunk and limbs are interrupted causing a decrease in total peripheral resistance, venous return, and cardiac output. In normal parturients, this insult induces a reflex cardiovascular response directed toward maintaining systemic blood pressure. Preload of an adequate intravenous crystalloid infusion, keeping the parturient on her side, and minimizing the dose of the local anesthetic all minimize the adverse decrease in blood flow to the pelvis and its structures.

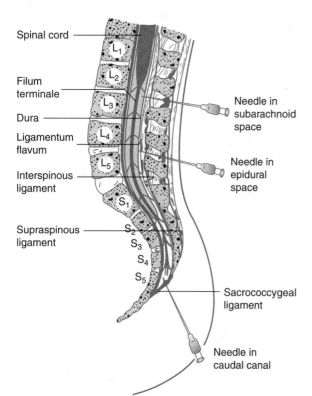

Spinal cord — L_1

Filum terminale — L_2

Dura — L_3

Ligamentum flavum — L_4

Interspinous ligament — L_5

Supraspinous ligament — S_1 S_2 S_3 S_4 S_5

Needle in subarachnoid space

Needle in epidural space

Sacrococcygeal ligament

Needle in caudal canal

FIGURE 20-4. Lumbosacral anatomy showing needle depth for epidural and subarachnoid injections.

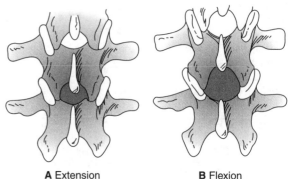

A Extension   **B** Flexion

FIGURE 20-5. Lumbar vertebrae. When patient is fixed, the interlaminar space enlarges, increasing the ability to enter the epidural/subarachnoid space.

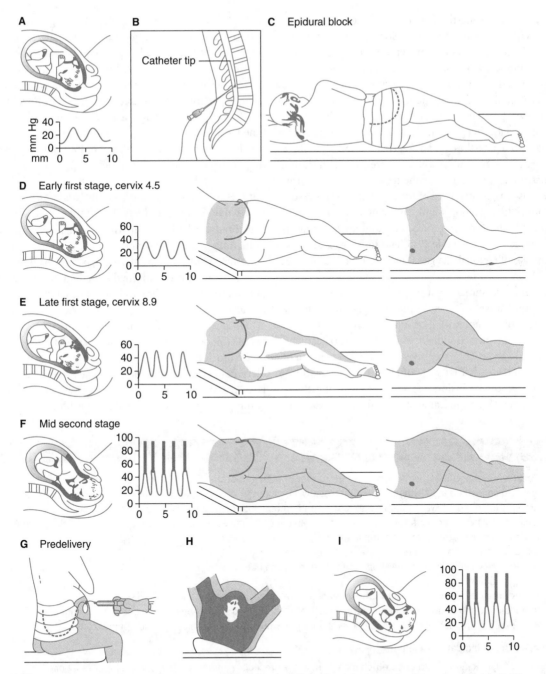

FIGURE 20-6. Lumbar epidural analgesia. **A-C.** Epidural catheter may be placed early in the first stage of labor **D.** When the patient experiences labor pain, local anesthetic may be injected to achieve a T_{10}-L_1 neuroblockade. **E-F.** In late first stage and mid-second stage of labor, the patient should be elevated 15°-20° to allow caudad spread of local anesthetic to achieve a T_{10}-S_5 block. **G-I.** To ensure sacral root dispersion of local anesthetic, once flexion and internal rotation of baby's head occurs, more local anesthetic can be injected with the patient in the seated upright position with a left tilt to the pelvis.

High epidural anesthesia that extends to T_4-S_5 is associated with a significant interruption of vasomotor segments resulting in significant hypotension. Again, fluid preload and lateral tilt of the parturient can augment the reflex corrective responses of the cardiovascular system in this situation. Extending the epidural blockade above spinal level T_{10} is unnecessary and counterproductive for the normal laboring patient. If epidural analgesia needs to be changed to anesthesia for a cesarian section, then these risks are necessary and measures to prevent them should be instituted. In addition, ephedrine, in most circumstances, is the best vasopressor to augment blood pressure without reducing blood supply to the uterus.

Contraindications to lumbar epidural analgesia/anesthesia are reviewed in Table 20-5. The advantages and disadvantages of regional analgesia/anesthesia are outlined in Table 20-6.

A combined spinal/epidural analgesia technique provides rapid onset of spinal opioid analgesia, plus the flexibility of the epidural blockade. Sufentanil 10 µg or fentanyl 25 µg injected spinally when the epidural catheter is inserted can reliably give several hours of analgesia to patients in the early first stage of labor (<5 cm dilation). The continuous infusion of a weak local anesthetic (0.125%/0.0625% bupivicaine or 0.2%/0.1% ropivacaine) with a low-dose narcotic (sufentanil 1-2 µg/cc or fentanyl 5-10 µg/cc) can provide good perineal analgesia for later stages of labor. If needed, higher concentrations of bupivacaine or lidocaine can be bolused for more complete nerve blockade. Less motor blockade, less hypotension, less local anesthetic administered with inherent toxicity risk, and faster onset of analgesia are all benefits of this combined technique.

The side effects of intrathecal opioids and corresponding treatment are listed in Table 20-7.

Fetal Bradycardia in Epidural Analgesia and Combined Spinal/Epidural Techniques

Fetal bradycardia is a nonreassuring fetal heart rate after induction of neuraxial anesthesia that may be due to maternal hypotension or uterine hyperactivity. It is mostly associated with the combined spinal/epidural technique but can be seen with any technique which produces profound analgesia.

The placental circulation is dependent on the maternal systolic blood pressure, and with a sudden onset sympathetic block from the local anesthetic, this can decrease placental perfusion and therefore cause fetal bradycardia. Local decreases in perfusion can occur without ever ascertaining a drop in the maternal systolic blood pressure.

■ TABLE 20-5. Contraindications to Lumbar Epidural Analgesia/Anesthesia

- Parturients who refuse the block or have great fear of puncture of the spine. In our experience, many patients who are concerned initially about epidural block will consent to be managed with this technique provided they are properly informed. However, if they still refuse, it is an absolute contraindication to the technique.
- Lack of skill by the administrator, not only in carrying out the procedure, but in the management of the parturient and in the prompt treatment of complications.
- Infection at the puncture site or in the epidural space.
- Severe hypovolemia from hemorrhage, dehydration, or malnutrition.
- Coagulopathies.
- Lack of resuscitation equipment in the immediate area ready for *prompt* use.
- In addition to the above, absolute contraindication to continuous caudal epidural anesthesia are infection or cyst in the area of the sacrococcygeal region and having the presenting part close to the perineum.

Relative Contraindications Include:

- Lack of appreciation by the obstetrician as to how the procedure influences the management of labor.
- A very rapid or precipitate labor, or in any case which requires immediate anesthesia. On the other hand for the anesthesiologist who is very skilled and has had extensive experience, extension of the epidural block in patients who have had the catheter in place during labor can be done as rapidly as getting things ready for anesthesia.
- Cephalopelvic disproportion unless the block is used for a trial of labor prior to cesarean section.

Source: Reproduced with permission from John J. Bonica. *Principles and Practice of Obstetric Analgesia and Anesthesia.* 2nd ed. Malvern, PA: Williams & Wilkins; 1995.

■ **TABLE 20-6. Advantages and Disadvantages of Regional Analgesia/Anesthesia**

Advantages

- In contrast to opoids, regional analgesia produces complete relief from pain in most parturients.
- The hazards of pulmonary aspiration of gastric contents that is inherent in general anesthesia is diminished and can be even eliminated.
- *Provided it is properly administered* and no complications occur, regional analgesia/anesthesia causes no serious maternal or neonatal complications.
- Administered at the proper time, it does not impede the progress of labor at the first stage.
- Continuous techniques can be extended for delivery and may even be modified for cesarean section if this becomes necessary.
- Regional analgesia permits the mother to remain awake during labor and delivery so that she can experience the pleasure of actively participating in the birth of her child.
- Regional anesthesia for cesarean section also permits the mother to be awake and immediately develop bonding with the newborn.
- Provided the mother is doing well, the anesthesiologist can leave her and resuscitate the newborn if this is necessary.

Disadvantages

- Regional techniques require greater skill to administer than do administration of systemic drugs or inhalation agents.
- Technical failures occur even in experienced hands.
- Certain techniques produce side effects (eg, maternal hypotension) that if not promptly and properly treated can progress to complications in the mother and fetus.
- Techniques that produce perineal muscle paralysis interfere with the mechanism of internal rotation and increase the incidence of posterior positions and thus require instrumental deliveries.
- These procedures can only be carried out in the hospital.

Source: Reproduced with permission from John J. Bonica. *Principles and Practice of Obstetric Analgesia and Anesthesia.* 2nd ed. Malvern, PA: Williams & Wilkins; 1995.

■ **TABLE 20-7. Intrathecal Opioids Side Effects and Recommended Treatment**

Side effect	Treatment
Itching	Benadryl, 25 mg IV
	Propofol, 10 mg IV
	Naloxone, 40 µg IV
Nausea and vomiting	Reglan, 10 mg IV
	Propofol, 10 mg IV
	Naloxone, 40 µg IV
	Zofran, 4 mg IV
Hypotension	IV fluids
	Ephedrine
Urinary retention	Catheterization
	Naloxone, 400 µg IV

Another proposed explanation is that the fetal bradycardia is due to intrathecal opioid-induced uterine hypertonus. The uterine tetany is thought to be due to rapid onset of analgesia, which causes a sudden decrease in maternal plasma epinephrine and subsequent withdrawal of epinephrine's β-sympathomimetic relaxant effects on the myometrium. This is followed with decreased placental blood flow, fetal asphyxia, and fetal bradycardia.

Preanalgesic adequate hydration of the patient must be achieved, as well as, the prevention of overdosing with high blocks beyond that necessary to achieve analgesia for the nerve roots involved with the labor pains, With this physiological understanding of the dynamics occurring, treatment is based on relaxing the uterus. Uterine hypertonus may be reversed with one or two doses of intravenous nitroglycerin (60-90 µg). The hypotension that results is treated with ephedrine (5-10 mg) or phenylephrine (40-800 µg). Persistent hypertonus can be treated with another dose of nitroglycerin or a β-agonist, such as terbutaline 0.25 mg intravenously; however, terbutaline results in an extended period of uterine relaxation and maternal tachycardia. Some studies have entertained the idea of "pretreating" all patients prior to neuraxial analgesia with ephedrine intravenously, and they had more resultant fetal tachycardia than the group without pretreatment and is not recommended.

■ OTHER REGIONAL ANALGESIC/ ANESTHETIC TECHNIQUES

There are two important techniques to discuss that may be used by the obstetric care provider to provide analgesia when obstetrical anesthesia coverage is unavailable. Although these techniques are relatively easy to execute, a thorough knowledge of the anatomy, physiology, and effects of local anesthetics on mother and fetus is paramount.

Bilateral Pudendal Nerve Block

This block is an effective blockade for the second and third stages of labor, blocking the sacral nerves S_3-S_4-S_5 (Fig 20-7). The transvaginal approach points the needle behind the sacrospinous ligament aiming toward the ischial spine. Up to 5 mg/kg of lidocaine (1% solution with or without 1:200,000 epinephrine) total dose provides relief of perineal pain within 3 to 5 minutes (Figs 20-8 and 20-9).

Bilateral Paracervical Block

Paracervical block interrupts uterine nociceptive pain pathways T_{10}-L_1, effecting complete relief from pain of the first stage of labor (Fig 20-10). This does not, however, relieve any perineal pain of the second and third stages of labor. Using up to 5 mg/kg of lidocaine in a 1% solution total dose will give good pain relief for approximately 2 hours. Associated transient fetal bradycardia has been reported with the use of paracervical blockade and therefore should be used with caution. Local anesthetics with epinephrine should not be used since the fetal head is so close to the injection site and the proximate location of the uterine artery and venous plexus that it may increase the risk of epinephrine uptake by mother and/or fetus.

■ ANESTHESIA FOR CESAREAN SECTIONS

Spinal Anesthesia

The advantages of spinal anesthesia responsible for its current popularity include relative simplicity, rapidity,

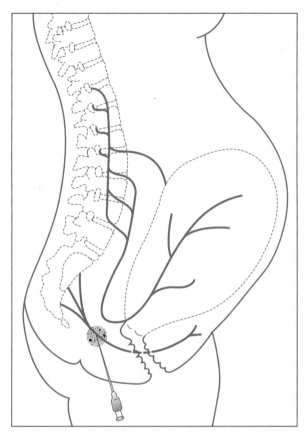

FIGURE 20-7. Demonstration of the pudendal nerve block involving only S_{3-5} for the pain associated with the second stage of labor.

certainty, duration, low failure rate, and minimal side effects. It also offers the lowest drug exposure since local anesthetic is being exposed directly to nerve fibers with minimal systemic uptake of the drug.

The primary disadvantages of spinal anesthesia are the effects of high T_{2-4} blockade with maternal hypotension and postural puncture headaches (Table 20-8). The risk of the high spinal includes sympathectomy with resultant unopposed parasympathetic stimulation. This leads to hypotension, increased gastric motility, increased nausea/vomiting, and instability of uterine perfusion. In parturients with severe asthma or reactive airway disease, this may precipitate bronchospasm. Also, the high motor blockade may inhibit motor fibers of the respiratory muscles impairing normal ventilation.

The postdural puncture headache risks are directly related to the size and type of needle used. With the 24/26 G Sprotte (blunted) needles now in use, the risk is <1% in this age group of patients. An important factor in the

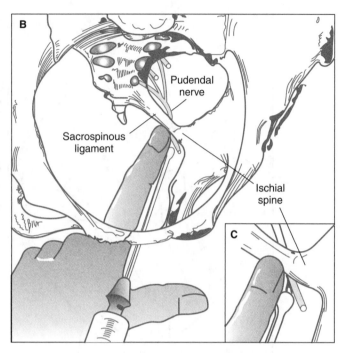

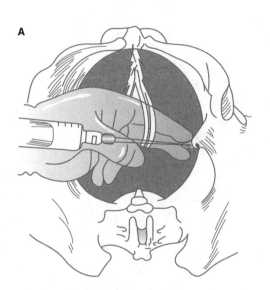

FIGURE 20-8. The transvaginal approach to pudendal neuroblockade. **A-C.** This technique is performed bilaterally. The needle passes behind the sacrospinous ligament and posterior to the ischial spine. Aspiration, prior to injection of the local anesthetic drug, is prudent to avoid inadvertent intravascular administration.

dispersion of the local anesthetic is the position of the patient. As shown in Fig 20-11, the lowest point of the spine is T_5. Care therefore should be directed toward raising the patient's head in an effort to reduce the inadvertent

FIGURE 20-9. Stippled area illustrates the extent of analgesia/anesthesia provided by pudendal neuroblockade—sufficient for the second stage of labor pain.

cephalad spread of the drug. Complications of subarachnoid block include

- Physiological: Hypotension, bradycardia, or possible cardiac arrest
- Nonphysiological: Respiratory arrest and toxicity reactions
- Neurological: Paraplegia, arachnoiditis, or postdural puncture headache

General Anesthesia for Cesarean Section

General anesthesia is reserved for life-threatening situations including severe fetal distress, cord prolapse, shoulder dystocia, intrauterine exploration for retained placenta or a twin, and replacement of an inverted uterus. In obstetrical anesthesia, the anesthesiologist is responsible for two lives: the mother and the baby.

Preanesthetic preparation includes a history and physical examination with emphasis on cardiac and pulmonary disease, evaluation of the airway, height/weight comparison, allergies, current medications, intravenous access, and blood product availability. Every pregnant woman beyond the first trimester is considered to have a full stomach and is at risk for aspiration of gastric contents. This demands

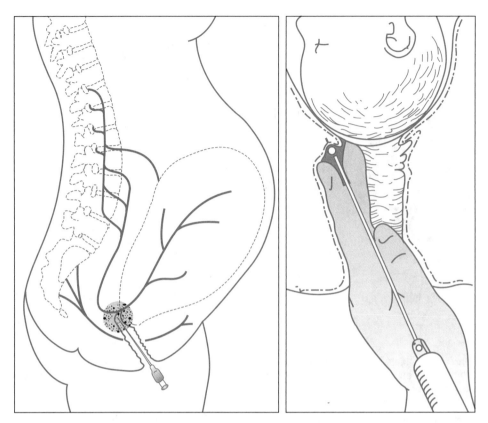

FIGURE 20-10. A technique for bilateral paracervical block. Neuroblockade involving T_{10}-L_1 when accomplished is adequate for the pain associated with the first stage of labor. Injections are made into the bilateral fornices of the vagina. Note the proximity of the presenting part, as well as, the deeper pelvic plexus with uterine arteries and ureters.

prophylaxis with a nonparticulate antacid, an H2-blocker, and metochlorpropamide (Reglan). The most common cause of maternal death related to general anesthesia is aspiration pneumonia secondary to inability to secure the airway with an endotracheal tube.

Induction of Anesthesia

The patient should be placed on the operating table with a leftward pelvic tilt to prevent aorto-caval compression with monitors applied. She should receive a 500 cc to 1000 cc lactated Ringer bolus while preoxygenation is performed. Cricoid pressure should be applied as the Sellick maneuver is achieved to prevent regurgitation of stomach contents into the lung. The obstetrician who is prepared and ready to make an incision with one hand may place the other hand on the patient's epigastric area. Intravenous induction (using the patient's ideal body weight) with thiopental (3-5 mg/kg), propofol (1-2 mg/kg), ketamine

(1 mg/kg), or Etomidate (0.2-0.3 mg/kg) may be used. Succinylcholine 1 mg/kg IV is given to achieve muscle relaxation to facilitate endotracheal intubation. Once the endotracheal tube is placed, the first breath given by the anesthesiologist should *not* be felt by the obstetrician's hand over the stomach. If a belch of air is perceived, the ETT may not, in fact, be in the trachea. This team approach assures maximal security of a protected, intubated airway prior to surgical incision. Maintenance of a balanced general anesthesia with both inhalational agents and intravenous muscle relaxants is performed until delivery of the baby. At this time, narcotics may be given to reduce the concentration of inhalational drugs needed.

The patient should be completely awake and in control of her airway protective reflexes before extubation occurs. It is important to understand that the risk of aspiration at the end of surgery (extubation) is just as great as at the start (intubation).

■ TABLE 20-8. The Primary Disadvantages of the Use of Spinal Anesthesia and the Contraindications

Primary disadvantages

Frequency of hypotension
Postdural puncture headaches

Contraindications

Infection at the site of puncture
Disease of the central nervous system
Severe hypovolemia due to hemorrhage, dehydration, or malnutrition
Fetopelvic disproportion unless the block is used for a trial of labor prior to cesarean section
Parturient refusal or fear of the procedure, or emotional unsuitability for regional anesthesia
Severe hypotension or hypertension
Lack of skilled physicians
Lack of resuscitation equipment in the immediate area

Source: Reproduced with permission from John J. Bonica. *Principles and Practice of Obstetric Analgesia and Anesthesia.* 2nd ed. Malvern, PA: Williams & Wilkins; 1995.

Figure 20-12 is a guide to failed intubation events with/without a known difficult airway, with/without the ability to ventilate, and with/without fetal distress.

■ SPECIAL CONSIDERATIONS

Preeclampsia

Preeclampsia is a multisystem disease. Although its hallmarks are hypertension and proteinuria, patients may develop renal failure, thrombocytopenia, hemolysis, liver dysfunction, and CNS involvement. For labor, epidural or epidural/spinal with narcotic/local anesthetic combinations are optimal to reduce the added stress related to pain. For cesarean section delivery, controversy remains whether epidural or general anesthesia is best. Epidural anesthesia for cesarean section requires a high block-T_4 with the associated risk of maternal hypotension. General anesthesia requires intubation, which with tracheal stimulation may result in dangerous hemodynamic aberrations including hypertension, increased mean pulmonary artery pressure, and increased pulmonary capillary wedge pressure. With adequate invasive monitors such as an arterial line with or without a pulmonary artery catheter, careful hydration, use of Ephedrine and slow onset of the block, epidural blockade can be safely conducted. Also, the use of β-blocker agents (preinduction) or lidocaine to blunt the tracheal stimulation of intubation can also be safe. Magnesium sulfate interacts with both depolarizing and nondepolarizing neuromuscular blocking drugs, so dosages must be altered accordingly. Close monitoring of the patient and open discussion of the patient's preoperative status with the obstetrician is helpful in determining the optimum anesthetic plan for mother and baby (see Chap 5).

Preterm Birth

Patients with preterm labor, for whatever reason, will most likely have been on tocolytic drugs. If β-adrenergic drugs were used to secure uterine relaxation, care must be taken to observe for tachycardia, hypertension, chest pain, myocardial ischemia, arrhythmias, pulmonary edema, anxiety, nausea/vomiting, hyperglycemia, or hypokalemia that may be exaggerated by general anesthetics. In parturients on intravenous magnesium sulfate as a tocolytic

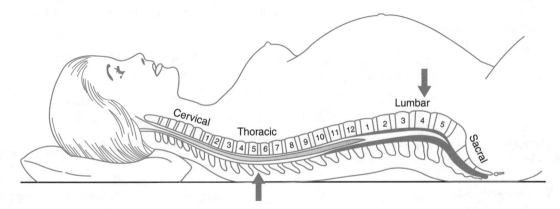

FIGURE 20-11. The natural curves of the female spine in the supine position. Gravity tends to ascend the level of anesthetic spread to T_3-T_5, therefore, an early head-up tilt would assure a lower level of blockade.

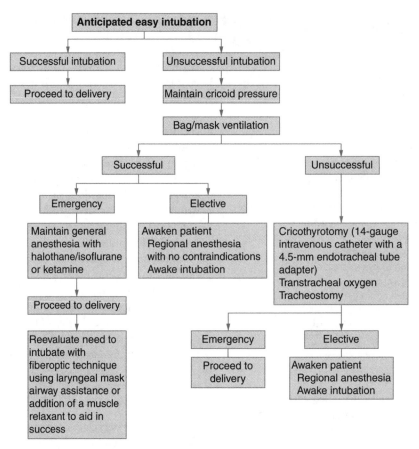

FIGURE 20-12. Guide for failed intubation.

agent, potentiation of muscle relaxant drug activity should be anticipated. Since preterm fetuses are often low birthweight, with diminished compensatory reserve, special attention should be directed at maintaining uteroplacental perfusion (see Chap 22).

HIV-Infected Parturients

Concern has been voiced in published literature that HIV positive parturients may not be candidates for regional anesthesia. The fear of spreading the infection to the central nervous system, adverse neurological sequelae, or attenuation of the immunological status of the patient has been questioned. To date, the available data support the use of epidural anesthesia in these patients with no substantiated evidence that these concerns are valid (see Chap 26).

Coagulopathies

The preoperative laboratory tests recommended in a parturient with a suspected coagulopathy include:

hemoglobin, hematocrit, platelet count, prothrombin time (PT), partial thromboplastin time (PTT), fibrinogen, and fibrin degradation products. There is no one source (authority) which specifies the best test or laboratory value in determining risk for epidural hematoma. The following are examples when epidural anesthesia is not recommended.

- Parturient on heparin therapy with elevated PTT or heparin level >0.24/mL
- Parturient with known factor deficiency, for example, von Willebrand with low Factor 8 levels
- Parturient with severe HELLP syndrome
- Parturient with disseminated intravascular coagulopathy
- Parturient actively bleeding and hemodynamically unstable

Many examples of stable, but abnormal laboratory values may be amenable to an epidural technique. However, discussion with the obstetrician as to whether active bleeding is occurring and an overall risks versus benefits discussion of general anesthesia as compared to conduction anesthesia, in a given high-risk circumstance, may help to determine the parturient's best overall anesthetic management.

CARDIAC DISEASE: CONGENITAL HEART DISEASE

The degree of shunting of blood in women with intracardiac defects is primarily determined by the balance of resistances in the systemic (systemic vascular resistance) and pulmonary vascular beds (pulmonary vascular resistance). During pregnancy, these resistances decline proportionally during the various stages of pregnancy. With atrial septal defect (ASD), ventricular septal defect (VSD), or patent ductus arteriosus (PDA) with a left to right shunt, these parturients usually tolerate pregnancy, anesthesia, and delivery well. Reminders are to be aware of arrhythmias, systemic embolism, right ventricular hypertrophy and failure, and pulmonary hypertension. These concerns are especially problematic in the postpartum period when placental shunting is gone (increased blood volume) resulting in an increased preload that places a strain on the shunt balance. Parturients with right-to-left shunts such as uncorrected Tetralogy of Fallot or Eisenmenger syndrome can be exacerbated by hypoxemia, hypercarbia, and decrease in systemic vascular resistance.

In right or left ventricular outflow obstruction such as valvular stenosis or coarctation of the aorta, volume depletion, or decrease in systemic vascular resistance can significantly exacerbate symptoms. With careful monitoring and attention to the specifics of the cardiac lesion and resultant cardiopulmonary pathophysiology, anesthesia and analgesia can be safely conducted in the high-risk parturient (see Chap 8).

PULMONARY DISEASE: PULMONARY EDEMA

Pulmonary edema, when it occurs during pregnancy invariably has a predisposing etiology (Table 20-9). Basic management of this condition includes establishing the cause and reversing the effects of hypoxemia. The use of hemodynamic monitoring in the form of a pulmonary artery catheter and arterial line can be extremely useful in elucidating the etiology and most appropriate treatment for pulmonary edema (see Chap 12).

Anesthetic management for delivery of the baby, in most circumstances, may be in the form of a conduction anesthetic. However, the parturient with severe respiratory

■ TABLE 20-9. Causes of Pulmonary Edema

Cardiac (high pressures)

Cardiac dysfunction	Decreased left ventricular contractility, mitral stenoses
	Mitral regurgitation, intravascular volume overload, dysrhythmias
Pulmonary venous dysfunction	Venous occlusive disease, neurogenic pulmonary vasoconstriction
Pulmonary embolization	Amniotic fluid, thrombus, fat, air
Airway obstruction	Edema, asthma, foreign body
Preeclampsia	Pulmonary hypertension
Miscellaneous	Pneumothorax, tumor, one lung anesthesia (down lung syndrome)

Noncardiogenic (permeability)

Adult respiratory distress syndrome
Aspiration syndromes
Pulmonary embolization
Abruptio placentae
Dead fetus syndrome
Sepsis

Source: Reproduced with permission from John J. Bonica. *Principles and Practice of Obstetric Analgesia and Anesthesia.* 2nd ed. Baltimore, MD: Williams & Wilkins; 1995.

failure may require general anesthesia with endotracheal intubation to obtain stability.

■ CONCLUSION

In conclusion, once an understanding of the nature of the parturient's pain is recognized, with techniques available to the anesthesiologist and obstetrician, an optimal care plan can be attained, even for high-risk parturients.

SUGGESTED READINGS

Avroy A. Fanacoff. *Neonatal-Perinatal Medicine: Diseases of the Fetus and Infant.* 5th ed. St. Louis, MO: Mosby; 1992.

Birnbach D. Ostheimer's *Manual of Obstetric Anesthesia.* 3rd ed. New York, NY: Churchill Livingstone; 2000.

Cascio M, Pygon B, Bernett C, Ramanathan S. Labour analgesia with intrathecal fentanyl decreases maternal stress. *Can J Anaesth.* 1997 Jun;44(6):605-609.

Collis RE. Randomized comparison of combined spinal—epidural and standard epidural analgesia in labour. *Lancet.* 1995;345(8962):1413-1416.

Dalton ME, Gross I. Seminars in Perinatology, April 2002. Vol 26, No 2. West Philadelphia, PA: W B Saunders.

Wallace D. Randomized comparison of general and regional anesthesia for cesarean delivery in pregnancies complicated by severe preeclampsia. *Obstetrics & Gynecology.* 1995;86 (2): 193-199.

Guyton AC, Hall JE. *Textbook of Medical Physiology.* 9th ed. West Philadelphia, PA: W.B. Saunders; 1996.

Hughes S. Parturients infected with human immunodeficiency virus and regional anesthesia. *Anesthesiology.*1995;82(1): 32-37.

IARS 2002 Review Course Lectures. Birnbaum, p. 12, Butterworth, pp. 22, 38, 54.

John J. Bonica. *Principles and Practice of Obstetric Analgesia and Anesthesia.* 2nd ed. Baltimore, MD: Williams & Wilkins; 1995.

Kreiser D, Katorza E, Seidman DS, Etchin A, Schiff E. The effect of ephedrine on intrapartum fetal heart rate after epidural analgesia. *Obstet Gynecol.* 2004 Dec;104(6):1277-1281.

Mark C. Norris. *International Anesthesiology Clinics.* Hagerstown, MD: Lippincott Williams & Wilkins; 1994;32(2):69-81.

Mercier FJ, Dounas M, Bouaziz H, Lhuissier C, Benhamou D. Intravenous nitroglycerin to relieve Intrapartum fetal distress related to uterine hyperactivity: a prospective observational study. *Anesth Analg.* 1997 May;84(5):1117-1120.

Seminars in Perinatology, New Techniques & Drugs for Epidural Labor Analgesia. Philadelphia, PA: W.B. Saunders; April 2002:100, Table I.

Sol M. Shnider. *Anesthesia for Obstetrics.* 3rd ed. Baltimore, MD: Williams & Wilkins; 1993.

CHAPTER 21

Psychiatric Emergencies in Pregnancy

• *Marlin D. Mills and Paul Berkowitz*

Psychiatric disorders in women of child-bearing years are common, given that the vast majority of psychiatric conditions declare themselves during this stage of life. Pregnancy, and the events surrounding this unique life experience, is filled with significant emotional and psychological stress. Even in cases where the pregnancy is planned, these stresses affect all involved, including the pregnant mother, her husband/birth-partner, family, friends, and health-care providers.

What constitutes a psychiatric emergency? Psychiatric presentations can occur in a variety of ways and obstetricians and obstetric staff caring for high-risk pregnant patients (and their families) are often confronted with behaviors that can quickly devolve into crisis situations. While each obstetric clinician will have their own set of personal reactions to various disruptive behaviors or personality types, the common thread for all of these providers comes from the most empiric goal of obstetric medicine—to assure the well-being of the mother and the baby. Therefore, a more structured, cohesive, and organized schema for identifying and managing these patients is necessary.

Although much has been written regarding women's mental health issues and psychiatric complications during pregnancy, it is scattered among a variety of subspecialty resources.[1] Postgraduate training programs in obstetrics offer very little in the way of formal education in this arena.[2]

Over the remainder of this chapter, we hope to provide clear and easy-to-follow guidelines for problem solving and triaging psychiatric emergencies that arise in pregnancy, including preexisting psychiatric conditions, those with new symptoms/behaviors, as well as those caused by other medical interventions (ie, delirium). Approaches to the patient at risk for harming themselves or others and the agitated or angry patient will be discussed. The use of psychotropic medications and specific nonpharmaceutical treatments in pregnancy will also be reviewed.

■ DANGER TO SELF OR OTHERS

Perhaps, the most anxiety generating crisis in the gravid patient is the patient who threatens to harm herself, her baby, or those around her. A patient's allusion to suicide is sometimes the only cue for an emergent psychiatric consultation request.[3] Suicide is the 11th leading cause of death in the United States.[4] About 5% of all female suicides occur during the child-bearing years. Additionally, nearly 2% of completed suicides in this group were by pregnant women. Rates of suicide increased with first trimester miscarriage or termination. (Table 21-1)

Despite previous beliefs, women are just as likely to complete a suicide attempt as their male counterparts thus indicating an increase in suicide completion rates in women.

Assessing for suicidality, or risk of harm to others (including the fetus), is of utmost importance and must be carried out in a prompt, yet professional and sensitive manner. While there are numerous suicide risk screening tools available, by far the most valuable tool one can employ involves respectful and open dialogue with the patient (and her immediate supports). A common misconception about suicide screening is that one may actually increase the risk of the patient attempting suicide

■ TABLE 21-1. Suicide After Pregnancy[5]

	(Rates per 100,000)
• Mean annual rate	11.3
• Rate assoc with birth	5.9
• Rate with miscarriage	18.1
• Rate with induced abortion	34.7
• 5.4% of all suicides in women in this age group	
• 1.7% of all suicides in women were pregnant at the time	

■ TABLE 21-3. Safety Assurance Interventions

Outpatient setting
- Don't leave the patient alone—engage with office staff, crisis team, family members, or friends to accompany the patient until the crisis is resolved.
- If her safety cannot be appropriately assured, safe and secure transportation to an ER (or crisis evaluation center) is indicated.
- Can the crisis team come to the obstetric office?
- If there are concerns about immediate harm or danger then consider calling 911.
- If there is an established outpatient mental health provider, engage with them promptly for guidance and support.

Inpatient setting
- Don't leave the patient alone—utilize companions (as per hospital policy).
- Engage other supports—family, friends, spiritual leaders, etc.
- Request psychiatry consultation.

(or implanting the suicidal notion into a patient's mind) simply by inquiring about these thoughts. There is evidence to support exactly the opposite; empathic questioning of a patient about her possible thoughts of self-harm may actually alleviate some of the related emotional distress and may even serve to reduce the risk for a suicide attempt. An honest, open, and gentle probing of a patient's thoughts and feelings about harming herself (or others) will often yield a wealth of useful information (Table 21-2).

Some women may actually experience the simple expression of their thoughts of suicide as the necessary tool to relieve their emotional tension, while others may use this as an arena to generate a heightened level of emotional support from their family or other supports. Not all women who express thoughts of suicide will go on to attempt or commit suicide. But given the potential cost is so great, each and every eruption of suicidal thinking deserves appropriate consideration.

Arrange for a safe environment! There are no limitations as to when and where we may encounter a suicidal patient, and there is no reason to limit the most basic of interventions—assure her safety. Examples of techniques that can be used to assure safety are listed in Table 21-3.

■ TABLE 21-2. Examples of Empathic Questions About Suicidal (or Self-Harm) Thinking

a. Have you been having thoughts about hurting yourself?
b. Are you having any thoughts about hurting the baby?
c. Have you ever tried to hurt yourself before?
d. Do you feel that you can be safe right now?

■ ANGER/AGITATION

The expression of anger often follows a recognized pattern. Just as dealing with a suicidal patient can elicit strong emotional reactions within the health-care provider, so too can the interactions with an angry, confrontational, enraged, aggressive, assaultive, or caustic patient (or family member). Being aware of this pattern can guide the health-care provider to diffuse a potentially explosive situation. The genesis of anger must begin with a stressor. While it may not always be possible to specifically identify the particular stressor, fear is one of the painful core feelings often expressed as anger. Continuing with the explosion analogy, there is often a triggering event (such as a comment, action/inaction, or event) that will release a cascade of emotions that can become expressed as anger. Anger is an ubiquitous human emotion. Yet, the source of the anger is often difficult to clarify as we can tend to focus more on the behavior demonstrated during the acting out phase of the anger process (Table 21-4).

When faced with an escalating situation, the initial response should be to remain calm (both emotionally and physically) and maintain good eye contact (remembering that in some cultures direct eye contact may be viewed as

■ **TABLE 21-4. The Process of Anger**

- Stressor
- Painful core feelings
- Trigger statements
- Anger
- Acting out

aggression). The patient is attempting to communicate something to you (which may not be clear to anyone, including the patient, at this point). Your job at this point, which is to gather as much data as possible, will prove fruitful toward the goal of a uneventful resolution. Some

■ **TABLE 21-5. Understanding the Angry Patient**

- The initial response should be to pause, acknowledge the emotions, and try to find a common point of agreement.
- "Step back" from the emotionally charged situation and try to analyze what is happening.
- Ask the patient to sit down and try to adopt a similar position (the mirroring strategy) without taking an aggressive pose. Establishing eye contact may be useful; however, in some cultures this may seem aggressive.
- Address the patient (or relative) appropriately. Avoid use of nicknames or too familiar terms until rapport has been established.
- Be calm.
- Appear comfortable and in control of your own emotions.
- Be interested and genuinely concerned about the patient and the problem.
- Use clear, firm, nonemotive language.
- Listen!
- Allow the patient to ventilate their feelings and help to relieve their burdens.
- Give appropriate reassurance (but do not go overboard to appease the patient).
- Allow time (at least 20 minutes).
- Try to identify any hidden agendas.
- Recognize the relationship between anger and fear.

helpful steps toward understanding the patient's needs are outlined in Table 21-5.

The following examples of techniques that can be used in these situations as a process of deescalating a crisis situation can be found in many counseling resources such as *Behavioral Medicine: A Guide for Clinical Practice* by Feldman (2007).[6]

Modeling
- Slow, steady breathing
  - Monitor the pace and tone of your voice.
- Open body language
  - Monitor your body language to avoid closed, aggressive postures. Sitting directly in front of someone can appear confrontational. Consider sitting at a 45° angle, or if safe, facing the same direction.

Rapport building
Listen with attention and intention.
Make empathic statements.
"I can appreciate how you feel."
"It concerns me that you feel so strongly about this."
"Tell me how I can make it easier for you."

Confrontation (difficult to do until rapport has been established)
"You seem very angry?"
"It's unlike you to be like this."
"I get the feeling that you are upset with..."
"What is it that's upsetting you?"
"What really makes you feel this way?"

Reflection, facilitation, clarification
Do not parrot patient statements or phrases, but try to accurately reflect or rephrase what you think the patient is trying to communicate.
"I find it puzzling that you are angry with me."
"So you feel that....."
"You seem to be telling me...."
"If I understand you correctly..."
"Tell me more about this."
"I would like you to enlarge on this point...it seems important."

Searching
"Do you have any special concerns about you or your baby's health?"
"Tell me more."
"How are things at home, work?"
"How are you sleeping, eating?"

"Do you have any special dreams?"

"Can you identify anyone who has a problem like you have?"

SELF CARE/PROVIDER SAFETY ASSURANCE

- Always position yourself with an easy exit.
- Watch for premonitory signs (fist clenching, use of profanity, violence to inanimate objects, actual verbal threats).
- Assess for access to a weapon.
- *A past history of violence* is the greatest predictor of future violence.
- Do not hesitate to call for security support.

In cases where the patient refuses to respond, or cannot respond, further investigation is necessary. It is impossible to predict with 100% certainty when a patient will become violent, however, relying on one's own self-preservation instincts can be a useful guide in determining the next management step. A patient who remains upset yet is responsive to your efforts will be managed differently than a patient who continues to display escalating hostile behavior.

When the anger begins to control physical behavior (ie, agitation), a process for evaluating other potential sources is necessary to make sure that an underlying cause (intoxication, delirium, psychosis, mania, etc) is not overlooked. Table 21-6 describes some potential causes of agitation, while a guideline for the evaluation for causes of altered mental status is shown in Table 21-7.

Part of the goal of controlling an erupting situation is to assure the safety to the patient as well as to the staff and others in the immediate area. Given that such scenarios are often highly emotionally charged (on both sides of the bed) utilizing basic crisis management techniques must occur so as to have the greatest likelihood of a smooth resolution. Table 21-8 describes the conceptualization of managing such situations.

ANXIETY

The pregnant patient may present with anxiety symptoms that predate the pregnancy or are specific to her current status. This can be related to realistic, or unrealistic, fears

---

■ TABLE 21-7. Mnemonic for Evaluation of Causes of Altered Mental Status

I WATCH DEATH

I = Infection
W = Withdrawal syndromes
A = Acute metabolic changes
T = Trauma
C = CNS pathology
H = Hypoxia
D = Deficiencies
E = Endocrinopathies
A = Acute vascular
T = Toxins or drugs
H = Heavy metals

■ TABLE 21-6. Potential Causes of Agitation

- Intoxication (ethyl alcohol [EtOH], illicit substances, pharmaceuticals)
- Withdrawal syndromes (EtOH, opiates, illicit substances)
- Delirium
- Psychosis
- Mania

■ TABLE 21-8. Management of Agitation in Pregnancy

- Reassessment:
  - Plan of approach
  - Engagement
  - Limit number of people involved/communicating with patient
  - One spokesperson
- Interventions
  - Establish rapport/trust
  - Clarification of patients wants/needs
  - Clarification of what you want/need from patient (what will and won't be tolerated)
- Security assistance: when to request, visible or not, restraints
  - Knowledge of state laws and hospital policies regarding specific security procedures and use of restraints is mandatory.
  - Assure proper documentation regarding use of restraints.

about the pregnancy. The health of the baby is a common fear, especially when additional worry is created by definite or suspected findings on ultrasound done during the pregnancy. There is the fear of the pain of a vaginal delivery or fear of failing to accomplish a vaginal delivery resulting in a cesarean delivery. Fears related to body image issues from the effects of the pregnancy or the resulting scar from cesarean delivery can also drive up anxieties. Having a new baby at home brings on fears of adequacy as a mother and/or wife. Other psychosocial issues such as financial strain and family tensions among other children, partners, and in-laws are examples of other anxiogenic sources.

Emergent situations related to anxiety can present as debilitating panic attacks, noncompliance in medical care, over-use of medical care, or the use of substances (self-medicating, illicit, misuse of prescribed medications).

Anxiety may present as an internal sense of nervousness, hostility, psychomotor agitation (fidgetiness, increase in purposeless movements), somatic complaints (chest pain, shortness of breath, diaphoresis, paresthesias, nausea, and other somatic preoccupations), or overt panic attacks. A calm and gentle first approach will often allow for the establishment of a good connection with the patient (and her supports). Careful initial evaluation (a review of systems, vitals, physical examination, and evaluation of the fetal status) can help properly rule-out medical causes (eg, hypoxia). A calm review of the reassuring elements of the preceding physical examination and fetal assessment along with the initiation of a basic behavioral psychotherapy technique (deep breathing exercises or serial muscle contraction/relaxation exercises) will often result in resolution of the acute anxiety symptoms. Pharmacologic strategies should be reserved for the most acute cases when all other interventions have failed. The proper selection of an anxiolytic agent will be based on the stage of pregnancy, current acuity level, and previous patient experience with the various pharmacologic options. Consultation with the pediatrician, or neonatologist, should be considered if this crisis evolves during labor.

The labor process can be very exciting yet equally distressing. If a patient's anxiety escalates such that she can no longer be an active participant in the delivery, maintenance of a clear line of communication is essential. The patient must be aware of the situation and able to cooperate and, if needed, be able to provide competent consent in case an emergent surgical situation arises. The delivery room can quickly become filled with chaos which can lead to a further disintegration of the patient's ability to participate. If possible, attempt to establish an advocate in

whom the patient can harbor trust, in order to maintain an open line of effective communication with the health-care team. Occasionally events can happen so quickly that the patient may lose her ability to perform properly in the delivery, in these cases using focus and direction interaction may actually allow for one to take advantage of the heightened state of awareness that can arise in such anxiety producing situations.

Some anxious patients will benefit by discussions that prepare them for potential complications. By knowing that there is an established plan of action to handle these unforeseeable events the patient may actually be more able to tolerate the growing anxiety and stay focused enough to allow for a good cooperation between patient and obstetrician. A debriefing session following these events will allow for the now postpartum patient to express her concerns, have questions addressed, and may even serve as a protective mechanism against acute posttraumatic stress reactions.

In summary, a close and trusting relationship with the obstetrician will prove useful to the patient, her family, and the treatment team. Preemptive strategies such as preparatory discussions about the patient's fears, establishing how communications will be handled in the event of an unintended outcome, and even allowing for cultural and religious input (such as a prayer before the start of the procedure) can have a calming influence on not only the patient but her family and health-care providers.

■ MOOD DISORDERS

Unipolar and bipolar spectrum mood disorders typically emerge in the late teens to early twenties which coincides with peak fertility years. There has been much work exploring the link between hormones and mood disorders with a strong focus on attempting to understand the post-partum mood state. Estimates on the incidence of post-partum mood disorders, ranging from mild and self-limited depressions (sometimes called "the baby blues") to severe depressions or manias or psychoses range from 10%-80%. The prevalence of mood disorders during pregnancy is less clear because these conditions are still poorly recognized in the community and the psychosocial stigma associated with psychiatric conditions in general tends to keep reporting low. The incidence of depression in the general population ranges from 2%-10% and estimates of perinatal depression has been as high as 20%-25% in a high-risk pregnancy population.

The obstetrician or perinatologist must assess for depression as part of the regular evaluation process.

Depression is often a condition intensified by psychosocial or emotional distress, thus it is not difficult to imagine that women with high-risk pregnancies will be at higher risk for developing this condition. Screening can start with as simple a question as "How has your mood been lately?" For a more formal process, the Edinburgh Postpartum Depression Scale (EPDS) is a commonly used tool,[7] although a number of screening tools are available (and can easily be implemented into an office or hospital-based perinatal practice).

The impact of depression is far reaching. Depression can result in muted emotional responses, diminished self-care, apathy, impaired compliance, substance misuse, and suicidality. Social, cultural, and even financial issues impact how depression is identified and addressed. Depression can, for many women, imply a sense of inadequacy or incompetence as a future mother; shame readily accompanies depression and only serves to more firmly anchor this disease and make for even more resistance and difficulty in seeking out appropriate treatment.

By far, the most important tool available to the clinician is awareness. Table 21-9 describes common risk factors for perinatal depression.

Depression can present in a variety of ways. Being able to engage with the patient to gather data and offer support enhances the therapeutic relationship. This should include establishing a connection with the birth partner and other family members/supports. These contacts can provide a wealth of information as well as allow for the further strengthening of support and comfort to the high-risk OB patient.

The presence of mania does not always signal the presence of bipolar disorder (BD). Substance induced mania is not uncommon and is typically associated with the misuse of illicit substances such as cocaine or methamphetamine. It has also been reported in cases of overuse of prescribed stimulants such as methylphenidate and dextroamphetamine. In the absence of such illicit drug use, manic eruption is then diagnostic for BD.

Mania refers to an escalated mood state and is characterized by an elated, expansive, or irritable mood, a diminished need for sleep, heightened impulsivity and recklessness, feelings of grandiosity, racing thoughts and rapid, hyperverbal, or pressured speech. Manic episodes can emerge spontaneously or in the face of heightened emotional distress. Psychotic symptoms can occur with mania (as well as with depression) and can lead to serious complications including violence and other dangerous behavior. Common management strategies when faced with a manic pregnant patient include assurance of safety

TABLE 21-9. Documentation Elements (Doc, You Meant)

- Maternal treatment indications.
  - Previous medications
- Review of alternatives.
  - Non-drug treatments
- Maternal consent to treatment.
  - Breastfeeding issues
- Discussions with consultants: psychiatrist, pediatrician.

and well-being to the mother and fetus and prompt initiation of psychiatric care. Gather collaborative data paying attention to the current medication regimen (if known) as well as previous history of violence or other unsafe acting out behaviors.

While a common response to the occurrence of a pregnancy in women on antidepressant medication is to immediately discontinue the medication, this has been associated with poorer outcomes, including exacerbations of the mood disorder. In a paper by Einarson (2001), over 70% of women abruptly discontinued use of antidepressants either because of fear of teratogenicity or on the advice of their physician.[8] Nearly 30% of these women experienced a worsening of their mood disorder resulting in suicidal ideation with 10% requiring psychiatric hospitalization. The consideration to use medications to treat a mood disorder, especially during pregnancy, is a complex

Guidelines for Use of Restraints in Pregnancy

- If restraints are needed, use them for the shortest time possible.
- Agitated pregnant mother may inadvertently injure herself/baby during restraining process or once in restraints if she continues to be agitated.
  - Dislocations, fractures, trauma to baby, OB complications
- Supine restraint position may obstruct venous return (supine hypertension syndrome), especially in advanced pregnancy.
- Electronic monitoring of fetal heart rate and uterine contractions may be indicated, based on gestational age, when the patient has been stabilized.
- Pharmacologic interventions
  - Pharmacologic management is *less* risky to patient and baby vs physical restraints. This is the preferred method for controlling agitation (over restraints) if other interventions have failed.

one that has implications to maternal and fetal well-being. Initiation of any psychotropic agent should never be done unilaterally and proper informed consent must occur. This discussion includes an explanation of known potential side effects, the FDA pregnancy category rating, any known teratogenic issues (such as the incidence of facial clefts) as well as any special precautions related to pregnancy (monitoring of lithium levels especially around the time of parturition).

Antidepressant medications are commonly used to treat unipolar depression. The selective serotonin reuptake inhibitors (SSRIs) are typically well tolerated and have high efficacy rates, becoming, the preferred first-line agent for many clinicians working with patients with depression. There are numerous anecdotal reports of medications of this class being used to treat depression during pregnancy. Recent reports suggest that the SSRI paroxetine may be associated with higher rates of ventricular septal defects in infants with first trimester in utero exposure while other reports fail to find a similar association.[9] The decision to treat a pregnant woman with any psychotropic agent must take into account the potential adverse effects of in utero exposure, weighed against the potential for psychiatric suffering (and its associated ill effects, including the heightened potential for suicide and neonaticide). Thorough and repeated discussions with the pregnant patient and her pregnancy partner (including family if indicated), including accurate documentation of these meetings, should be a standard part of any such intervention. Consultation with a psychiatrist, familiar with and skilled at working with the gravid patient, is preferred, but often such clinicians are not available in the community or the patient (or family) declines such encounters.

Side effects of the antidepressants can include nausea/GI distress, headache, dizziness, tremulousness, diminished appetite, insomnia or hypersomnia, and sexual dysfunction. The serotonin syndrome is a rare clinical entity that can be seen with the use of serotonergic antidepressants. It can occur in patients who, unbeknownst to the clinician, are concomitantly on other serotonergic agents (ie, St. John's Wort or even meperidine). The clinical presentation can range from very mild to quite severe and typically includes fever, skin flushing, agitation/restlessness or alterations in mental status, diaphoresis, GI cramping with diarrhea, hyperreflexia, rigors, autonomic instability, seizures, and gait disturbances. Supportive care is the treatment of choice.

Electroconvulsive therapy is a viable alternative particularly in cases that involve significant melancholia with poor self-care or refusal to eat or drink. It may also prove useful with patients who are actively suicidal or psychotic. Special considerations for the administration of this modality are described in Table 21-10.

Anderson (2009) reported on a review of 339 cases of electroconvulsive therapy (ECT) in pregnancy.[10] In the 339 cases reviewed there were 25 adverse fetal events and 20 adverse maternal events. Of the 25 fetal events, 11 (3.2%) were thought to be related to ECT. The most common was transient fetal bradycardia or deceleration, which occurred in 8 (2.7%) of cases. The others fetal events included one fetal death following an episode of status epilepticus, one first trimester miscarriage 24 hours after ECT, and one case of multiple brain infarcts after multiple ECT courses. Of the maternal adverse events, 18 (5.3%) were thought to be related to ECT. Uterine contractions or preterm contractions was the most common event and occurred in 12 (3.5%) of cases. Other complications thought to be related to ECT included status epilepticus, hematuria, miscarriage, vaginal bleeding, abdominal pain, and placental abruption. Where efficacy data were available, the results were similar to ECT in the nonpregnant patient with at least partial response reported in 84% of those treated for depression and in 61% of those treated for schizophrenia. Additionally, the response to ECT occured more rapidly compared to antidepressant medication.

The anticonvulsant mood stabilizer medications (valproic acid, carbamazepine, oxcarbazepine, lamotrigine, etc) are commonly used by psychiatrists to treat bipolar spectrum mood disorders. While generally very effective, their use in pregnancy is being studied very closely (in both epileptic and bipolar patients where it is felt, by the physician, patient, and her supports, if necessary for use of one of these medications during pregnancy) to watch for teratogenic effects. Valproic acid and carbamazepine, for example, have been associated with facial cleft anomalies and neural tube defects and other features (see Table 21-11). The risk of neural tube defects is even higher when valproate is used in combination with other anticonvulsant agents. Additional folic acid supplementation to women taking such medications given the known link between these medications in folic acid metabolic pathways has been recommended. However, the specific folic acid dose is still undetermined with recommendations from various experts ranging from 1 to 4 mg daily. Vitamin K supplementation of 20 mg daily (at 36 weeks' gestation) has also been suggested by some clinicians for patients on carbamazepine. To date, lamotrigine has shown to have the lowest incidence of anomalies to babies exposed in utero.

■ **TABLE 21-10.** Medications Used for Treatment of the Agitated Patient

Class	Group	Drug (generic)	Typical drug dose range (used as needed)	FDA risk category
Sedatives				
	Antihistamines			
		Diphenhydramine[a]	**25-50 mg q6h**	B
		Hydroxyzine[a]	**25-50 mg q6h**	C
	Benzodiazepines			
		Lorazepam[a]	**0.5-2 mg q8h**	D
		Alprazolam	.25-1 mg q6h	D
		Diazepam	2-10 mg q12h	D
		Oxazepam	10-30 mg q8h	D
		Clonazepam	0.5-2 mg q12h	D
Neuroleptics				
	Conventional			
		Haloperidol[a]	**2-10 mg q6h**	C
		Chlorpromazine	25-50 mg q8h	C
		Fluphenazine	2-10 mg q6h	C
		Thiothixene	2-5 mg q12h	C
		Perfenazine	4-8 mg q12h	C
		Trifluoperazine	2-5 mg q12h	C
	Atypical			
		Olanzapine[a]	**2.5-5 mg q8h**	C
		Risperidone	1-2 mg q12h	C
		Aripiprazole	2-5 mg q12h	C
		Ziprasidone	20 mg q12h	C
		Quetiapine	25-50 mg q8h	C

[a]Typically used as the first choice.

■ **TABLE 21-11.** Risk Factors for Perinatal Depression

Prenatal depression	Difficult family relationships
Child care stress	Work stress/new job, nightshift work
Life stress	Severe financial difficulties
Poor social support	Recent stressful events
Prenatal anxiety	Victim of violence or abuse
Poor marital relationship	Single marital status
Low confidence as a parent	Substance use disorders
History of previous depression	Family history of postpartum depression
Young children at home to care for	Teen or adolescent pregnancy
Complicated or difficult pregnancy	Prior stillborn
Thyroid disease	Medical/obstetric complications
Previous postpartum depression	Poor diet or severe morning sickness
Severe premenstrual syndrome (PMS)	Family history of depression
Early or recent loss of a parent/support	Other psychiatric disorders

When a decision is made to use an antiepileptic to treat a bipolar spectrum mood disorder, striving for the lowest effective dose with a single agent is still the preferred approach. The Antiepileptic Drug Pregnancy Registry is currently gathering this data in an attempt to monitor the safety of these medications in pregnancy (http://www.aedpregnancyregistry.org/ or 1-888-233-2334). This registry is still open at the time of this chapter's preparation.

Lithium use has historically been avoided during pregnancy due to its link with Ebstein's anomaly. Lithium, a well-respected mood stabilizer, has been shown to provide mood stabilization, alleviation of depressive symptomatology, and reduction of suicidality. Although not typically used in the acute or emergent situation, lithium is the only agent shown to reduce suicidality in bipolar patients[11] and should receive appropriate consideration for its use. Further observation has shown that this fear may be overstated especially if the exposure occurs after the first trimester. The risk ranges from 1:1,000 to 1:20,000. Lithium, however, is not completely innocuous. Given the ever changing fluid balance states of the pregnant woman, serum lithium levels can fluctuate rapidly, especially around the time of delivery. Other factors associated with lithium toxicity are listed in Table 21-12.

Lithium can also be associated with neonatal complications (Table 21-13). The maternal and neonatal complications of

TABLE 21-13. Teratogenic Effects of Antiepileptic Agents

Valproic acid (VPA)
  Neural tube defects   5%: monotherapy
                          9%: combination VPA + another AED
  Neonatal toxicity
    Withdrawal symptoms
    Hepatotoxicity, hypoglycemia
Carbamazepine (CBZ)
  Neural tube defects: 0.5%-1%
  CBZ exposure syndrome
    Craniofacial defects, fingernail hypoplasia, developmental delay
  Maternal risk of agranulocytosis, hepatotoxicity, Stevens-Johnson syndrome

lithium therapy can be reduced by avoiding those factors associated with lithium toxicity, monitoring serum levels during the pregnancy (ideally a 12-hour trough level), discontinuing the medication at delivery (or 48 hours in advance of a scheduled delivery), and reinstitution of the medication at a lower dose after delivery. Table 21-14 outlines a basic guideline for management of the pregnant patient taking lithium (Newport 2005). Tables 21-15 and 21-16 describe more information on issues related to Lithium use in pregnancy.

■ PSYCHOSIS

Psychosis is a mental disturbance in which there is a loss of contact with reality evidenced by hallucinations, delusions,

TABLE 21-12. Guidelines for Pregnant Woman Receiving Electroconvulsive Therapy[12]

1. Consultation with an obstetrician and anesthesiologist before initiation of treatment.
2. Perform treatments in a facility with immediate access to obstetric care for emergencies.
3. Perform a complete detailed obstetrical ultrasound between 18 weeks and 22 weeks gestational age.
4. Document fetal heart rate before and after treatments. Once beyond what is considered a viable gestational age (generally 24 weeks), perform electronic fetal heart rate non-stress test before and non-stress test with uterine contraction monitoring after treatments to assess possible risk of placental abruption.
5. Use routine anesthetic measures (leftward tilt of trunk, adequate oxygenation, hydration, and muscle relaxation, non-particulate antacid, and consider intubation in the third trimester).

TABLE 21-14. Causes of Lithium Toxicity

Iatrogenic: over-ingestion/overdosing
Medication interactions
  ACE Inhibitors
  Antiemetics
  Calcium channel blockers
  NSAIDs
  Caffeine
Failure to reduce dose after delivery
Na-restricted diet
Dehydration
Perinatal complications:preeclampsia
Fluid Loss: hyperemesis
Fluid shifts: oligo- or polyhydramnios

■ TABLE 21-15. Neonatal Complications Associated With Lithium Use

Hypotonia: floppy baby
Macrosomia
Lethargy
Diabetes insipidus
Cardiac dysfunction
Hepatic abnormalities
Respiratory difficulties

■ TABLE 21-17. Components of Psychosis

- Delusions
  - Fixed false beliefs
    - Paranoia, influence, religious, erotic, nihilistic
- Perceptual disturbances
  - Hallucinations
    - Auditory, visual, gustatory, olfactory, tactile, somatic/visceral
- Disorganization of thought
  - Formal thought disorder: circumstantiality, tangentiality, thought blocking, derailment, looseness of associations

or thought disorganization.[13] Psychotic disorders range from primary thought disorders (such as schizophrenia or schizoaffective disorder) to secondary disorders (due to a mood disorder or substance induced). Table 21-17 describes the salient features of psychosis.

Although denial of pregnancy is not unique to the psychotic patient, it is a fascinating phenomena that can occur in the patient with psychosis and can have serious implications to the mother, fetus, and family. Denial of pregnancy is associated with unexpected delivery of a viable fetus in 1:2455 pregnancies; denial of pregnancy until formally diagnosed at 20 weeks in 1:475; and unexpected delivery at home in 1:9821. Complications seen can include insufficient prenatal care, alcohol or substance exposure, prematurity, longer NICU stays, breech presentations, deliveries outside of a typical medical setting, and, in extreme cases, neonaticide with either

■ TABLE 21-16. Management of the Pregnant Patient on Lithium

1. With first trimester exposure
   a. Level II sono at 18-20 wk.
   b. Fetal echocardiogram 22-24 wk.

2. During pregnancy
   a. Maintain level: 0.8-1 mEq/L.
   b. Avoid causes of toxicity.
   c. Suspend lithium 24-48 h before scheduled delivery or at the onset of spontaneous labor.

3. During Labor
   a. Maintain adequate hydration.
   b. Monitor levels at presentation to the hospital.
   c. Restart lithium after delivery using the preconception dose.

unintentional drowning of the neonate who is delivered into a toilet or a panic-stricken mother dissociates and kills the neonate out of distress. Risk of intrauterine growth restriction is increased twofold, while the risk of stillbirth is quadrupled. Issues associated with denial include personally, socially, or culturally driven pressures which make the pregnancy unacceptable. These types of nonpsychotic denials of pregnancy are more commonly seen in unmarried, teenaged, or emotionally immature mothers. Other issues seen in pregnancies where the mother is psychotic include: a higher risk for maternal smoking, unplanned pregnancies, pregnancy termination, sexually transmitted diseases, and difficulty parenting and maintaining custody of the newborn.

New-onset psychosis in pregnancy is uncommon and should initiate a thorough workup for organic causes before concluding that it is a primary psychiatric condition. This workup would be akin to that performed when evaluating other alterations in mental status. This would also include engagement with the psychiatric team. This may include transfer to an inpatient psychiatric unit.

The treatment for psychosis will involve the use of antipsychotic medications. As noted previously, no medications in this class are specifically approved for use during pregnancy. Haloperidol remains the antipsychotic with the most extensive reproductive safety data, therefore it is typically used to manage new-onset psychosis during pregnancy.[13] Benzodiazepines can be useful in the treatment of psychotic agitation; however, these agents provide no antipsychotic benefit and can, in some cases, worsen the psychosis through disinhibition and further disorganization of thought. In patients with existing psychosis already on another neuroleptic (and has shown efficacy) continuation that agent would likely be preferred. As with treating mood disorders, the potential costs and benefits should be explored and properly documented.

Antipsychotic side effects can include the extrapyramidal syndrome (pseudoparkinsonism), akathisia, dystonias, tardive dyskinesia (TD), and, in more extreme cases, the neuroleptic malignant syndrome. These symptoms can be very distressing to patients. Pseudoparkinsonism may present as bradykinesia, rigidity, tremor, and masked fascies. This is typically managed by lowering the dose of the offending agent and/or institution of the anticholinergic agent benztropine 1 mg bid or trihexyphenidyl 5 mg tid.

Akathisia is the subjective sense of restlessness which can mimic worsening agitation. It is not difficult for the less-enlightened clinician to mistake akasthisia for agitation and attempt to treat this with more of the causative agent. While anticholinergics may offer some benefit, along with cessation of the neuroleptic, β-blockers (such as low-dose propranolol—10 mg tid) are the preferred intervention.

Dystonic reactions can be severe, painful, disfiguring, and frightening to the patient, family, and staff. Laryngospasm can be life threatening, while an occulogyric crisis can end in blindness due to retinal ischemia caused by kinking of the retinal artery that runs through the optic nerve, when the eye is dramatically deviated beyond its typical range of motion. Dislocations and even fractures have been reported. Diphenhydramine 50 mg or lorazepam 2 mg intramuscularly is the treatment of choice and usually results in a satisfactory relief of the spasm. OnabotulinumtoxinA has also been used to treat dystonic reactions of the sternocleidomastoid muscle.

Tardive dyskinesia (TD) is a permanent movement disorder that is associated with longer term use of antipsychotic medications. It is more commonly seen in the muscles of the mouth and face, but any skeletal muscle group can be afflicted. Abrupt cessation of the neuroleptic can actually result in an unmasking of the TD, while an increase in the dose may conceal the movement disorder temporarily. There does appear to be a lower incidence of TD with the newer atypical antipsychotics, but even so the risk is not zero. An effective treatment for this horrible disorder remains elusive.

The neuroleptic malignant syndrome (NMS) is a potentially lethal condition that is, functionally, a systemic dystonic reaction. The incidence of NMS has been reported to be as high as 0.5% to 1% of all patients on neuroleptics with a reported mortality rate approaching 5%. It is more commonly seen with the older conventional high-potency agents such as haloperidol or fluphenazine. The onset of NMS is usually shortly after initiating neuroleptization, and may be more frequent in the neuroleptic-naïve patient. The classic presentation consists of alterations in mental status, muscle rigidity (stove-pipe rigidity), and hyperpyrexia. Autonomic instability and derangements in laboratory studies such as leukocytosis, elevations in CPK levels, and even thrombocytopenia can be seen. In pregnancy this can be confused with thrombotic thrombocytopenic purpura (TTP) or maternal infection/sepsis.

A history of neuroleptic use should create high level of clinical suspicion in patients presenting with these symptom clusters. Intervention will include supportive care (hydration, electrolyte stabilization, cooling, airway protection, etc) and immediate cessation of any neuroleptics. In theory, dantrolene and bromocriptine can reverse these clinical syndromes; however, there is little evidence to support this. These patients are critically ill and should be treated as such. This will include prompt transfer to an intensive care environment as well as fetal monitoring, if indicated, based on gestational age. Lorazepam has been shown to offer some relief of the rigidity.

■ SUBSTANCE ABUSE IN PREGNANCY

Abuse of drugs in pregnancy continues to be a significant problem. The problem involves inappropriate use of over-the-counter medications, abuse and diversion of prescribed medication, and abuse of both legal (alcohol and tobacco) and illegal substances (illicits). Overall exposure of illegal substances is 11% with higher and lower incidences varying as much as 4.3% to 30% in different areas across the nation.[14,15] Maternal psychosocial effects include poverty, lack of prenatal care, unwanted pregnancy, sexually transmitted diseases, poor nutrition, physical abuse, stress, depression, and lack of social support. The treatment of chronic substance abuse is beyond the scope of this chapter. Many of these agents, however, have acute effects resulting in symptoms of agitation, delirium, and psychosis, which will be the focus of this section.

As outlined in the Algorithm for Altered Mental Status (Fig 21-1), the initial workup includes: a detail substance exposure history including both prescribed, over-the-counter, and illicit substances. Often the patient is unable to provide a coherent story so information from others

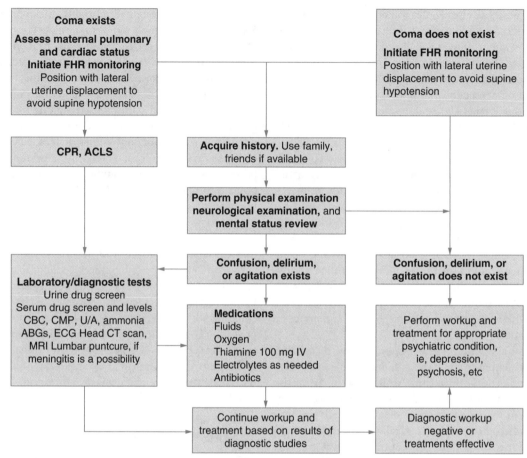

FIGURE 21-1. Algorithm for evaluation of Altered Mental Status.

accompanying the patient may be necessary. Details of the amount of drug used needs to be specified clearly. The consequences, medically, to a patient who states that she only drinks a glass of vodka daily is entirely different if the glass is only a small tumbler mostly filled with ice compared to a full 16-ounce glass. Also, multiple agents may be abused, which further complicates the workup and treatment.

After a detailed history, evaluation with laboratory studies to confirm both the type of exposure and to assess the pathophysiologic effects are necessary. Urine drug screen, serum drug levels, and targeted functional tests of the potential organs affected should be done.

While laboratory studies are processed, assessing and treating the patient's behavior should be done as described in the section on the agitated patient. Drugs with significant behavioral effects include alcohol, phencyclidine

(PCP), opioids, cocaine, and methamphetamine. Methamphetamine, particularly, has been associated with paranoid psychosis, delusions, hallucinations, and suicidal ideation.

With the exception of fetal alcohol syndrome, none of the illicit agents have been associated with a consistent pattern of anomalies. The vasoconstrictive agents cocaine and methamphetamine have been associated with anomalies presumed to be the result of loss of circulation to the developing organ that subsequently develops abnormally. But, no consistent pattern of anomalies has emerged.

The vasoconstrictive agents, especially cocaine, tobacco, and methamphetamine are the only agents to consistently be associated with reducing fetal growth and premature labor and delivery. Cocaine and methamphetamine may also increase the risk of placental abruption.

Long-term effects of prenatal exposure to illicit substances have not shown the profound developmental effects once feared. However, subtle developmental effects have been demonstrated and there is still much to be learned about the impact on societal resources for large populations. These risks, however, do not compare currently with the known developmental risks of alcohol and tobacco exposure. Both of these agents are common agents associated with multiple substance exposure.

Heavy alcohol use results in fetal alcohol syndrome which is characterized by pre- and postnatal growth restriction, cranial dysmorphology, and cognitive deficits. Prenatal smoking is also related to intrauterine growth restriction (IUGR) and behavioral problems during childhood.

Fetal assessment during pregnancy, when careful substance use history indicates exposure, includes

- Cessation of substance use, education, and counseling
- Careful pregnancy dating
- Detailed anatomical evaluation by ultrasound at 18 to 20 weeks gestation
- Serial ultrasound assessment of fetal growth
- Antepartum fetal assessment if IUGR is demonstrated
- Prompt response to indicators of acute changes in the pregnancy such as placental abruption

Neonatal evaluation includes

- Careful physical examination for features associated with substance exposure, for example, fetal alcohol syndrome
- Structured observation for evidence of withdrawal with treatment as needed
- Careful assessment of the neonatal home environment with appropriate family education
- Scheduled developmental follow-up

■ POSTPARTUM STATES

The postpartum period has been shown to be a time of heightened risk for mood and psychotic disorder eruption. Around 400 BC, Hippocrates described the relationship between mental illness and the postpartum period. Diagnosis and treatment will follow the same pattern as in assessing patients in other phases of life. However, a heightened level of mindfulness is necessary, particularly with women with a preexisting psychiatric condition. This mandates good communication with and education of the patient and her family to report any changes in mood or cognition.

The risk factors for postpartum depression (PPD) are similar to those listed on the mood disorders, see Table 21-11. Postpartum blues can occur in as many as 50% to 70% of postpartum women, but symptoms are usually mild and resolve spontaneously within the first 1 to 2 weeks. In patients where symptoms persist beyond 2 weeks, or if the severity escalates quickly, a more thorough evaluation is indicated. Evaluation for suicidality or thoughts to harm the baby, or others, must occur.

Differing from PPD, postpartum psychosis can evolve quickly (typically within the first few days postpartum) and is a true psychiatric emergency! The psychotic symptoms may not necessarily differ from symptoms seen in other life stages; however, careful evaluation as to the theme or content of the psychosis is vital. Risk factors for postpartum psychosis include a previous history of postpartum psychosis, family history of psychosis, and a history of bipolar disorder (100 × risk). Often the neonate is actively included within the psychotic process, therefore increasing the risk for infanticide which has been reported to occur in up to 4% of patients with postpartum psychosis. Despite the apparent certainty as to the accuracy of the diagnosis of a postpartum mood or psychotic state, a thorough organic workup (as noted above) is indicated.

Treatment is similar to treatments in the antepartum period; however, given the high potential for lethality, prompt psychiatric hospitalization may be indicated in cases that involve suicidal or homicidal thoughts. The mother's desire to continue with breast-feeding must be addressed, especially in cases where psychotropic medications are indicated. In patients with milder forms of a postpartum mood disorder, psychotherapy such as interpersonal or cognitive-behavioral has been demonstrated to improve outcomes. However in cases with greater symptom severity psychotropic medications are usually necessary. Electroconvulsive therapy has been shown to provide rapid and effective relief from symptoms and is considered, by some, as first line in treating postpartum psychosis or conditions that include suicidal or homicidal ideations.

Upon delivery, 20% to 30% of neonates exposed to SSRIs may experience what has been described as a neonatal adaptation disorder. This disorder generally is self-limited and resolves in about 2 weeks. More common symptoms include tremors, jitteriness, feeding problems, fussiness, irritability, hyperreflexia, and sleep disturbances. The more severe symptoms of seizures, hyperpyrexia, dehydration, and respiratory distress requiring intubation are rarely encountered.

Careful documentation is a significant component of the care provided to the patient with psychiatric or behavioral problems. Accurate recording of the elements of care are necessary whether the patient is seen for preconceptional counseling, care during the antepartum period, during labor and delivery, or in the postpartum period. Elements to be included in the documentation are described previously in Table 21-9.

■ PEARLS

Gather collaborative data whenever possible. Patients may consciously or unconsciously not provide all of the pertinent information to you. Additionally, having the perspective of someone else who is close to the patient may shed a new light on the situation.

Always screen for suicidality or thoughts to harm others when evaluating a patient with a mood or psychotic disorder.

The interpersonal relationship you have with your patient can prove invaluable especially when the time comes to inquire about delicate or sensitive information. A patient who trusts her doctor will be more open to engaging with her when rough times come.

Do not underestimate the power of being kind and empathic.

Screen for substance abuse.

Ask about access to guns just as you would inquire about smoking or wearing seat belts. It's important information to have, so gather it.

Be really sure that the patient and her supports/family understand the important points about psychotropic medications you may prescribe to her; make sure they have adequate time to ask questions.

Use psychiatric consultants.

Document your rationale for doing something.

Rely on your countertransference feelings—if you are uncomfortable or uneasy with a particular situation it's probably for a good reason. Seek advice.

REFERENCES

1. Stowe Z. Psychiatric Disorders in Pregnancy. *Clinical Obstet and Gynecol.* 2009;52:423-529.

2. Weissberg M. The meagerness of physcians' training in emergency psychiatric interventions. *Acad Med.* 1990;65:747-750.

3. Stotland N. *Obstetrics and Gynecology; Textbook of Consultation Liaison Psychiatry.* Washington, DC: American Psychiatric Press; 1996.

4. Heron M, Hoyert D, Murphy S, et al. National Vital Statistics Report. Vol 57, Number 14. Hyattsville, MD: Center for Disease Control and Prevention; 2009.

5. Gissler M, Hemminki E, Lönnqvist J. Suicides after pregnancy in Finland, 1987-94: register linkage study. *BMJ.* 1996 Dec 7;313(7070):1431-1434.

6. Feldman MD, Christensen JF. *Behavioral Medicine: A Guide for Clinical Practice.* 3rd ed. Philadelphia, PA: McGraw Hill Lange Publications; 2007.

7. Cox, JL, Holden, J, Sagovsky, R. Detection of postnatal depression: development of the 10-item Edinburgh Postnatal depression Scale (EPDS). *Brit J Psychiatry.* 1987;150: 782-786.

8. Einarson, A, Selby P, Koren G. Abrupt discontinuation of psychotropic drugs during pregnancy: fear of teratogenic risk and impact of counseling. *J Psychiatry Neurosci.* 2001;26(1):44-48.

9. Yonkers KA, Wisner KL, Stewart DE, et al. The management of depression during pregnancy: a report from the American Psychiatric Association and the American College of Obstetricians and Gynecologists. *Obstet Gynecol.* 2009;114(3); 703-713.

10. Anderson EL, Reti IM. ECT in pregnancy: a review of the literature from 1941 to 2007. *Psychosom Med.* 2009;71: 235-242.

11. Tondo, L. Baldessarini RJ, Hennen J, et al. Lithium treatment and risk of suicidal behavior in bipolar disorder patients. *J Clin Psychiatry.* 1998 Aug;59 (8):405-414.

12. Pinette MG, Santarpio C, Wax J,. Blackstone J. Electroconvulsive therapy in pregnancy. *Obstet Gynecol.* 2007 Aug; 110(2 Pt 2):465-466.

13. Watkins ME, Newport J. Psychosis in pregnancy. *Obstet Gynecol.* 2009;113:1349-1353.

14. Curet LB, His AC. Drug abuse during pregnancy. *Clin Obstet Gynecol.* 2002;45(1):73-88.

15. Schempf AH. Illicit drug use and neonatal outcomes: a critical review. *Obstet Gynecol Survey.* 2007;62:749-757.

SUGGESTED READINGS

Anderson EL, Reti IM. ECT in pregnancy: a review of the literature from 1941 to 2007. *Psychosom Med.* 2009;71(2): 235-242.

Cox J, Holden J. Perinatal Psychiatry: use and misuse of the Edinburgh Postnatal Depression Scale. Gaskell, London: The Royal College of Psychiatrists; 1994 (Reprinted 1996).

Diagnostic and Statistical Manual of Mental Disorders (DSM-IV-TR). Washington, DC: American Psychiatric Association; 2000.

Feldman MD, Christensen JF. *Behavioral Medicine: A Guide for Clinical Practice*. 3rd ed. Philadelphia, PA: McGraw Hill Lange Publications; 2007.

Newport DJ, Viguera AC, Beach, AJ, Ritchie, JC, Cohen, LS, Stowe, ZN. Lithium placental passage and obstetrical outcome: implications for clinical management during late pregnancy. *Am J Psychiatry*. 2005 Nov; 162:2162-2170.

Watkins ME, Newport J. Psychosis in pregnancy. *Obstet Gynecol*. 2009;113:1349-1353.

Yonkers KA, Wisner KL, Stewart DE, et al. The management of depression during pregnancy: a report from the American Psychiatric Association and the American College of Obstetricians and Gynecologists. *Obstet Gynecol*. 2009;114(3); 703-713.

CHAPTER 22

Fetal Considerations in the Critical Care Patient

• *Thomas J. Garite*

Virtually any pathologic process which affects the mother has the potential to affect the fetus. The type and severity of the fetal impact will depend on many variables among which are whether the insult is acute or chronic, how the insult affects fetal oxygenation via oxygen delivery and uterine perfusion, and the ability to intervene based on gestational age and the hemodynamic and respiratory status of the mother. Critical to decision making in these situations is a basic understanding of the fetal physiology as it relates to these functions.

■ FETAL PHYSIOLOGY

The fetal impact of most critical diseases in the mother will depend on how well the mother is able to continue to deliver oxygen to the fetus while at the same time dealing with her own compromised state. Fetal oxygen delivery depends on placental blood flow, differences in partial pressure of oxygen between mother and fetus, oxygen content (a function of oxygen carrying capacity of the maternal blood), and the placental surface area, and is inversely proportional to the thickness of the placental diffusing membrane. In diseases that primarily affect the mother, except for those that may lead to abruptio placentae, placental issues remain constant and the critical issues become blood flow and oxygen pressure and content.

The fetus functions at a much lower oxygen tension than its air breathing counterpart. Its ability to do so is based on an hemoglobin/oxygen dissociation curve that is to the left of its mother (Fig 22-1) allowing a considerably higher oxygen saturation at lower partial pressures of oxygen. This is absolutely essential in the human placental model which has a type of parallel flow that has been described as "concurrent." In this flow model (Fig 22-2), the maximum fetal Po_2 will be a few torr less than that of the mother's venous Po_2. This is because at the end of the exchange loop for oxygen to be continually exchanged in the direction of mother to fetus, the fetal Po_2 can never exceed that of maternal venous blood. Thus in the healthy, normally perfused placenta, fetal venous blood (the oxygenated side of the fetal circuit) will have a maximum Po_2 of about 35 given that mother's venous Po_2 is 35 to 40. At this Po_2 the fetal blood is about 70% saturated with oxygen. The fetus will maintain aerobic metabolism at saturations above 30% to 35% corresponding to a Po_2 of 15 to 20. This is important information when trying to understand the impact of maternal hypoxia with alterations in uterine blood flow, such as with the mother with acute respiratory illnesses and especially with a mother on a ventilator. Maternal anemia will significantly alter the level at which anaerobic metabolism and acidosis may occur since reduced levels of hemoglobin will reduce the absolute amount of oxygen the blood will carry at a given saturation and Po_2. Conversely in the absence of maternal hypoxemia, the fetus may become hypoxic due to anemia alone at severely low levels. (Fig 22-3) The exact level at which this may occur is not well known and is probably variable.

In other maternal critical care situations blood flow will be the determinant of whether adequate fetal oxygenation is occurring. Uterine blood flow is generally a function of maternal cardiac output. Normally during the late second and early third trimester, maternal cardiac output reaches its maximal level and peaks at about 6 L/min. Maternal blood volume is similarly increased. Approximately 750 cc/min of the maternal cardiac output flows through

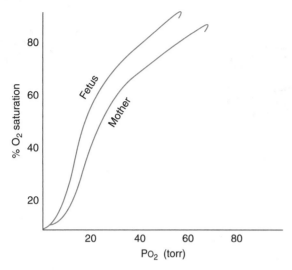

FIGURE 22-1. The oxygen hemoglobin saturation curves for maternal and fetal human blood. (*Adapted from Hellegers AD, Schruefer JJ. Am J Obstet Gynecol. 1961;81:377.*)

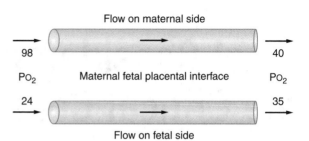

FIGURE 22-2. Oxygenation based on concurrent model of maternal and fetal blood flow within the placenta, with actual values based on normals found at cordocentesis in the mid–third-trimester period.

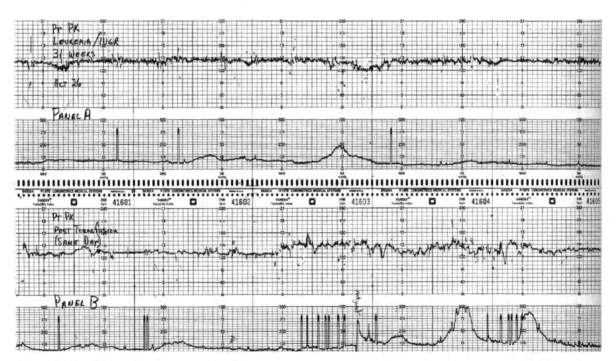

FIGURE 22-3. Although not an example of an acute anemia due to injury or other acute illness, this case demonstrates the potential fetal effects of maternal anemia and decreased oxygen-carrying capacity. This patient had anemia with a hematocrit of 26. The fetus on the upper panel exhibits absent reactivity and late decelerations. After 3 units of packed red blood cell transfusion, the fetal heart rate on the lower panel recovered with return of normal accelerations and disappearance of late decelerations.

the low resistance placental bed. Uteroplacental perfusion is critical to the maintenance of fetal oxygen and even minor alterations may result in fetal hypoxia. Several potential alterations may occur in the critically ill patient that can result in decreased placental perfusion. A large amount of occult blood loss (eg, intraperitoneal) may not be as readily apparent in pregnancy because of the marked increase in blood volume and the ability of the mother to redistribute blood away from the uterus. As much as 2000 cc (30%) of maternal blood volume may be lost without significant changes in vital signs as opposed to only about 1000 cc (20%) in the nonpregnant female. The placental bed is neurologically linked to the maternal splanchnic (sp) bed and the physiologic response to decrease in blood volume in the mother is diversion of blood away from the placenta when other vital organs (brain, heart, adrenals) must be preserved. In such situations, the fetus may even become hypoxic even before shock occurs. Hypovolemia may result in decreased cardiac output further decreasing placental perfusion. While it may seem paradoxical, hypertension is also associated with decreased placental perfusion and the more severe the blood pressure elevation, the more likely one will face an underperfused placenta associated with fetal hypoxia. And finally, often critical situations result in the premature onset of contractions which further decrease uterine blood flow during the contractile epochs.

■ CRITICAL CARE PATIENTS WITH ACUTE INSULTS

In almost all critically ill patients, as compared to immediate delivery of the compromised fetus, the better choice is to improve maternal condition in a way in which maternal benefit will result in improved fetal condition. While the fetus may often demonstrate signs of hypoxia as a result of the maternal compromise, the temptation to proceed with delivery can result in destabilization of the mother, unnecessary surgery (ie, cesarean section), and often the unnecessary delivery of a premature infant with the inherent complications of prematurity. One glaring exception to this is in the case of cardiopulmonary arrest, where delivery of the fetus may be the only way to allow adequate maternal resuscitation.

■ INITIAL EVALUATION AND CARE OF THE FETUS

There are some general elements that are common to evaluating and caring for the fetus when there is a critical

illness in the mother. The first issue is to determine the gestational age and potential viability of the fetus. The approach to subsequent evaluation and management will always depend on this issue. To maximize fetal well-being in general, be sure the mother has some left uterine displacement usually best accomplished with a roll under the right buttocks. Administer oxygen by face mask using a tightly fitting nonrebreathing mask whenever possible. Determine as quickly as possible the general condition of the mother including especially her primary diagnosis, her vital signs, and hemodynamic status and include pulse oximetry to quickly determine her oxygen saturation. Maternal evaluation will include palpation of the uterus for size, fetal position, tenderness, and contractions, and, where appropriate, may also include a perineal or even pelvic examination to assess for bleeding, rupture of membranes, and cervical dilation. At that point, if the fetus is of a viable gestational age, cardiotachometry is the critical next step. This modality will assist in determining the fetal oxygen status and uterine perfusion and whether there are contractions present. The ultrasound evaluation of the fetus should be reserved until the fetal well-being has been assured and contraction status has been determined. The level of detail required for the ultrasound will be determined by the preceding evaluations. Ultrasound will be important in being sure there is not an obvious lethal anomaly (eg, anencephaly) making the fetal evaluation moot. It may be important to confirm the gestational age and fetal viability to make the correct decision regarding timing and route of delivery. Ultrasound may be used as a tool to further evaluate fetal condition if the fetal heart rate (FHR) is not reassuring with biophysical profile including amniotic fluid volume assessment. And in some situations, more sophisticated fetal assessment such as Doppler flow studies may also become useful. (Fig 22-4)

■ FETAL EVALUATION AND MANAGEMENT IN SPECIFIC CRITICAL SITUATIONS

Trauma

The leading cause of death and adverse outcome in the patient with major trauma is death of the mother. Thus the initial evaluation and management, other than the steps outlined in the previous section, will be to ensure that the mother is appropriately assessed and stabilized. Major hemorrhage in the mother may lead to decreased placental perfusion and fetal hypoxia and must be controlled. Occult intra-abdominal hemorrhage may lead to

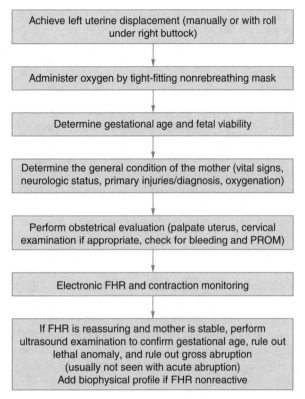

FIGURE 22-4. Initial evaluation of the fetus in the critical care mother.

diversion of blood away from the uterus and late decelerations may be the earliest sign of this problem even before major changes in maternal vital signs.

Evaluation for intra-abdominal hemorrhage may be more difficult because the enlarged uterus makes abdominal examination more difficult and the tenting of the peritoneum and anti-inflammatory effects of progesterone may dampen normal tenderness. Ultrasound can be useful in detecting intraperitoneal bleeding and open peritoneal lavage has been used with success in pregnancy. In the hemodynamically compromised patient who is tachycardic and hypotensive, aggressive fluid management is critical. In those patients, where in addition vasopressors are needed, care should be taken to consider the effects on the fetus. Low-dose dopamine, which in the mother is effective primarily due to increased cardiac output, has been shown in animals to decrease uterine perfusion, so careful fetal monitoring is warranted. Norepinephrine and isoproterenol may have similar fetal effects. Ephedrine may be considered as it is one agent known not to adversely affect uterine circulation.

The obstetric complications of major blunt trauma include abruptio placentae, fetal-maternal hemorrhage (with or without abruption), labor (and premature labor in the preterm gestation), and very rarely, uterine rupture and fetal trauma.

In patients without obvious clinical abruption (ie, uterine contractions, pain, tenderness, and vaginal bleeding) the fetal heart rate monitor may be the most sensitive tool to detect abruption placentae. The characteristic findings in abruption placentae include a tachysystolic contraction pattern and late decelerations (Fig 22-5). Ultrasound will usually not reveal an acute abruption as the ultrasonic density of fresh bleeding is virtually identical to the placenta. Evaluation of the patient should also include laboratory assessment of hematocrit, fibrinogen, and platelet count for retroplacental consumptive coagulopathy, and a Kleihauer-Betke to rule out major fetal-maternal hemorrhage and determine whether and how much Rh-negative immune globulin is needed.

Delivery is generally the only option for patients with abruption. There is often a conflict, as the trauma teams wants to be sure the mother has adequate diagnostic studies to rule out intracranial or other injuries. The obstetrician must become the advocate for the fetus and open communication is essential. Tocolysis for premature labor associated with trauma induced abruption should be approached with extreme caution. If considered at all, it should be limited to patients with very early gestational ages (ie, <32 weeks) and in those who are hemodynamically stable with reassuring fetal status, no active bleeding, and no coagulopathy. Corticosteroids for lung maturity should be used concurrently. (Table 22-1)

Rarely a patient will have a major fetal maternal hemorrhage without a significant clinical abruption. Fetal heart rate findings may include tachycardia, decreased variability, late decelerations, and/or sinusoidal patterns. A biophysical profile may reveal a depressed fetus. Betke-Kleihauer will reveal the size of the fetal hemorrhage. Whether middle cerebral artery Doppler studies will be diagnostic in this situation is unknown at this time. In the very early gestation emergency intrauterine transfusion can be an alternative to delivery.

Following the initial evaluation, there should be a more prolonged period of FHR and contraction monitoring. (Fig 22-6) The duration of monitoring will depend on the severity of the injury, presence of contractions, and/or vaginal bleeding, and other clinical findings. Following any significant abdominal trauma, the fetus should be observed

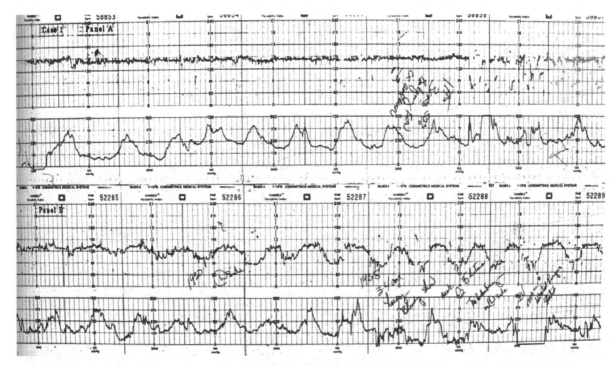

FIGURE 22-5. Abruptio placentae. This tracing demonstrates the characteristic contraction patterns (tachysystole: frequent contractions with short or absent relaxation period) and, beginning on the lower panel persistent late decelerations. At the last half of the lower panel, this patient who previously had not been bleeding began actively hemorrhaging from her vagina and immediate cesarean section revealed an acute 50% abruption.

■ TABLE 22-1. Candidates for Tocolysis and Corticosteroids with Suspected Abruptio Placentae

1. Actively contracting
2. Cervical dilation appropriate for tocolysis (≤4 cm)
3. Gestational age appropriate for tocolysis and corticosteroids (24-34 wk)
4. No vigorous active bleeding
5. Reassuring FHR pattern
6. No evidence of significant coagulopathy (fibrinogen >100 mg%, platelet count >100,000)
7. No medical contraindications to tocolysis

on the monitor for a minimum of 4 hours and if any signs of abruption exist for at least 24 hours. (Fig 22-7)

Hypoxia

Maternal hypoxemia may obviously lead to fetal hypoxia. Situations where acute hypoxia may present a challenge for fetal assessment and management may include an acute asthmatic episode, acute respiratory distress, often associated with sepsis (pyelonephritis, appendicitis), pulmonary edema with preeclampsia/eclampsia, cranial injuries with respiratory failure, amniotic fluid or pulmonary embolism, cardiac decompensation (eg, pulmonary edema associated with mitral stenois), pneumonia, and irritant inhalation or burns.

Therapy is directed to the primary condition of the mother. FHR monitoring will be useful in assessing how the fetus is tolerating any reduced oxygen delivery. In the absence of uterine contractions a hypoxic fetus will develop tachycardia and loss of variability, and prolonged decelerations will only be seen preterminally. If contractions are present, late decelerations may be seen. A general goal for optimizing fetal oxygenation is to keep maternal Po_2 above 60 mm Hg and O_2 saturation above 90%. Levels below this on supplemental oxygen with rebreathing mask may require ventilator therapy. The goal should also be to avoid either hypercarbia or hypocarbia. The pregnant women normally hyperventilates and a Pco_2 of 35 is normal in pregnancy and lower levels may be associated with decreased placental perfusion. The goal should be maintaining Pco_2 between 35 and 40.

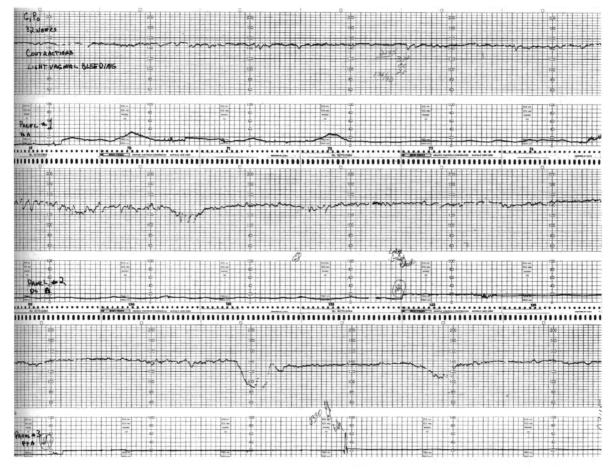

FIGURE 22-6. This patient at 32 weeks had been in an automobile collision and sustained mild abdominal trauma. Her uterus was not tender and there was minimal but present vaginal bleeding. The electronic fetal monitor revealed irregular and infrequent contractions which the patient was not feeling and on the lower two panels late decelerations. It is critical to be able to recognize late decelerations even without apparent contractions. Immediate cesarean section revealed a 30% abruption.

While colloid oncotic pressure may play a role in maintaining intravascular volume, and logically situations like pulmonary edema would be reduced with intravenous colloid administration, this should not be used in such situations, especially in acute situations. The problem is that the protein may leak into the pulmonary interstitium and further aggravate the ventilation-perfusion mismatch. Severe anemia, however, should be corrected with packed red cells as maximizing oxygen-carrying capacity is critical to fetal oxygen delivery.

Delivery is rarely indicated in situations of maternal respiratory failure unless the mother cannot be adequately oxygenated on full ventilatory settings. One other rare situation which may require delivery, especially in the third trimester is in the mother with a muscle weakness situation (eg, spinal muscular atrophy) where the elevation of the diaphragm compromises breathing and only delivery provides adequate relief.

Sickle Cell Crisis

While not truly a hypoxemic event, patients with sickle cell crises have compromised oxygen-carrying capacity. Often patients who present with sickle cell crisis in the late second or third trimester will have fetal signs of hypoxia on the FHR monitor. Evaluation and management of the fetus will be virtually identical to patients with acute asthmatic episodes or other examples of respiratory failure. Thus aggressive maternal therapy aimed at maximizing

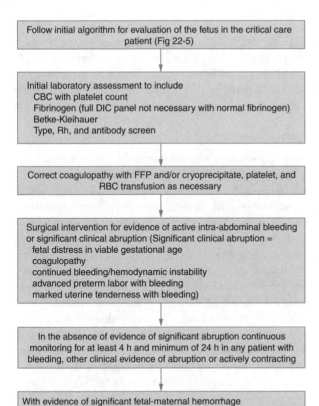

FIGURE 22-7. Evaluation of the pregnant patient with blunt abdominal trauma.

oxygenation and uterine perfusion is important. Rarely will intervention for fetal compromise be necessary. Transfusion may be more important for the fetus in such situations than for mother alone, as increasing oxygen-carrying capacity improves fetal oxygen transfer. Improvement in the FHR should be expected as the crisis is resolving.

Anaphylaxis

Anaphylaxis is an acute allergic reaction with systemic manifestations that can include urticaria, respiratory distress, and cardiovascular collapse. The inciting agent may be food or medication.

With either respiratory compromise or shock or both, fetal hypoxia would be expected. The treatment is similar to the nonpregnant patient. Urgent resuscitation includes maintenance of an airway, oxygen administration, epinephrine, diphenhydramine, and intravenous hydration.

The FHR may manifest late decelerations with or without tachycardia. Correction of maternal hypoxia and blood pressure should restore placental perfusion and correct the fetal hypoxia and the accompanying FHR pattern, although there may be a time lag of up to 2 hours before the FHR returns to complete normalcy.

Hypertensive Crisis

Acute hypertensive crisis in pregnancy may occur for reasons similar to those in the nonpregnant patient such as poorly controlled chronic hypertension and pheochromocytoma, or may occur as a result of severe preeclampsia/eclampsia. In either case, the principles of maternal therapy and the fetal considerations are similar. The blood pressure must be lowered to less dangerous levels to avoid severe secondary complications in the mother, principally intracranial hemorrhage. The obstetrical benefit of lowering blood pressure at these high levels may also be to avoid abruption placentae. However, acute reduction of the blood pressure must be done very carefully, as in these cases, the fetus may not tolerate too large a drop in pressure, especially if accomplished too rapidly. This is true regardless of the agent used. The goal should be to lower pressure gradually over 30 to 60 minutes and to not reduce the pressure to normotensive levels. For example, the patient with an admission blood pressure of 220/130 should be gradually reduced to a pressure of approximately 160 to 170/100 to 105. Medications such as apresoline, labetalol, or even nitroprusside may be used in either small boluses or by slow intravenous infusion as these drugs allow titration of blood pressure without overshooting if used appropriately.

In the case of the chronic hypertension, especially early in pregnancy, where delivery is not immediately planned, blood pressure should also be controlled with care not to overcorrect the levels. The fetus may demonstrate growth restriction or even hypoxia if blood pressure levels in severe hypertensives are overly corrected.

Maternal Acidosis

Rarely situations of maternal metabolic acidosis in the absence of hypoxemia or shock will present an extraordinary management challenge from a fetal perspective. Most commonly this will be seen with diabetic ketoacidosis (DKA), but other situations such as drug or toxin-induced acidosis (eg, aspirin overdose) may also present similarly. Generally speaking, the fetus will become acidotic slowly as buffers, including especially HCO_3^-, move slowly across the placenta from the fetal to the maternal intravascular compartment. This buffer depletion in the fetus then results in fetal acidosis. The fetus will demonstrate loss of variability with or without late decelerations on the FHR monitor and biophysical parameters including fetal movement, breathing, and tone will be reduced or absent. In such situation maternal correction of the acidosis will improve the fetal condition and delivery is usually not warranted. The key point is that the fetal condition will require several hours or more beyond correction of the acidosis in the mother for its acidosis to clear as well. (Fig 22-8) Again the reason is that the fetal buffer must equilibrate back from the maternal to the fetal side of the placenta and because these are either very large or negatively charged buffers, this process occurs at a very slow rate. Continuous fetal heart rate monitoring during the correction of the maternal acidosis will provide information as to when the fetus is recovering. Rarely the fetus may deteriorate before the maternal acidosis can be corrected to the point of developing a preterminal prolonged deceleration/bradycardia. In this situation, if maternal condition permits and the fetus is of a viable gestational age, emergent cesarean section may be required.

In the situation of DKA, and perhaps in other such non-hypoxic metabolic acidoses, the mother will be severely dehydrated as well. This may result in underperfusion of the placenta and hypoxia may compound the metabolic acidosis. Therefore, it is equally important to correct the dehydration with aggressive fluid administration.

Seizures

Maternal seizures, whether due to eclampsia, epilepsy, or even metabolic disturbances, will usually result in major alterations in the parameters used to assess fetal well-being, especially the FHR. Seizures may alter placental perfusion and hence fetal oxygenation in several ways. Maternal hypoxia often results from suspended breathing. Diversion of blood flow away from the uterus will occur because of the intense maternal muscular activity. And finally, probably as result of the intense uterine ischemia, there will often be titanic or prolonged uterine contractions occurring during the seizure. All of these factors together will most often result in the anticipated changes in the FHR. Usually a prolonged deceleration or deep late decelerations will occur during the seizure. Once the seizure resolves, the deceleration(s) will resolve, but a period of tachycardia and reduced

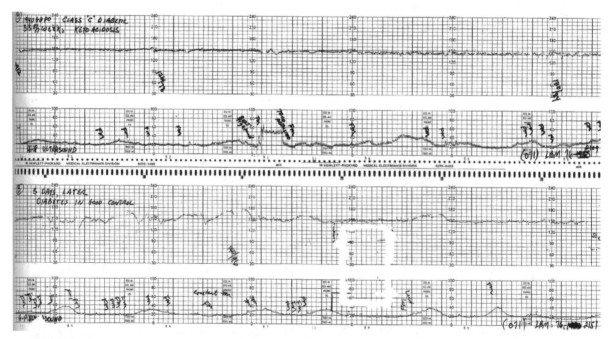

FIGURE 22-8. This patient at 33 weeks was admitted in diabetic ketoacidosis. On the upper panel this fetal heart rate demonstrates the characteristic pattern of this problem with decreased to absent variability on the external monitor, although there are no late decelerations. After correction of the DKA, the fetal heart rate pattern returned to normal with acceleration and normal variability seen on the lower panel.

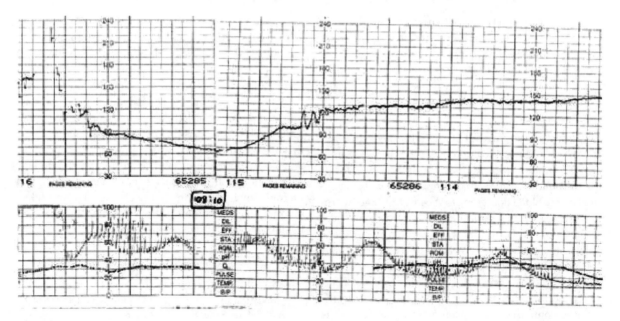

FIGURE 22-9. Illustrates the characteristic fetal heart rate and contraction pattern associated with an acute eclamptic seizure. Note the prolonged deceleration with loss of variability and the titanic contraction during the seizure and the development of tachycardia and loss of variability following the seizure. This fetus was also being monitored with fetal pulse oximetry and the oxygenation saturation falls to 30% during the seizure and returns to normal values (50%) following its cessation.

FHR variability will occur, often lasting 30 minutes to 2 hours. If the FHR was normal preceding these changes and the mother is now well oxygenated and seizure free, the FHR will gradually return to normal. (Fig 22-9)

Therapy is directed at maternal condition. The keys as with nonpregnant patients are to maintain the airway and avoid maternal injury. Tilting the mother to her left side will avoid aortocaval compression. Once the seizure is resolved, treatment is aimed at preventing further seizures with medication and then treating the cause when possible. The choice of medications for treatment of acute seizures, or with status epilepticus, must be made with the fetus in mind. Azodiazepams should be used cautiously if there is a chance the baby will need to be delivered, especially if the fetus is premature, as these drugs alter thermoregulation and are neurodepressive. In such cases, short-acting barbiturates (eg, pentobarbital) are reasonable alternatives. Delivery is rarely needed for the FHR changes due to the seizure and in most situations it is better to allow the placenta to resuscitate the fetus even if immediate delivery is warranted, such as with eclampsia.

Thyrotoxicosis

Acute thyrotoxicosis and especially thyroid storm are obstetrical emergencies that have significant fetal implications. Potential complications include asphyxia, premature labor, preeclampsia, and fetal hyperthyroidism. The mechanisms of the potential fetal compromise are multifactorial. The maternal hyperdynamic state will divert blood flow away from the uterus. Uterine ischemia may lead to intrauterine growth restriction (IUGR), fetal hypoxia, and premature contractions. Superimposed preeclampsia may further aggravate the placental hypoperfusion. Thyroid immunoglobulin is an IgG and crosses the placenta potentially causing fetal hyperthyroidism increasing metabolic demands of the fetus. With thyroid storm, besides being a more intense hyperdynamic state amplifying the potential fetal compromise, there may also be maternal heart failure and pulmonary edema superimposing maternal hypoxemia.

The FHR may be altered in any number of ways depending on which of these complex factors are involved at any one time. Tachycardia may be due to either the maternal disease or fetal hyperthyroidism. Late decelerations may occur if placental hypoperfusion is severe. Treatment, as with other similar situations where correction of maternal condition will usually improve fetal condition, thus does not require immediate delivery.

Cardiac Arrest

The presence of an enlarged uterus, especially with a gestational age >24 weeks, compromise the ability to resuscitate the mother with cardiac arrest occurs. This is primarily due to aortocaval compression but is also aggravated by the blood flow going to the low resistance uteroplacental bed which is critically needed by the vital organs of the mother. Furthermore, the potential for fetal asphyxia in the case of maternal cardiac arrest is very high.

Cardiopulmonary resuscitation in the pregnant woman thus involves two principal differences. The first is to assure left uterine displacement. Tilting the maternal trunk may not be the best option as this may compromise the efficiency of chest compression. It is recommended that either the entire backboard be tilted or that an assistant manually displaces the uterus to the left. The second issue is the timing of the delivery. Katz et al performed a large review of cardiopulmonary arrest in pregnancy. Fetuses delivered within 5 minutes of maternal death all survived and appeared to be neurologically intact. Given this information and the knowledge that the pregnancy compromises the resuscitation, it is recommended that bedside cesarean section be begun if the resuscitation has not restored cardiac function within 4 minutes, so as to accomplish delivery within 5 minutes.

Brain Death and Life Support

A few cases of prolongation of pregnancy in an effort to reach a viable or near mature gestation have been reported in the mother who is brain dead but remains on cardiopulmonary life support. In these cases delivery was required for sepsis, fetal distress, or maternal hypotension. Thus it is critical to use continuous fetal monitoring once viability is reached, maintain adequate uteroplacental perfusion with aggressive hemodynamic monitoring and fluid management, and avoid infection. Tocolysis can be considered as needed. Setup at bedside for immediate cesarean section should be available at all times.

■ SUMMARY

The principles of fetal evaluation and management for maternal critical care situations are remarkably similar for most conditions. Correction of the maternal condition and/or stabilization of maternal cardiorespiratory status should always be the first goal. Whenever possible, if the condition can be reversed, the ultimate goal should be to correct the maternal condition without the necessity for premature delivery. If delivery will improve the maternal condition, as in severe preeclampsia/eclampsia, the mother should still be stabilized before delivery should occur. A thorough understanding of the physiologic changes in pregnancy, how these affect maternal evaluation, and how pathologic conditions affect fetal oxygen delivery and uteroplacental perfusion are the critical steps in understanding the fetal component of evaluation and management of the critical care pregnant patient.

SUGGESTED READING

Behrman RE, Lees MH, Peterson EN, et al. Distribution of the circulation in the normal and asphyxiated fetal primate. *Am J Obstet Gynecol.* 1970;108:956.

Bernstein IM, Watson M, Simmons GM, et al. Maternal brain death and prolonged fetal survival. *Obstet Gynecol.* 1989; 74:434.

Bickers RG, Wennberg RP. Fetomaternal transfusion following trauma. *Obstet Gynecol.* 1983;61:258.

Bocka J, Courtney J, Pearlman M, et al. Trauma in pregnancy. *Ann Emerg Med.* 1988;17:829.

Boehm FH, Growdon JH. The effect of eclamptic convulsions on the fetal heart rate. *Am J Obstet Gyncol.* 1974;120:851.

Buchsbaum HJ. Splenic rupture in pregnancy: report of a case and review of the literature. *Obstet Gynecol Surv.* 1967; 22:381.

Cantee RW, Thompson JP, Staggers BA. Neurological injuries in pregnancy. In: Haycock CE, ed. *Trauma and Pregnancy.* Littleton, MA: PSG Publishing Co; 1985.

Connolly AM, Kate VL, Bash KL, et al. Trauma and pregnancy. *Am J Perinatol.* 1997;14:331.

Cruz AC, Spellacy WN, Jarrell M. Fetal heart rate tracing during sickle cell crisis: a cause for transient late decelerations. *Obstet Gynecol.* 1979;54:647.

Dias MS. Neurovascular emergencies in pregnancy. In: Pitkin RM, Scott JR, eds. *Clinical Obstetrics and Gynecology.* Philadelphia, PA: JB Lippincott Co; 337:1994.

Dildy GA, van den Berg PP, Katz M, et al. Intrapartum fetal pulse oximetry: fetal oxygen saturation trends during labor and relation to delivery outcome. *Am J Obstet Gynecol.* 1994;171:679.

Freeman RK, Garite TJ, Nageotte MP. *Fetal Heart Rate Monitoring.* 3rd ed. Baltimore, MD: Williams & Wilkins; 2003.

Goodwin TM, Breen MT. Pregnancy outcome and fetopmaternal hemorrhage after noncatastrophic trauma. *Am J Obstet Gynecol.* 1990;162:665.

Higgins SD, Garite TJ. Late abruptio placenta in trauma patients: implications for monitoring. *Obstet Gynecol.* 1984;63:105.

Hilman BC, Aitken ML, Constantinescu M. Pregnancy in patients with cystic fibrosis. *Clin Obstet Gynecol.* 1996;39:70.

Hurd WW, Miodovni KM, Hertzberg V, et al. Selective management of abruptio placentae: a prospective study. *Obstet Gynecol.* 1983;61:467.

Jaffe R, Mock M, Abramowicz J, et al. Mytonic dystrophy and pregnancy: a review. *Obstet Gynecol Surv.* 1986;41:272.

Katz VL, Dotters DJ, Droegemueller W. Perimortem cessarean delivery. *Obstet Gynecol.* 1986;68:571.

Kuhlmann RS, Cruikshank DP. Maternal trauma in pregnancy. In: Pitkin RM, Scott JR, eds. *Clinical Obstetrics and Gynecology.* Philadelphia, PA: JB LippincottCo; 274:1994.

Lavin JP, Polsky SS. Abdominal trauma during pregnancy. *Clin Perinatol.* 1983;10:423.

Lees MM, Scott DB, Kerr MG, et al. The circulating effects of recumbent postural change in late pregnancy. *Clin Sci.* 1967;332:453.

LoBue C, Goodlin RC. Treatment of fetal distress during diabetic ketoacidosis. *J Reprod Med.* 1978;20:101.

Marx G. Shock in the obstetric patient. *Anesthesiology.* 1965;26:423.

Modanlou HD, Freeman RK. Sinusoidal fetal heart rate pattern: its definition and clinical significance. *Am Obstet Gynecol.* 1982;142:1033.

Nyberg DA, Cyr DR, Mack LA, et al. Sonographic spectrum of placental abruption. *AJR.* 1987;148:161.

Paul RH, Koh KS, Bernstein SG. Changes in fetal heart rate: uterine contraction patterns associated with eclampsia. *Am J Obstet Gynecol.* 1978;130:165.

Pearlman MD, Tintinalli JE, Lorenz RP. Blunt trauma during pregnancy. *N Engl J Med.* 1990;323:1609.

Pritchard J, Mason R, Corley M, Pritchard S. Genesis of severe placental abruption. *Am J Obstet Gynecol.* 1970;108:22.

Pritchard JA, Brekken AL. Clinical and laboratory studies on severe abruption placenta. *Am J Obstet Gynecol.* 1967;97:681.

Rigby FB, Pastorek JG. Pneumonia during pregnancy. *Clin Obstet Gynecol.* 1996;1:107.

Rolbin SH, Levinson G, Shnider DM, et al. Dopamine treatment of spinal hypotension decreases uterine blood flow in the pregnant ewe. *Anesthesiology.* 1979;51:36.

Rothenberger DA, Quattlebaum FW, Zabel J, et al. Diagnostic peritoneal lavage for blunt trauma in pregnant women. *Am J Obstet Gynecol.* 1977;129:479.

Schatz M, Zeiger RS. Asthma and allergy in pregnancy. *Clin Perinatol.* 1997;24:407.

Sheldon RE, Peeters LLH, Jones MD Jr, et al. Redistribution of cardiac output and oxygen delivery in the hypoxic fetal lamb. *Am J Obstet Gynecol.* 1979;135:1071.

Sholl JS. Abruptio placentae: clinical management of nonacute cases. *Am J Obstet Gynecol.* 1987;156:40.

Poisoning in Pregnancy

• *Alfredo F. Gei and Victor Suarez*

Poisoning is a morbid state produced by the exposure to a toxic agent (poison) that because of its chemical actions causes a functional disturbance and/or structural damage.

Although the majority of poisonings during pregnancy are accidental, up to one-fifth can be intentional as part of a suicide gesture or attempt.

Two general principles should be kept in mind when treating pregnant women who are poisoned.

1. With rare exception, we save the baby by treating the mother.
2. More harm and damage result from withholding needed therapy from the mother.

Excluding drugs of abuse, the three most common intentional poisonings during pregnancy are those by acetaminophen (APAP), nonsteroidal anti-inflammatory medications (NSAIDs), and selective serotonin reuptake inhibitors (SSRIs). This chapter specifically addresses the perinatal concerns and management of these three poisonings and that of iron, which because of its availability to pregnant women can also be implicated in an acute poisoning in this group of patients.

■ ACETAMINOPHEN

Excluding alcohol and drugs of abuse, APAP is the most common drug taken in overdose during pregnancy.

Maternal Concerns

Pathophysiology

Most APAP is metabolized in the liver by being conjugated with sulfate or glucuronide to form nontoxic metabolites that are excreted in the urine (Fig 23-1). Approximately 7% of APAP, however, is metabolized in the liver and kidneys by cytochrome P450 to form a toxic metabolite,

N-acetyl-*p*-benzoquinoneimine (NAPQI). NAPQI is an extremely reactive molecule that covalently binds to macromolecules, leading to cell injury and death. NAPQI normally undergoes detoxification by combining with glutathione to form a nontoxic mercapturic acid metabolite that is excreted in the urine. With APAP overdose, however, so much NAPQI is formed that glutathione stores become depleted resulting in NAPQI-induced cytotoxicity. Acetaminophen poisoning principally affects the liver and, to a lesser extent, the kidneys.

Toxic Doses and Clinical Course

Patients *acutely* ingesting >140 mg/kg of acetaminophen are at risk for hepatotoxicity. One can predict the risk for developing hepatotoxicity after an *acute, single* ingestion by obtaining a serum APAP concentration at least 4 hours after ingestion. Plotting the resulting level on a standard nomogram estimates the risk for hepatotoxicity (Fig 23-2). If an antidote is not given within 8 hours and hepatotoxicity develops, it is associated with prolonged prothrombin time (PT) and elevation of transaminases (commonly into the thousands). Enzyme values usually peak between 72 and 96 hours after ingestion. Jaundice is uncommon. Seriously poisoned patients occasionally suffer from pancreatitis, oliguria, hypotension, myocardial ischemia, and, possibly, necrosis. Persons who take massive overdoses may present in the first few hours (before the onset of liver failure) with coma and severe metabolic acidosis with elevated lactate concentrations.

While nausea and vomiting commonly develop early in APAP poisoning, patients who ingest fatal doses may suffer no symptoms until the onset of symptomatic liver failure, which can occur 1 to 4 days later. Therefore, a serum APAP value must be obtained from both symptomatic and asymptomatic patients in order to properly assess the severity of the overdose.

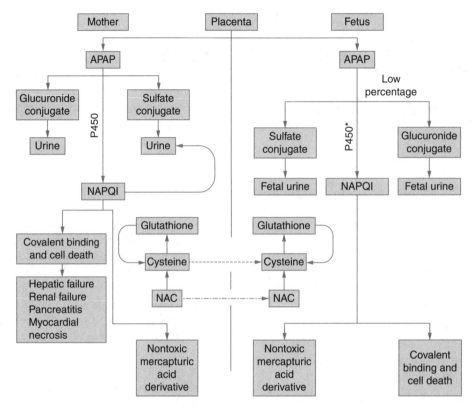

FIGURE 23-1. Pathophysiology of acetaminophen poisoning. APAP, acetaminophen; NAC, *N*-acetylcysteine; NAPQI, *N*-acetyl-*p*-benzoquinoneimine. *Steadily increases after 14 weeks of life.

Patients who habitually take excessive doses of acetaminophen (usually well in excess of 4 g per day) are more likely to develop renal failure along with hepatotoxicity. Serum APAP concentrations in these patients cannot be correlated with severity of illness or risk of hepatotoxicity.

Acetaminophen can cross the placenta and has the potential for fetal hepatotoxicity and in acute intoxications of spontaneous abortion and stillbirth.

Treatment

Supportive therapy, including IV fluids, oxygen, cardiac monitoring, and electronic fetal monitoring (if appropriate for the gestational age of the pregnancy).

Decontamination procedures: Induced emesis may be indicated for home treatment of a large dose (>100 mg/kg). Gastric lavage and activated charcoal (1 g/kg in water) can prevent further absorption of acetaminophen. Oral activated charcoal (AC) avidly adsorbs acetaminophen

and should be administered if the patient presents within 1 hour of ingestion. The network of pores present in activated charcoal adsorbs 100 to 1000 mg of drug per gram of charcoal.

In pregnancy oral AC may be of benefit greater that 1 hour after the ingestion as the gastric emptying is delayed. Oral activated charcoal administered with NAC greater than 4 hours after ingestion has been shown in one case series to be effective in reducing the incidence of liver toxicity after toxic acetaminophen ingestion.

Antidote: The antidote for APAP poisoning is *N*-acetylcysteine (NAC, Mucomyst) (Fig 23-3). *N*-Acetylcysteine undergoes conversion to cysteine, which, in turn, is metabolized to glutathione. *N*-Acetylcysteine's main effect is to maintain glutathione stores so that NAPQI can be detoxified. Started within 8 hours of ingestion, NAC prevents serious maternal hepatic and renal

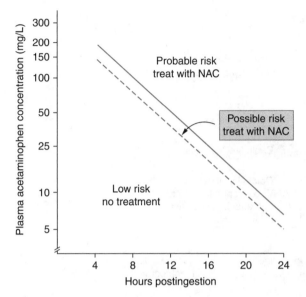

FIGURE 23-2. Acetaminophen nomogram. For use only after a single, acute ingestion in a patient who has not recently taken acetaminophen prior to ingestion. A level should not be plotted on the nomogram unless it was obtained at least 4 hours after ingestion. If a level falls above the lower line, N-acetylcysteine should be continued (if already started) or administered immediately.

toxicity from APAP. To ensure that NAC is started promptly after an acute ingestion, it is generally most prudent to begin NAC therapy immediately and discontinue it only if the serum APAP concentration is found to be in the nontoxic range when plotted on the nomogram. Therapy with NAC provides benefit by lessening the severity of hepatic necrosis and increasing chances for survival, even when begun more than 24 hours after ingestion. Therefore, it is never too late to begin NAC therapy; though efficacy begins to decrease if therapy is delayed beyond 16 hours.

A serum APAP concentration (measured at least 4 hours after ingestion) resulting in a value above the lower line of the nomogram necessitates a full course of NAC therapy (eg, 17 oral doses) be delivered. NAC therapy should not be stopped prematurely simply because a repeat serum APAP concentration falls to zero or plots below the lower line on the nomogram.

Patients commonly experience nausea and vomiting following APAP ingestion, sometimes making it difficult to administer oral NAC therapy. In these cases, NAC has been given intravenously. An intravenous formulation is prepared in the pharmacy by aseptically passing sterile

inhalable or oral NAC solution through a 0.2-μm filter and diluting it in 5% dextrose in water, to create an intravenous solution. An intravenous protocol commonly used in the United States is described in Fig 23-3.

Occasionally, patients suffer symptomatic histamine release from intravenous NAC and require treatment with antihistamines. On rare occasions, patients suffer life-threatening anaphylactoid reactions requiring fluids, epinephrine, antihistamines, and corticosteroids. If the pharmacy cannot timely prepare intravenous NAC, treatment should not be delayed and oral NAC therapy should be started immediately. Treatment for adjunctive complications (eg, liver failure, renal failure) is entirely supportive and identical to that for other pregnant patients.

Fetal Concerns

Fetal death from APAP overdose has been reported in all trimesters. Maternal NAPQI does not cross the placenta. Maternal APAP, however, does cross and has the potential to produce toxic fetal concentrations. The fetus's ability to produce NAPQI from APAP begins as early as 14 weeks intrauterine life and increases until term. The fetus's ability to detoxify APAP by conjugation with sulfate and glucuronide remains impaired until after birth, possibly shunting more APAP through cytochrome P450. The third-trimester fetus, therefore, appears to be at greatest risk for *direct* toxicity from APAP. Nevertheless, fetal loss appears to be most common in the first trimester—not because the fetus is necessarily poisoned, but because maternal illness is more likely to lead to fetal loss at that time.

Placental transfer of NAC (a class B medication) in humans has been documented with concentrations in the umbilical cord blood similar to maternal levels (Horowitz et al). Because considerations of lack of first-pass effect through the fetal liver (compared to the maternal intake of NAC), most authorities prefer the parenteral use of the antidote during pregnancy. When NAC is given intravenously at currently used therapeutic doses, serum levels are 10 to 100 times higher.

At least one authority has recommended consideration for delivery of the mature fetus by cesarean section so that NAC therapy can be administered directly to the baby at risk (ie, when maternal serum APAP concentrations are toxic). This has to be balanced against the maternal of the procedure because of a potential coagulopathy. Advocates of immediate delivery state that the maternal and fetal risk of late third-trimester cesarean section is extremely low in comparison to data from the several case reports describing

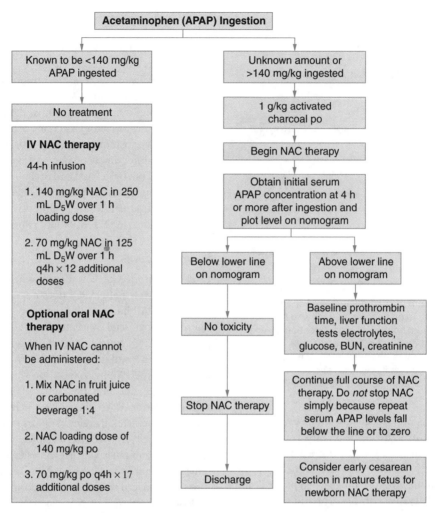

FIGURE 23-3. General guidelines for managing acetaminophen poisoning. Oral NAC should be used when IV NAC cannot be prepared by the pharmacy and promptly administered. NAC, *N*-acetylcysteine; APAP, acetaminophen. (See text for discussion on role of cesarian section.)

fetal death from APAP toxicity. The incidence correlates with delays in initiating therapy with NAC. Unfortunately, no animal or human studies have examined the benefits of immediate delivery followed by direct newborn NAC therapy. The published experience does not contain reports of fetal demise following acute single APAP ingestions if NAC therapy is begun promptly. No standard of care to guide clinicians who face this dilemma exists. Given the potential for a nonreassuring fetal condition, fetal monitoring of viable pregnancies is recommended

during therapy. Although it has not being proven, serial assessments of the fetal well-being are recommended upon discharge from a severe exposure to acetaminophen.

■ IRON

Large doses of iron are extremely toxic and may lead to multiorgan system dysfunction and death. Strong evidence indicates that the fetus is protected from elevated maternal iron levels. Iron poisoning is, almost entirely, a situation

■ TABLE 23-1. Pathophysiology of Iron Poisoning

1. Iron is corrosive to the gastrointestinal tract, producing nausea, vomiting, diarrhea, abdominal pain, gastrointestinal bleeding, and rarely perforations.
2. Systemically absorbed iron causes venodilatation and increased capillary permeability with associated third spacing of fluid.
3. Iron causes cell dysfunction and death by disrupting ATP formation in mitochondria and by catalyzing the formation of oxygen-free radicals that destroy cell membranes. The liver takes the brunt of the injury with potential for fulminant hepatic failure, but in massive iron poisoning, any organ can be affected.
4. Early after ingestion, high serum iron concentrations directly inhibit serine proteases (thrombin) and lengthen the prothrombin time, even in the absence of hepatic failure.

in which fetal survival depends on maternal survival. Table 23-1 and Fig 23-4 summarize the pathophysiology and management of iron toxicity, respectively.

Maternal Concerns

Toxic Doses

To determine how much iron was ingested, the elemental iron content must be calculated. On a milligram basis, ferrous sulfate contains 20% elemental iron; ferrous fumarate 33% elemental iron; and ferrous gluconate 12% elemental iron. Any patient who ingests more than 20 mg/kg of elemental iron, any patient with symptoms, and/or any patient in whom the amount of ingested iron is not known requires an evaluation. During pregnancy the prepregnancy weight should be used for calculation of the dose ingested. Keep in mind that if the mechanism of the poisoning was intentional, the history may be unreliable as patients may conceal or minimize the magnitude of the exposure.

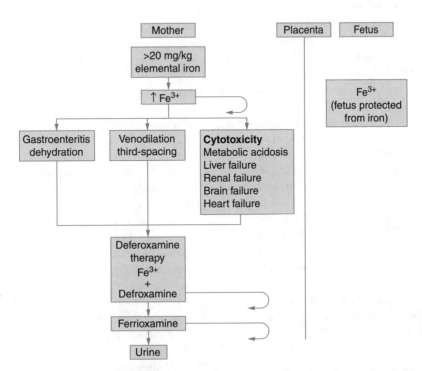

FIGURE 23-4. Pathophysiology of iron poisoning and rationale for treatment. (See text for conversion of iron salts to elemental iron.)

Clinical effects

Traditionally, clinical effects are considered in four stages, although the distinctions between stages are not always clear.

Stage 1 is characterized by abdominal pain, vomiting, and diarrhea, and results from the corrosive effects of iron on the gut. Stage 1 begins 1 to 6 hours after ingestion. Hematemesis is possible, and hypovolemia may result in hypotension and metabolic acidosis. Serum iron levels may be normal or elevated at this stage.

Stage 2 is not always seen, but, when present, lasts for about 2 to 24 hours or so after Stage 1. Stage 2 is characterized by resolution of gastroenteritis, and patients commonly lie in bed quietly. Pallor, metabolic acidosis, and in the face of uncorrected hypovolemia, tachycardia and hypotension may be noted. Physicians may be falsely reassured by the resolution of gastroenteritis in the face of ensuing systemic iron toxicity as tissue iron stores rise. Tachycardia and hypotension are common if hypovolemia has not been corrected. Metabolic acidosis and hypotension result from uncorrected hypovolemia, venodilation, third-spacing of fluid, and the cytotoxic effects of iron. Serum iron concentration may be elevated and liver enzyme values are normal. PT may be elevated if serum iron concentrations are high from a direct effect of iron on serum proteases such as thrombin. In severe iron poisoning, the patient may rapidly progress from Stage 1 to Stage 3.

Stage 3 comprises systemic organ damage or failure from the cytotoxic effects of iron. Its onset is observed at any time from ingestion through 48 hours. Stage 3 is characterized by hepatic failure, lethargy/coma/convulsions, renal failure, and, occasionally, heart failure. Hypoglycemia and coagulopathy reflect hepatic damage. In this setting, metabolic acidosis has numerous causes including hepatic failure, low cardiac output, and impaired oxidative phosphorylation. The liver is the major organ affected by the toxicity of iron and typically is the first organ to fail. Stage 3 toxicity is associated with spontaneous abortion, preterm delivery, and maternal death.

Stage 4 is characterized by gastric outlet or small bowel obstruction from gastrointestinal scarring several weeks after the poisoning.

Evaluation and Treatment

Serum Iron Concentrations While most patients who suffer iron poisoning of Stage 2 or greater are thought to have *peak* serum concentrations >350 µg/dL, the actual peak level is seldom observed as a consequence of mistiming. Serum iron levels peak sometime between 2 and 6 hours after ingestion. Normal or mildly elevated serum iron concentrations can be misleading, since they do not always reflect the tissue iron burden, which is the one responsible for the systemic toxicity. Therefore, as an isolated finding, a normal serum iron concentration cannot always be used to exclude iron poisoning in the symptomatic patient. Obtaining a normal or low iron level more than 6 hours after an ingestion may be misleading as the reason that the level is low is redistribution of iron in the tissues. Toxicity is still possible in these cases and the patient, not the numbers need to be treated. The measurement of total iron binding capacity (TIBC) does not assist in the treatment of acute iron poisoning since it is falsely elevated in the face of high serum iron concentrations by some methods and since serum iron concentrations may be quickly changing in their relationship to TIBC.

Asymptomatic Patients Ipecac emesis may be considered in the conscious patient within the first hour of exposure. Prolonged vomiting (>1 hour) should be attributed to iron toxicity rather than to the effects of ipecac. Generally, patients who remain completely asymptomatic for 6 hours after ingestion and have a normal physical examination do not require treatment for iron poisoning (Fig 23-5). Asymptomatic patients who ingest >20 mg/kg of elemental iron but are seen within 6 hours might benefit from gastric lavage with saline. If vomiting has already occurred, it is not thought that gastric lavage would be of further benefit. 1% bicarbonate (200-300 mL) after lavage or induced emeses may promote the conversion of ferrous iron to ferrous carbonate (less soluble). Alternatively a single oral dose of 8% magnesium oxide (Milk of Magnesia; 60 mL/g of elemental iron ingested) significantly reduces iron absorption in healthy volunteers.

Symptomatic Patients Patients are considered symptomatic when they present with more than minimal symptoms (eg, more than one emesis). These patients require treatment with fluids and deferoxamine mesylate, in addition to magnesium oxide (Table 23-2). When a patient has significant clinical symptoms, it is never prudent to wait for results of a serum iron concentration before beginning therapy, including deferoxamine.

Fetal Concerns

The placenta selectively transports maternal transferrin-bound iron only when it is required by the fetus. Animal

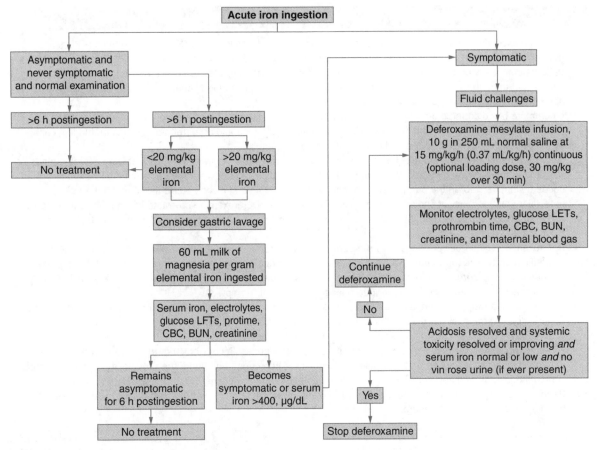

FIGURE 23-5. Treatment of acute iron ingestion.

models of iron poisoning in pregnancy, along with human experience, lead to the conclusion that the fetus does not develop elevated iron burdens in the face of maternal iron poisoning (Fig 23-4). Fetal demise appears to be due, entirely, to maternal illness or death. Fetal outcome depends on the well-being of the mother; it is in the interest of both mother and child that significant poisoning be treated promptly with deferoxamine. *Pregnancy or fetal concerns are never reasons to withhold deferoxamine therapy.*

In a review of 61 cases of iron overdose in pregnancy, Tran and colleagues noted that the degree of maternal toxicity was directly related to the risk of fetal loss. Fetal demise appeared to be related to the timing and severity of the maternal illness, rather than to fetal toxicity directly from iron.

Prior to discharging the patient, always evaluate the mechanism of the exposure and obtain other consultations as required by the particular case (Psychiatry; Social Services, etc).

■ SALICYLATE

Sources of salicylate include aspirin (acetylsalicylic acid), oil of wintergreen (methyl-salicylate), salicylic acid, and salsalate. All of these compounds are converted to salicylate after absorption. With the exception of aspirin's ability to inhibit platelet function, salicylate is responsible for most of the observed toxic effects.

Salicylate poisoning remains one of the most underestimated and mismanaged poisonings in medicine. This problem is further compounded by pregnancy, when only moderate maternal toxicity may result in fetal demise secondary to the ability of the drug to freely cross the placenta and the propensity of the drug to concentrate in the fetus, particularly the central nervous system (CNS).

■ **TABLE 23-2. Management: Symptomatic Iron Poisoning**

1. With rare exception, all symptomatic patients are hypovolemic. Administering 500-1000 mL fluid challenges (Ringer lactate or normal saline) to restore fluid volume and ensure urine output of 1-2 mL/kg/h is therapeutic. Patients commonly require maintenance infusions at twice the normal rates to keep up with gastrointestinal losses and third spacing. In addition, aggressive hydration aids in eliminating chelated iron by maintaining an appropriate urine output (see below).

2. A complete blood count, prothrombin time, electrolytes, serum glucose, liver function studies, arterial blood gases and blood urea nitrogen/creatinine, and serum iron concentration should be obtained. A total iron binding capacity is not useful in acute toxicity as it is frequently falsely elevated.

3. Deferoxamine mesylate is an iron-chelating agent that is given to remove iron from tissues. Deferoxamine binds with iron to form ferrioxamine, which is excreted in the urine over days or weeks. Ferrioxamine occasionally produces a vin rose color in the urine. This color change is unreliable and inconsistent; it should not be used to determine the adequacy of chelation or the need for treatment. Deferoxamine mesylate can be mixed in the crystalloid of choice and should be infused continuously at 15 mg/kg/h after optional loading dose of 30 mg/kg over 30 min (Fig 23-5)[a].

4. Deferoxamine should be continued until the serum iron concentration (levels every 4-6 h) is normal or low and systemic toxicity is resolved (eg, resolved acidosis, liver function studies normal or improving) and if it is present, obvious vin rose-colored urine disappears. Most patients require 12-24 h of deferoxamine infusion. Occasionally patients taking very large overdoses require a longer duration of therapy.

5. If renal failure develops, deferoxamine should be continued, but at much lower infusion rates. Assuming that therapeutic deferoxamine levels have been obtained, anuric patients should continue to receive infusions at about 1.5 mg/kg/h, based on the known prolonged half-life in renal failure.

6. For large intakes of iron consider a KUB after emesis and the possibility of whole-bowel irrigation in those patients with a radiopacity on KUB suspicious of remaining iron concretions until the radiopacity clears. Activated charcoal does not bind iron but should be utilized if coingestants are suspected.

7. General supportive care for attendant complications (eg, liver failure, gastrointestinal bleeding) is the same as that for any other pregnant patient.

---

[a]Many statements in the package insert for deferoxamine do not reflect common practice and are misleading or incorrect. Deferoxamine is not contraindicated in pregnancy for the treatment of acute iron poisoning. At 15 mg/kg/h, most patients will receive well over 6 g deferoxamine mesylate per day and this is safe for short-term treatment of iron poisoning. Intramuscular deferoxamine is not recommended.

Maternal Concerns

Pharmacokinetics and Toxic Doses

Significant salicylate toxicity is said to develop after the acute, single ingestion of at least 150 mg/kg of aspirin (or its equivalent). However, given the fetus's ability to concentrate salicylate, concern arises when an acute, single maternal ingestion exceeds 75 mg/kg. Salicylate levels may not peak until 24 hours after the drug is absorbed. Enteric-coated aspirin may not produce toxic serum concentrations for many hours after ingestion.

Salicylate exists in blood as an equilibrium between the ionized and the nonionized form (Fig 23-6). The nonionized, nonprotein-bound fraction of salicylate is in equilibrium with tissue stores. This nonionized form easily moves into body compartments because of its lipophilic nature.

As serum salicylate levels rise, protein binding becomes saturated, producing a higher free (nonionized) fraction of the drug (from approximately 10% to 25%). As pH falls the nonionized fraction of salicylate increases. Therefore, rises in serum salicylate concentration or falls in blood pH result in an increase in the apparent volume of distribution of salicylate as salicylate moves from blood into tissue. This important concept is critical in understanding both the pathophysiology and the management of salicylate toxicity, since the serum salicylate concentrations can fall while tissue concentrations and severity of toxicity increase.

In salicylate poisoning, most salicylate is eliminated unchanged by the kidneys. Elimination half-lives can be as long as $1\frac{1}{2}$ to 2 days in untreated patients because of saturable elimination kinetics.

Salicylate poisoning

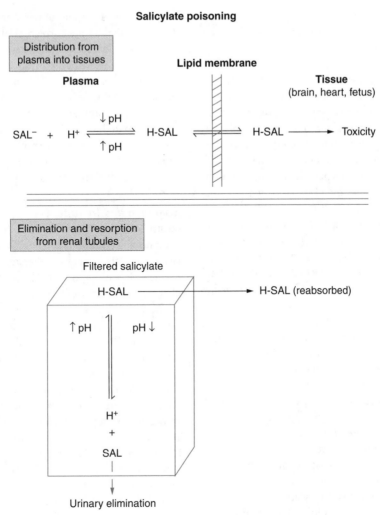

FIGURE 23-6. Salicylate distribution between blood, tissues, and urine. A smaller fraction of salicylate is protein bound at higher concentrations. A fall in pH increases the fraction of unionized salicylate. Therefore, falls in pH or rises in salicylate concentrations result in a greater fraction of the drug that can move into tissues, including the brain and fetus. Alkalinization of the blood helps prevent movement of salicylate into tissue. Alkalinization of urine traps salicylate in an ionized form so it cannot be reabsorbed, enhancing urinary elimination. H-SAL, unionized salicylic acid; SAL$^-$, ionized salicylate anion.

Pathophysiology and Clinical Effects

Salicylate produces numerous actions that produce various effects in many organ systems. These diverse clinical manifestations result, in part, because of impaired adenosine triphosphate (ATP) formation from salicylate's actions on cellular metabolism.

Gastrointestinal Irritation Direct corrosive injury to the gut is responsible for abdominal pain, nausea, vomiting, gastrointestinal bleeding, and rare reports of gastric perforation.

Respiratory Alkalosis Salicylate directly stimulates the brain stem to cause hyperventilation. However, the onset of coma may mask hyperventilation, and can even produce hypoventilation and hypercapnia.

Metabolic Acidosis Salicylate affects numerous metabolic pathways to inhibit ATP formation. Salicylate inhibits the Krebs' cycle, uncouples oxidative phosphorylation, and enhances lipolysis. All of these actions serve to produce metabolic acidosis. Ketonuria is usually present, and lactate levels are usually normal. The anion gap can be normal or frequently elevated.

Glucose Metabolism Increased glucose demand accompanied by glycogenolysis explains occasional hyperglycemia seen early in poisoning. However, salicylate inhibits gluconeogenesis so when glycogen stores become depleted, hypoglycemia is possible.

Fluid and Electrolytes Dehydration from gastrointestinal losses and hyperventilation is common. Patients may lose 1 to 2 L/h from severe diaphoresis, alone. The average patient with moderate to severe salicylate poisoning has a 6-L fluid deficit. Both hypokalemia and hyperkalemia may be observed. Hypokalemia results from gastrointestinal losses and obligatory urinary excretion of potassium with organic acids (eg, salicylate). Hyperkalemia usually reflects acidosis, severe dehydration, and prerenal azotemia, sometimes with rhabdomyolysis.

Pulmonary Noncardiogenic (low pressure) pulmonary edema can develop with salicylate poisoning; however, hydrostatic (high pressure) pulmonary edema may also occur in persons with chronic heart disease or salicylate-induced heart failure, or in those whose fluid therapy has not been carefully monitored for fluid balance.

Cardiovascular The metabolic insult to myocardium induced by salicylate results in tachycardia, ventricular arrhythmias, heart failure, hypotension, and sudden death. In the absence of heart disease, metabolic acidosis and neurotoxicity almost always precede severe cardiac dysfunction and shock if the patient has been adequately fluid resuscitated.

Central Nervous System Impaired ATP production produces neurotoxicity which is manifested by hallucinations, agitation, delirium, lethargy, coma, convulsions, malignant cerebral edema, and brain death.

Coagulation and Platelets Salicylate impairs vitamin K–dependent coagulation factors to prolong PT in a manner similar to Coumadin. Aspirin (acetylsalicylic acid) also inhibits platelet function, though this is rarely responsible for major morbidity.

Miscellaneous Hyperthermia may be observed, but is the exception. When present, it portends a poor prognosis. Acute tubular necrosis has been reported. Rhabdomyolysis contributes to hyperkalemia, coagulopathy, and renal failure. Tinnitus is common when serum salicylate levels exceed about 25 mg/dL.

Clinical Presentation

Patients who present shortly after an overdose are usually awake and complain of tinnitus, abdominal pain, nausea, and vomiting. Other abnormalities include tachypnea, respiratory alkalosis with alkalemia, hypovolemia, hypokalemia, and gastrointestinal bleeding.

Progression of the poisoning is characterized by diaphoresis, tachycardia despite correction of hypovolemia, metabolic acidosis and acidemia, progressively severe neurotoxicity, alterations of glucose homeostasis, elevated PT, pulmonary edema, and cardiotoxicity. The combination of acidemia and neurotoxicity carries a grave prognosis unless aggressive treatment is initiated promptly.

As compared to acute salicylate poisoning, serum salicylate concentrations are lower for any given degree of toxicity in chronic poisoning because of larger tissue burdens of salicylate, reflecting a larger volume of distribution.

Evaluation and Treatment

Serum Salicylate Concentrations Interpretation of serum salicylate concentrations can be difficult. Similar levels can have varied effects because of changing tissue burdens of the drug depending on blood pH, protein binding, and other factors. Because of these factors, tissue concentrations of salicylate can actually rise while serum levels are falling, causing the patient's condition to deteriorate while the physician is falsely reassured by falling serum drug concentrations. It is always more important to treat the patient than the serum salicylate concentration.

Basing treatment and disposition on a single serum salicylate concentration can be misleading and is to be discouraged. Though a serum salicylate level less than 30 mg/dL (and known to be falling) would be reassuring for an asymptomatic mother, because the fetus develops higher serum salicylate concentrations than the mother, it is possible for fetus to develop significant toxicity.

Hyperbilirubinemia can cause falsely elevated salicylate concentrations when levels are measured using a colorimetric method. In these cases, serum salicylate concentrations should be measured by an immunoassay or by a chromatographic method.

General Principles All patients with salicylate poisoning should be admitted to an intensive care setting, whether in labor and delivery or in a medical intensive care unit. Successful maternal management of acute salicylate poisoning hinges on intensive and attentive medical care (Fig 23-7). Specifically, frequent attention to fluid balance, electrolyte and acid-base status, bedside examination, and rapid institution of hemodialysis at the earliest signs of central nervous system deterioration are required. It is also recommended that hemodialysis be performed earlier during pregnancy, given ability of the fetus to concentrate salicylate.

Airway As with many patients, immediate attention to airway and adequate oxygenation are mandatory. If a

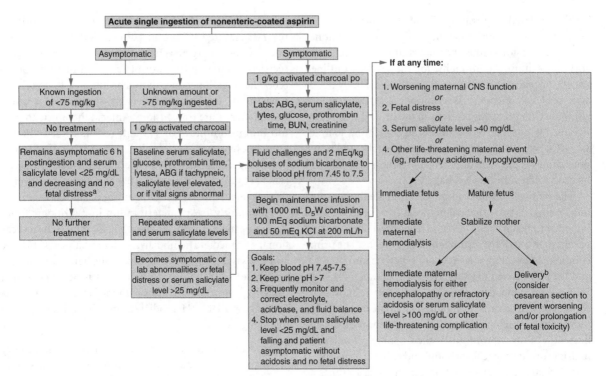

Acute single ingestion of nonenteric-coated aspirin

Asymptomatic

- Known ingestion of <75 mg/kg
  - No treatment
  - Remains asymptomatic 6 h postingestion and serum salicylate level <25 mg/dL and decreasing and no fetal distress[a]
  - No further treatment

- Unknown amount or >75 mg/kg ingested
  - 1 g/kg activated charcoal
  - Baseline serum salicylate, glucose, prothrombin time, lytes, ABG if tachypneic, salicylate level elevated, or if vital signs abnormal
  - Repeated examinations and serum salicylate levels
  - Becomes symptomatic or lab abnormalities or fetal distress or serum salicylate level >25 mg/dL

Symptomatic

- 1 g/kg activated charcoal po
- Labs: ABG, serum salicylate, lytes, glucose, prothrombin time, BUN, creatinine
- Fluid challenges and 2 mEq/kg boluses of sodium bicarbonate to raise blood pH from 7.45 to 7.5
- Begin maintenance infusion with 1000 mL D$_5$W containing 100 mEq sodium bicarbonate and 50 mEq KCl at 200 mL/h
- Goals:
  1. Keep blood pH 7.45-7.5
  2. Keep urine pH >7
  3. Frequently monitor and correct electrolyte, acid/base, and fluid balance
  4. Stop when serum salicylate level <25 mg/dL and falling and patient asymptomatic without acidosis and no fetal distress

If at any time:

1. Worsening maternal CNS function
   or
2. Fetal distress
   or
3. Serum salicylate level >40 mg/dL
   or
4. Other life-threatening maternal event (eg, refractory acidemia, hypoglycemia)

Immediate fetus → Immediate maternal hemodialysis

Mature fetus → Stabilize mother

Immediate maternal hemodialysis for either encephalopathy or refractory acidosis or serum salicylate level >100 mg/dL or other life-threatening complication

Delivery[b] (consider cesarean section to prevent worsening and/or prolongation of fetal toxicity)

[a]Enteric-coated aspirin may not produce toxic serum salicylate concentrations until well after 6-h postingestion.
[b]See text for discussion.

FIGURE 23-7. Treatment guidelines for salicylate poisoning.

patient receives narcotics or sedatives, including when used for endotracheal intubation and mechanical ventilation, a drop in an elevated minute ventilation (from salicylate-induced hyperventilation) to normal values can precipitate a rapid decline in blood pH, movement of salicylate into tissues and fetus, and rapid deterioration. Therefore, close attention must be given to maintaining alkalemia (ABGs + potassium every 2-4 hours) with additional doses of IV sodium bicarbonate when sedation or mechanical ventilation is instituted.

Glucose Abnormalities Patients must be monitored for hypoglycemia (every 2 hours), especially in the face of any mental status changes. Treatment comprises IV boluses of 50% dextrose and infusions of dextrose solutions to keep the glycemia above 90 mg/dL.

Gastrointestinal Decontamination A single dose of 1 g activated charcoal per kilogram body weight should be given initially if it is immediately available, no contraindications are present and the patient is not vomiting. Most patients suffering from acute salicylate poisoning vomit repeatedly, rendering further attempts at gastric emptying

(lavage and ipecac) unnecessary. If salicylate levels continue to rise, repeated doses of 0.25 g activated charcoal per kilogram body weight, every 4 to 6 hours until levels begin to fall, may be considered if the patient has normal gastrointestinal motility. Phenothiazines are to be discouraged, as they usually are ineffective and lower the seizure threshold.

Fluid and Electrolyte Therapy Most patients are moderately to severely dehydrated and require immediate fluid challenges with normal saline or Ringer lactate until urine output is 2 to 3 mL/kg/h. Initial sodium bicarbonate boluses of 2 mEq/kg are given, if needed, to raise arterial blood pH from 7.45 to 7.5. A typical patient with moderate to severe salicylate toxicity has a 6-L fluid deficit on presentation.

A recommended *initial* regimen for maintenance fluid therapy *after* fluid resuscitation and establishment of good urine flow is a continuous infusion of 1000 mL of 5% dextrose in water to which is added 150 mEq sodium bicarbonate (3 ampules of 8.4% NaHCO$_3$) and 40 mEq potassium chloride to run at 2 to 3 mL/kg/h. Hypokalemia must be treated aggressively. Urine alkalinity cannot be achieved in the setting of hypokalemia because the kidney will secrete protons rather than potassium ions when reabsorbing sodium. Additionally, for the reasons outlined above, the patient usually presents with a total body potassium debt, and ongoing losses continue as salicylate anions combine with potassium cations in the urine during elimination. Despite intravenous infusions containing 40 mEq/L of KCl, patients almost always require regular additional potassium supplementation. Oral potassium solutions can be used when vomiting has halted.

The rationale behind sodium bicarbonate therapy outlined below has two principal purposes (see Fig 23-6). Most important, alkalinization of blood helps prevent movement of salicylate out of the serum into target organs. The prime concern is preventing movement of salicylate into the CNS and the fetus. Blood pH should be kept between 7.45 and 7.50. A drop in blood pH from 7.45 to 7.20 can almost double the concentration of nonionized salicylate that is able to move into the brain and fetus. Of lesser importance, alkalinization of urine promotes "ionic trapping" of salicylate in urine, preventing reabsorption, and enhancing elimination. Urinary salicylate excretion can increase 15 times as urine pH increases to pH 8.0, above which there is no additional benefit. Monitoring the urinary ph every hour during treatment is recommended.

Fluid and electrolyte infusions are modified as needed to prevent hypovolemia, fluid overload, normalize electrolytes, ensure adequate urine output, and prevent acidemia and hypoglycemia. Because of fluid losses through hyperventilation, diaphoresis, vomiting, and sometimes, hyperthermia, it is common for moderately to severely ill patients to require more than 500 mL/h of intravenous fluid to maintain euvolemia and prevent the rises in serum creatinine, sodium, and hematocrit typical of hemoconcentration.

Serum salicylate concentrations should be obtained every 2 hours until a declining trend is noted and the levels fall under 30 mg/dl, with findings interpreted in the context of the patient's condition.

Noncardiogenic Pulmonary Edema Adult respiratory distress syndrome (ARDS) is more common in chronic toxicity and should be treated with oxygen and continuous positive airway pressure (CPAP) or positive end-expiratory pressure (PEEP), if required. Only cautious use of diuretics is recommended, as these patients are usually volume depleted. If mechanical ventilation is required hyperventilation (rates of 16-20/min) might be needed to keep the $Paco_2$ around 35 mm Hg.

Miscellaneous A 10-mg parenteral dose of vitamin K_1 reverses elevated PT produced by salicylate over several hours. In an emergency, fresh frozen plasma rapidly corrects coagulopathy (but not platelet dysfunction). Serial blood hemoglobin values should be followed to determine if gastrointestinal bleeding develops and becomes severe enough to require transfusions. Antacid therapy with proton pump inhibitors or H2 antagonists are commonly used, but have not been studied in the setting of salicylate poisoning. Serial measurements of serum creatine kinase (CK) activity should be evaluated to rule out rhabdomyolysis, which, if present, will require specific therapy.

Hemodialysis Any deterioration in neurologic function, especially if associated with acidemia, is an indication for immediate hemodialysis. Hemodialysis is effective and life saving in that it removes salicylate and corrects acid-base electrolyte abnormalities. It is best performed using high-flux hemodialysis with the largest-surface area cartridge available. Hemodialysis may be indicated in the following situations:

1. Moderately to severely ill patients with renal insufficiency
2. Seizures or other severe CNS symptoms or worsening neurotoxicity, even if serum salicylate concentrations are falling
3. Other life-threatening complications (pulmonary edema) accompanied by elevated serum salicylate concentrations
4. Salicylate level greater than 90 mg/dL (or 60 mg/dL with a chronic overdose)
5. No improvement of acidemia with decontamination and urine alkalinization.
6. Hypotension refractory to optimal supportive care
7. To ensure fetal survival (see below)

Fetal Concerns

Salicylate crosses the placenta and concentrates in the fetus at higher levels than in the mother, at least in part, by differences in protein binding. The relative acidemia of the fetus also contributes to a higher relative volume of distribution and, therefore, higher tissue levels for a given serum salicylate concentration. In addition, the fetus has a lower capacity to buffer the acidemic stress imposed by salicylate and, relative to the mother, a reduced capacity to excrete the toxin. Collectively, this places the fetus at greater risk for death and forms the basis for the subsequent recommendation of hemodialysis and/or possible cesarean section.

Premature Fetus

Given that the fetus concentrates salicylate and suffers greater toxicity than the mother, it seems wise to institute hemodialysis for lesser degrees of maternal toxicity than would be done in nonpregnant patients. Unfortunately, there are no studies to guide clinicians in this setting. It would be advisable to recommend immediate hemodialysis in the face of any signs of fetal distress, in the face of chronic maternal salicylate poisoning (where high tissue levels predominate), or whenever maternal serum salicylate concentrations exceed 40 mg/dL.

In term pregnancies, it has been proposed that delivery should be considered when deemed safe for the mother. However, there are no studies that have addressed this issue, and decisions must be made on an individual basis. It is possible that hemodialysis would result in falls in both maternal and fetal salicylate concentrations from the redistribution of salicylate across the placenta. Fetal monitoring is certainly part of the adequacy assessment of the supportive measures implemented.

■ SELECTIVE SEROTONIN REUPTAKE INHIBITORS

Commonly used selective serotonin reuptake inhibitors (SSRIs) include fluoxetine (Prozac), sertraline (Zoloft), paroxetine (Paxil), and citalopram (Celexa). There has been an increase in exposures reported to US poison control centers involving SSRIs. Besides its neurotransmitter action in the central nervous system, SSRIs act directly on the myometrium via 5-HT2a receptors.

In most instances, isolated SSRI poisoning has no significant clinical. At very high doses, SSRIs may trigger serotoninergic syndrome with or without signs of the anticholinergic syndrome. Most fatalities have been reported with either large doses (>150 times the daily dose) or with the presence of coingestants such as ethanol, benzodiazepines, or tricyclic antidepressants. Transplacental transference of SSRIs has been documented.

Serotoninergic syndrome is characterized by the simultaneous presence of at least three of the following signs: confusion, agitation, delirium, hallucinations, mania, coma, seizures, slow, continuous, horizontal, eye movements (referred to as ocular clonus), myoclonus, hyperreflexia, sweating, shivering, trembling, diarrhea, hyperthermia, or lack of motor coordination. Myoclonus is the most specific sign.

The anticholinergic syndrome is characterized by agitation, delirium, tremor in the extremities, mydriasis, dryness of the mucous membranes, urinary retention, constipation, and sinusal tachycardia.

During pregnancy, particularly in the third trimester, intense uterine contractions and fetal heart rate anomalies have been reported as a consequence of SSRI intoxication.

Supportive care and decontamination are the most important aspect of treatment.

All pregnant patients with suicidal intent or SSRI abuse should be admitted.

Following initial patient stabilization, administer activated charcoal (1 g/kg; standard adult dose is 50 g). Greatest benefit from charcoal decontamination occurs if given within 1 to 2 hours following the ingestion. Do not induce emesis. The use of oral activated charcoal can be considered since the likelihood of SSRI-induced loss of consciousness or seizures is small. As for most toxic agents a specific SSRI-antidote does not exist. There is no role for hemodialysis.

Secure airway, breathing, and circulation; intubate as clinically indicated.

If a patient is clinically sick or comatose, consider the presence of coingestants or an underlying nontoxicologic condition. Significant toxicity in an isolated SSRI ingestion is unlikely.

If patient is hyperthermic (>104°F [>40°C]), use benzodiazepines and external cooling measures.

Seizures generally are best treated with benzodiazepines (Lorazepam 1-2 mg IV every 5 minutes prn). Drug-associated agitated behavior is generally best treated with benzodiazepine administration, supplemented with high potency neuroleptics (haloperidol) prn. Agitation associated with the anticholinergic syndrome may be best treated with physostigmine (initial dose: 0.5-2.0 mg slow IV over 3-5 minutes).

If hypotension does not respond to intravenous fluids, vasopressors will be required. Direct-acting vasopressors, such as norepinephrine can be used safely in pregnancy. If severely hypertensive, use nifedipine or labetalol. Ventricular tachycardias are generally treated with lidocaine. Symptomatic bradyarrhythmias (with hypotension for example) should be treated with atropine or temporary pacing).

L&D management: Tocodynamometry must be maintained during the first 12-24 hours following ingestion. Prophylactic tocolysis (calcium channel blocker) to reduce the strength of uterine contractions and reduce risk of preterm delivery has been advocated.

Fetal heart rate abnormalities: Unless persistently nonreassuring (category III) tracing is present, expectant management is recommended given that premature birth will likely be complicated by severe neonatal withdrawal syndrome (irritability, vomiting, and convulsions, etc).

Antenatal steroids is recommended if fetus is viable and at less than 34 weeks' gestation. With SSRI use during pregnancy, there is the additional risk of persistent pulmonary hypertension.

■ USEFUL REFERENCES

United States Poison Control Centers can be reached through a toll-free line (1-800-222-1222).

The World Health Organization provides a listing of international poison centers at its website: www.who.int/ipcs/poisons/centre/directory/en.

SUGGESTED READING

Berkovitch M, Uziel Y, Greenberg R, et al. False-high blood salicylate levels in neonates with hyperbilirubinemia. *Therap Drug Monitor.* 2000;22:757-761.

Boyer EW, Shannon M. The serotonin syndrome. *N Engl J Med.* 2005;352:1112-1120.

Bronstein AC, Spyker DA, Cantilena LR Jr, Green JL, Rumack BH, Giffin SL. 2008 Annual Report of the American Association of Poison Control Centers' National Poison Data System (NPDS): 26th Annual Report. *Clinical Toxicology.* 2009;47:911-1084.

Chyka PA, Erdman AR, Christianson G, et al. Salicylate poisoning: an evidence-based consensus guideline for out-of-hospital management. *Clin Toxicol (Phila).* 2007;45 (2):95-131.

Curry SC, Bond GR, Raschke R, et al. An ovine model of maternal iron poisoning in pregnancy. *Ann Emerg Med.* 1990;19:632-638.

Gray TA, Buckley BM, Vale JA. Hyperlactataemia and metabolic acidosis following paracetamol overdose. *Q J Med.* 1987;65:811-821.

Harrison PM, Keays R, Bray GP, et al. Improved outcome of paracetamol-induced fulminant hepatic failure by late administration of acetylcysteine. *Lancet.* 1990;335:1572-1573.

Horowitz RS, Dart RC, Jarvie DR, et al. Placental transfer of *N*-acetylcysteine following human maternal acetaminophen toxicity. *J Toxicol Clin Toxicol.* 1997;35:447-451.

Johnson D, Simone C, Koren G. Transfer of *N*-acetylcysteine by the human placenta. *Vet Hum Toxicol.* 1993;35:365.

Lacoste H, Goyert GL, Goldman LS, Wright DJ, Schwartz DB. Acute iron intoxication in pregnancy: case report and review of the literature. *Obstet Gynecol.* 1992 Sep;80(3; Pt 2):500-501.

Levy G. Clinical pharmacokinetics of aspirin. *Pediatrics.* 1978; (5 Part 2 Suppl):867-72.

Loebstein R, Koren G. Clinical relevance of therapeutic drug monitoring during pregnancy (protein binding changes in fetus). *Therap Drug Monitor.* 2002;24:15-22.

Manoguerra AS, Erdman AR, Booze LL, et al. Iron ingestion: an evidence-based consensus guideline for out-of-hospital management. *Clin Toxicol (Phila).* 2005;43(6):553-570.

Moses-Kolko EL, Bogen D, Perel J, et al. Neonatal signs after late in utero exposure to serotonin reuptake inhibitors: literature review and implications for clinical applications. *JAMA.* 2005; 293:2372-2383.

Mills KC, Curry SC. Acute iron poisoning. *Emerg Med Clin North Am.* 1994;12:397-413.

O'Malley GF. Emergency department management of the salicylate-poisoned patient. *Emerg Med Clin North Am.* 2007 May;25(2):333-346.

Riggs BS, Bronstein AC, Kulig K, et al. Acute acetaminophen overdose during pregnancy. *Obstet Gynecol.* 1986;74:247-253.

Rollins DE, von Bahr C, Glaumann H, et al. Acetaminophen: potentially toxic metabolite formed by human fetal and adult liver microsomes and isolated fetal liver cells. *Science.* 1979;205:1414-1416.

Selden BS, Curry SC, Clark RF, et al. Transplacental transport of *N*-acetylcysteine in an ovine model. *Ann Emerg Med.* 1991;20:1069-1972.

Smilkstein MJ, Bronstein AC, Linden C, et al. Acetaminophen overdose: a 48-hour intravenous *N*-acetylcysteine treatment protocol. *Ann Emerg Med.* 1991;20:1058-1063.

Smilkstein MJ, Knapp GL, Lulig KW, et al. Efficacy of oral *N*-acetylcysteine in the treatment of acetaminophen overdose. Analysis of the national multicenter study (1976-1985). *N Engl J Med.* 1988;319:1557-1562.

Tenenbein M. Poisoning in pregnancy. In: Koren G, ed. *Maternal-Fetal Toxicology.* 3rd ed. New York, NY: Marcel Dekker; 2001:233-256.

Tixier H, Feyeux , Girod S, et al. Acute voluntary intoxication with selective serotonin reuptake inhibitors during the third trimester of pregnancy: therapeutic management of mother and fetus. *Am J Obstet Gynecol.* 2008 Nov; 199(5):9e-12e.

Tran T, Wax JR, Philput C, et al. Intentional iron overdose in pregnancy—management and outcome. *J Emerg Med.* 2000; 18:225-228.

Wallace KL, Curry SC, LoVecchio F, et al. Effect of magnesium hydroxide on iron absorption following simulated mild iron overdose in human subjects. *Acad Emerg Med.* 1998; 5:961-965.

Wolf SJ, Heard K, Sloan EP, Jagoda AS. Clinical policy: critical issues in the management of patients presenting to the emergency department with acetaminophen overdose. *Ann Emerg Med.* Sep 2007;50(3):292-313.

CHAPTER 24

Neonatal Resuscitation: Pathophysiology, Organization, and Survival

• *Keith S. Meredith and Pranav Patel*

Each year, an estimated 19% of the 5 million neonatal deaths that occur worldwide are the result of birth asphyxia. In the United States, approximately 4.25 million children are born annually, with a reported perinatal mortality rate of 6.64 for the year 2008.[1] This suggests that every year, among US children who reach 28 weeks' gestation, over 28,000 die prior to their *seventh day of life*. A significant portion of those infants who succumb do so from birth asphyxia. Further, among children reaching term gestation, 2 to 3 per 1000 live term births suffer hypoxic ischemic encephalopathy (HIE), (0.3 per 1000 severe HIE). (Table 24-1) Up to 80% of infants who survive severe hypoxic-ischemic encephalopathy develop serious complications and 10%-20% develop moderately serious disabilities. In addition, it is widely accepted that 10% of all newborns require some assistance to begin and maintain normal breathing and that 1% require aggressive resuscitation. Thus, using the national birth rate data, annually 400,000 newborns need some help during the perinatal period, 40,000 per year require expert assistance to reverse profound cardiorespiratory depression, and 1200 per year develop severe HIE. Although there is some evidence that therapeutic hypothermia is beneficial to term newborns with moderate to severe hypoxic ischemic encephalopathy, and that cooling decreases death without increasing major disability in survivors, this therapy is not available at all centers yet as further research is being compiled. (Table 24-2).

Since, for those caring for mothers and their babies, the goal for each pregnancy is to optimize short-term and long-term outcome of both patients, steady increase in rate of late preterm births (34-36 weeks' gestational age [GA]) has also become concerning because current data clearly point out that late preterm infants are not only likely to have much higher rate of immediate morbidity and mortality but they are also at a higher risk for developmental delay and school-related problems compared to full-term infants. There is also an escalating concern that some late preterm births occur not for medical but logistic reasons and it must be acknowledged that if not for medical reasons, it is much more beneficial for elective deliveries to occur at full term.

You need only to relate previously listed statistics to your own practice to appreciate the frequency with which you may encounter an infant in need of neonatal resuscitation and at risk for long-term neurodevelopmental sequelae. Unfortunately, despite best efforts by care providers, this goal is often challenged by the expected, or, even more challenging, unexpected delivery of a neonate who requires urgent medical attention for a disorder(s) threatening his/her life. Obstetrical providers are, by training and experience, more skilled in adult than neonatal emergency care. As a consequence, without standards in place that direct personnel, training, and equipment, an obstetrical practitioner may find himself/herself ill prepared to effectively respond to a neonatal emergency. The objective of this chapter is to offer an overview of the pathophysiology, organization, and provision of emergency medical care to the newly born patient for the obstetrical primary care provider.

■ **TABLE 24-1. ACOG and American Academy of Pediatrics (AAP) Task Force on Neonatal Encephalopathy and Cerebral Palsy**

Part 1 Four essential criteria (all four must be met)
- Evidence of metabolic acidosis in fetal umbilical cord arterial blood obtained at delivery (pH<7 and base deficit of ≥12 mmol/L)
- Early onset of severe or moderate neonatal encephalopathy in infants born at 34 or more weeks of gestation
- Cerebral palsy of the spastic quadriplegic or dyskinetic type
- Exclusion of other identifiable etiologies, such as trauma, coagulation disorders, infectious conditions, or genetic disorders

Part 2 Criteria that may suggest intrapartum timing, but nonspecific for an asphyxial insult
- A sentinel (signal) hypoxic event occurring immediately before or during labor. A serious pathologic event has to occur for a neurologically intact fetus to sustain a neurologically damaging acute insult
- A sudden and sustained fetal bradycardia or the absence of fetal heart rate variability in the presence of persistent late or persistent variable decelerations, usually after a hypoxic sentinel event when the pattern was previously normal
- Apgar scores of 0 to 3 beyond 5 min
- Onset of multisystem involvement within 72 h of birth
- Early imaging study showing evidence of acute nonfocal cerebral abnormality

Source: http://www.acog.org/from_home/Misc/neonatalEncephalopathy.cfm?printerFriendly=yes.

■ **TABLE 24-2. Criteria for Hypothermia Therapy**

Infant born ≥ 36 weeks' gestation and <6 h
- One or more of the following
  - Apgar score of 5 or less at 10 min
  - Continued need for resuscitation at 10 min after birth
  - Severe acidosis:
    - pH level of <7 or base deficit of ≥16 mmol/L from cord blood gas or patient gas obtained within first hour

- Evidence of moderate to severe encephalopathy at birth
  - Clinically determined by one or more of the following
    - Lethargy, stupor, or coma
    - Abnormal tone or posture
    - Abnormal reflexes (suck, grasp, Moro, gag, stretch reflexes)
    - Decrease or absent spontaneous activity
    - Autonomic dysfunction (including bradycardia, abnormal pupils, apneas)
    - Clinical evidence of seizures
    - Moderately or severely abnormal aEEG background or seizures

This chapter is not meant to replace the information found in references such as the *Textbook of Neonatal Resuscitation*. Instead, the reader will be guided through an approach of creating an environment conducive to facilitating optimal neonatal emergency care. This will include a brief discussion of the pathophysiology of brain injury, a description of the organization of neonatal resuscitation teams and equipment, and a review of resuscitation guidelines. Readers interested in more detail will find additional resources in the selected list of suggested readings. All obstetrical clinicians will find completing Neonatal Resuscitation Program (NRP) certification useful and are encouraged to do so.

■ PATHOPHYSIOLOGY OF HYPOXIC ISCHEMIC ENCEPHALOPATHY

The onset of an aberration in fetal well-being marked by concerning changes in vital signs, like fetal heart rate, is a common herald of a potentially deteriorating fetus. Clinicians respond to this with measures designed to improve oxygen and energy substrate (glucose) delivery to the fetus. Ominous changes in fetal heart rate and the clinician's response to it highlight, in great measure, one of the most concerning disturbances in homeostasis occurring to the unborn child—ischemia and hypoxemia. The result of worsening oxygen and energy delivery to the fetus is the onset of a series of changes in fetal status that must be reversed to avoid an untoward neurodevelopmental outcome. The scope of this chapter is not intended to cover prepartum management, but the same sequence of events can continue into the immediate postpartum period prompting the need for infant management. A brief review of the fetal response to hypoxia is useful (Fig 24-1).

Studies in newly born animals describe the importance of both low oxygen states and decreased cerebral flow in the development of perinatal depression and, if uninhibited, HIE. The addition of absent breathing and resulting respiratory acidosis common to clinical events distinguishes the human experience from animal research. However, from limited studies in nonhuman primates, we know that complete asphyxia results in a series of fetal responses. Initially, there is an increase in muscular activity with tachypnea followed by a period of muscular quiet and apnea (primary apnea). The apnea lasts for about 1 minute, is followed by a few minutes of gasping respirations, and simple stimulation of the baby is usually adequate to restore normal breathing. During this time the

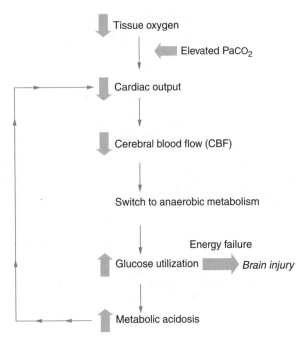

FIGURE 24-1. Schematic, relative to time, of physiological events resulting in neonatal birth depression and leading to brain injury.

fetal heart rate is less than the allowed threshold, 100 beats per minute (bpm). After 4 to 5 minutes without resolution, secondary apnea with progressive fetal bradycardia occurs. This is unresponsive to simple stimulation. Fetal arterial blood pressure, and as a consequence, cardiac output and cerebral blood flow have also been decreasing coincident with the lowered heart rate (Fig 24-1).

As tissues receive less and less oxygen from the combination of low fetal oxygen content and decreased cardiac output (low heart rate not compensated for by an increase in stroke volume), glycolytic pathways switch from aerobic to anaerobic. This results in increasing metabolic acidosis followed by primary energy failure from inefficient glucose utilization (recall that under aerobic conditions a unit of glucose produces 16 times more high-energy phosphate ATP than under anaerobic conditions). This further inhibits the effectiveness of myocardial contractility and a positive feedback loop develops with disastrous consequences (Fig 24-2). As this sequence of events continues, the fetus or newborn infant develops a deepening derangement in vital functions and the opportunities for recovery

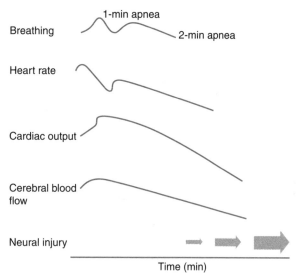

FIGURE 24-2. Pathophysiological events leading to brain injury and positive feedback loop.

without sequelae rapidly diminish. The key ingredients to this are depression of fetal oxygenation, impaired cardiac output, altered central nervous system and myocardial energy stores, and neural cell death. Resuscitative efforts designed to mitigate this process as it develops are discussed in Resuscitation section. The essentials needed to develop and implement the resource capabilities required to assure state-of-the-art neonatal resuscitation are shown in Table 24-3, and will form the blueprint for the remainder of this discussion.

■ TABLE 24-3. Organization of Neonatal Resuscitation

Identification of peripartum risk factors for fetal/ neonatal depression
- Antepartum
- Intrapartum

Personnel
- Team identification
- Team training
- Intra-team communication

Equipment
- Inventory
- Maintenance

■ ORGANIZATION

Identification of Peripartum Risk Factors

Anticipating the specific clinical circumstances leading to the need for neonatal resuscitation in the delivery room is very helpful. Not enough can be said for the value of time to prepare for a sick newborn. In addition, while the basics of resuscitation do not vary from one patient to the next, certain clinical situations will require the resuscitation team to be prepared to provide specific medical care beyond the usual. For example, the needs of an uncomplicated 28-week premature infant delivered for worsening maternal preeclampsia will be quite different from a term infant with particulate meconium stained amniotic fluid, or a 36-week-old child with nonimmune hydrops fetalis. Table 24-4 shows many of the more common ante- and intrapartum conditions likely to result in the initiation of neonatal resuscitation. Some of the additional requirements of children presenting under these circumstances are shown in Tables 24-5 and 24-6. An unusual example of this is the EXIT procedure (ex utero intrapartum treatment). This operating room procedure is used when a prenatal diagnosis is made of a fetus with airway anatomy likely to make endotracheal tube intubation difficult. The delivered infant's umbilical cord blood flow is not interrupted until airway access is secured. This allows the intubation to proceed without immediate concern for asphyxia. In addition, if a tracheotomy is anticipated, the provision of anesthetic to the maternal circulation can provide the fetus with pain relief adequate for the procedure to be performed. Thus, advance preparation will optimize even the most complex and dire delivery room events.

Team Identification

In order to function properly, each member of the resuscitation team (and back up members in the event of simultaneous resuscitations, eg, multiple gestation) should be identified for each shift. All team members should respond to high-risk deliveries and to urgent calls from the delivery room. In addition, it is standard of care for the team to attend all cesarean deliveries. A recommended team composition and delineation of responsibilities are listed in Table 24-7. Note the considerable overlap of duties. The nature of a neonatal delivery room emergency requires that all team members are capable of performing multiple tasks, as the circumstance requires. Indeed, a child who needs a thoracentesis for a spontaneous pneumothorax or

■ **TABLE 24-4. Clinical Conditions Commonly Leading to Neonatal Resuscitation**

Antepartum	Intrapartum
Maternal conditions	**Maternal conditions**
Age <16 y or >35 y	Vaginal breech
Substance abuse (recreational or prescribed)[a]	Vacuum extraction
Chronic illness	Forceps delivery
Endocrine[a]	Prolonged rupture of membranes
Cardiac	Chorioamnionitis
Autoimmune[a]	Medications
Pulmonary	Anesthesia/analgesia[a]
Renal	Placenta previa[a]
Central nervous system	Abruptio placentae[a]
Oligohydramnios[a]	Vasa previa[a]
Polyhydramnios[a]	Umbilical cord prolapse
Premature rupture of membranes	Meconium stained amniotic fluid[a]
Multiple gestation	**Neonatal conditions**
Medications	Preterm birth
β-blockers[a]	Nonreassuring fetal heart rate pattern
Magnesium sulfate[a]	Congenital diaphragmatic hernia[a]
Anesthesia/analgesia[a]	Esophageal atresia[a]
Diabetes	Omphalocele/gastroschisis[a]
No prenatal care[a]	Congenital hydrops fetalis[a]
Fetal conditions	Suspected airway compromise[a]
Decreased fetal movement	Campomelic dysplasia
Fetal malformation[a]	Severe micrognathia
Anemia	
Isoimmunization	
Infection	
Intrauterine growth retardation	
Macrosomia	

[a]Conditions which usually require additional peripartum neonatal management measures (see Table 24-5).

large pleural effusion will need the most skilled practitioner to perform this procedure. Usually, this clinician is the one managing the airway. He/she will have to relinquish that responsibility to another to be free to emergently evacuate the chest of air or fluid. Team flexibility is a requirement rather than a luxury.

Team Training

In addition to completing and maintaining NRP certification, each team member should be responsible for participating in periodic *mock codes*. These training exercises are extremely valuable for evaluating the team member knowledge of resuscitation procedures, adequacy of communication systems and response times, and for identifying general logistical problems unique to each institution (reliability of elevators, distance to operating rooms and delivery rooms, location of personnel and adequacy of equipment, etc). After each mock and real code, a debriefing to evaluate team performance is strongly recommended. This activity creates the methodology to systematically identify and correct deficiencies noted during the code.

Communication

Critical to successfully completing a neonatal resuscitation is getting the resuscitation team to the delivery. This may seem a trite comment to make, and, therefore, one not worth making. However, once the delivering department

■ **TABLE 24-5. Maternal Conditions Requiring Additional Neonatal Resuscitative Measures**

Maternal conditions	Neonatal issues
Substance abuse	Avoid naloxone
Endocrine	
Graves disease	Thyrotoxicosis: propranolol, PTU
Diabetes	Hypoglycemia: glucose, glucagon
Autoimmune (systemic lupus erythematosus)	Neonatal third-degree heart block: pace maker
Multiple gestation	More babies than resuscitators
Oligohydramnios	Airway obstruction: tracheal suction
Polyhydramnios	Presence of anomalies: anomaly specific
Medications	
β-blockers	Hypoglycemia: glucose
Magnesium sulfate	Respiratory depression/hypotonia
Anesthesia/analgesia	Respiratory depression/drug specific
No prenatal care	Hepatitis B or C exposure, etc
Placental abnormality (previa, abruption, vasa previa)	Hypovolemia: volume replacement
Meconium stained amniotic fluid	Meconium aspiration syndrome: selective tracheal suctioning, management of syndrome

of a hospital comes to rely upon a designated team of individuals to provide a service, no one else is likely to provide it. A simple and effective communication means becomes the backbone of the team's function, notifying members

■ **TABLE 24-6. Fetal Conditions Requiring Additional Neonatal Resuscitative Measures**

Fetal conditions	Neonatal management or problem
Congenital diaphragmatic hernia	Lung hypoplasia, bowel in thorax: orogastric tube placement
Esophageal atresia	Excessive oral secretions: secretion drainage
Omphalocele/ gastroschisis	Heat/fluid loss: sterile moist inclusive cover, avoid vascular compromise to gut
Congenital hydrops fetalis	Large pleural, pericardial, peritoneal effusions: emergent fluid drainage
Suspected airway compromise	Difficult endotracheal intubation: EXIT procedure, ENT or pediatric surgery

of the timing and location of the anticipated need. This is accomplished by facilities in many ways.

Some utilize broadcast paging. This method allows multiple so-called *code pagers* to be accessed with a single pager number entry. This minimizes the time required for contacting multiple parties but is vulnerable to pager battery life and black out areas. Others employ overhead paging that disturbs uninvolved patients and staff, is vulnerable to ambient noise interference and areas not served with speakers, and can be confusing. Many institutions use both of the above. Recent technological communication advances have increasingly permitted direct voice communication between staff members. This is accomplished both by localized FM transmitted telephone communications (zone phones), direct voice-to-voice technologies (modified walkie-talkies), or by digital cellular telephones with web-based direct connection to on-call clinicians. The latter permits user to call one telephone number and access the communication device of the clinician(s) on call using a web-based system that also permits the entry of backup providers. While dependent upon battery life and signal adequacy, direct voice-to-voice communication allows clinicians to share critical case-specific information while simultaneously proceeding to the location required (ie, time waiting for someone to return their page is mitigated).

TABLE 24-7. Resuscitation Team Composition and Duties (Suggested)	
Team member	**Responsibility**
Neonatologist Pediatrician Neonatal nurse practitioner	• Obtain perinatal history • Lead resuscitation • Endotracheal intubation • Manage airway (bagging, suctioning, etc) • Order/administer medications • Perform chest compressions • Obtain vascular access
Neonatal nurse	• Evaluate neonatal heart rate: air entry
Obstetrical nurse	• Documentation • Administer medications • Apply patient identification • Perform chest compressions • Obtain intravenous access • Apply monitoring equipment • Endotracheal intubation
Respiratory care practitioner	
Additional personnel	• Manage airway (bagging, suctioning, etc) • Evaluate air entry: heart rate • Administer surfactant replacement • Perform chest compressions • Documentation • Apply patient identification • Apply monitoring equipment

■ TABLE 24-8. Equipment and Supplies for Neonatal Resuscitation

Suction equipment
Bulb suction syringe
DeLee mucous trap with No. 10 French catheter
Wall or mechanical suction
Suction catheters, No. 5, 8, 10 French

Bag and mask ventilation equipment
Infant resuscitation bag with pressure gauge/ release valve
Face masks, newborn and premature sizes (cushioned rim preferred)
Oral airways, newborn and premature sizes
Oxygen with flow meter and tubing
Air-oxygen blender
Stethoscope

Intubation equipment
Laryngoscope and straight blades, No. 0 (premature) and No. 1 (term)
Extra light bulbs (unless fiberoptic) and batteries
Endotracheal tubes, sizes 2.5, 3.0, 3.5, 4.0 mm I.D.
Stylet (optional)
Scissors, skin barrier, and adhesive tape
Gloves
Pedi-Cap/CO_2 detector

Vascular access equipment
Umbilical vessel catheters, 3.5 and 5.0 Fr.
Umbilical vessel catheterization kit
24- and 26-gauge peripheral intravenous catheters

Thoracentesis equipment
18- and 20-gauge intravenous catheters
20- and 30-mL syringes
Three-way stopcock

Once alerted, the team should be familiarized with the details of the case to allow them to adequately prepare for any needs particular to each circumstance (Tables 24-5 and 24-6). Again, adequate preparation should not be undervalued.

■ EQUIPMENT

Inventory and Maintenance

A list of standard equipments needed for neonatal resuscitation is presented in Table 24-8. Medications for resuscitation and their doses and indications are listed in Table 24-9. These items should be placed in the same order and in the same place at all resuscitation stations. The identification of individuals responsible for ensuring that each equipment and medication store is adequately stocked is critical. Confirmation of adequate supplies should be accomplished in each shift and after each resuscitation. Documentation of this confirmation is strongly encouraged. Inadequate supplies noted during a resuscitation are inexcusable.

■ RESUSCITATION

Since the preparation has been accomplished and the clinician is now armed with a fundamental understanding of the pathophysiology of perinatal asphyxia and has advanced warning about the clinical scenario of each case, he/she is prepared to provide emergency care to a recently delivered depressed newborn. Figure 24-3 depicts the

■ TABLE 24-9. Medications for Neonatal Resuscitation

Medication	How supplied	Dose and indication
Epinephrine	1:10,000; 3- or 10-mL ampules	0.1-0.3 mL/kg, IV or IT: bradycardia not responsive to stimulation or adequate ventilation
Normal saline	250-mL bag	10 mL/kg IV: push or over 10-30 min if hypovolemia suspected
Ringer lactate		
Sodium bicarbonate	4.2% (0.5 mEq/mL); 10-mL ampule	1-3 mEq/kg: after adequate ventilation established, if persistently poor perfusion noted and hypovolemia not suspected
Dextrose	10% 250-mL bag	2 mL/kg: once resuscitation completed and poor perfusion persists (not responsive to other measures)
Naloxone HCl (neonatal Narcan)	0.02 mg/mL; 2-mL ampule	0.5 mL/kg: for respiratory depression with known recent maternal narcotic treatment[a]

[a]Do not use in newborns whose mother has known narcotic addiction.

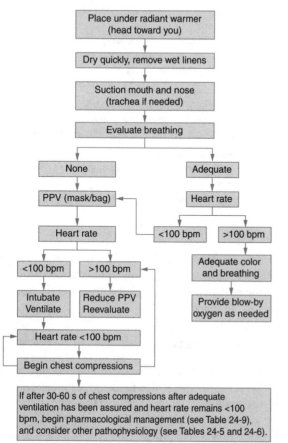

FIGURE 24-3. Algorithm for neonatal resuscitation.

general considerations of performing essential tasks. It is imperative not to underestimate the importance of a patent airway and adequate gas exchange. The overwhelming proportion of newborns requiring the institution of life-sustaining support in the delivery room will respond to proper oxygenation and ventilation alone. No amount of external cardiac compressions or intravenous/intratracheal epinephrine will adequately restore the heart rate and perfusion if appropriate gas exchange cannot be achieved. Medications for resuscitation and their doses and indications are shown in Table 24-9. The interested reader is again encouraged to complete NRP certification.

■ SURVIVAL

Tables 24-10 and 24-11 show survival and outcome data for in excess of 56,000 infants born recently in the United States. The first of the two tables (Table 24-10) shows pure survival by both birth weight and estimated gestational age (EGA). The second (Table 24-11) demonstrates survival without two significant disorders that are predictive of impaired long-term neurological development (severe intraventricular hemorrhage and retinopathy of prematurity). This format is particularly useful to the obstetrical clinician since at the bedside, gestational age is more often used to discuss pregnancy status than is birth weight. If both birth weight and gestational age are known, then the

■ TABLE 24-10. Survival without Severe IVH or ROP, by Estimated Gestational Age and Birth Weight[a]

Birth weight (gm)	Estimated Gestational Age (weeks)														Total
	23	24	25	26	27	28	29	30	31	32	33	34	35	36	
250 to 500	46	138	295	233											168
501 to 750	212	361	508	591	711	771	822								469
751 to 1000		473	595	728	836	898	912	974	987	1000					786
1001 to 1250				788	848	934	948	972	970	971	1000	932			932
1251 to 1500					825	926	953	971	980	988	991	992	991	1000	972
1501 to 1750						957	965	966	986	991	994	999	998	995	989
1751 to 2000								981	979	993	995	997	998	993	994
2001 to 2250								1000	994	994	997	998	999	994	997
2251 to 2500									962	1000	997	998	1000	999	999
2501 to 2750										949	997	998	1000	999	999
2751 to 3000											1000	1000	999	997	998
3001 to 3250											1000	1000	1000	993	995
3251 to 3500												980	1000	1000	997
3501 to 3750												1000	989	996	994
3751 to 4000													1000	984	990
4001 to 4250														1000	1000
4251 to 4500														1000	1000
4501 to 4750															1000
4751 to 5000															1000
GT5															1000
Total	177	362	540	688	819	911	943	971	981	991	996	997	999	997	955

[a]The outcomes of 56,701 non-anomalous neonates born at, cared for in, and discharged from 234 hospitals in 28 states from 2005 to 2006. Minimum cell sample size was 20 patients. Data presented as survival per 1000 discharged patients. These numbers represent an estimate. The likelihood of a good outcome is influenced by many variables, only two of which are estimated gestational age and birth weight.

Source: Pediatrix-Obstetrix Outcomes Data: Survival without severe IVH or ROP by estimated gestational age (EGA) and birth weight. NATAL U Clinical Research Center (http://www.natalu.com/clinical_research_center.asp?log=1) 2008, Pediatrix Medical Group, Inc. Used with permission.

TABLE 24-11. Survival by Gestational Age and Birth Weight[a]

Birth weight (gm)	Estimated Gestational Age (weeks)														Total
	23	24	25	26	27	28	29	30	31	32	33	34	35	36	Total
250 to 500	138	288	477	300											293
501 to 750	374	572	721	743	855	865	889								648
751 to 1000		651	811	863	910	945	967	987	987	1000					888
1001 to 1250				894	936	961	973	985	985	975	1000	955			965
1251 to 1500					860	966	976	983	997	991	993	992	991	1000	985
1501 to 1750						957	977	982	992	994	997	1000	998	1000	993
1751 to 2000								994	990	996	997	998	999	996	996
2001 to 2250								1000	994	996	998	999	999	994	998
2251 to 2500										1000	999	999	1000	1000	999
2501 to 2750									962	949	997	999	1000	999	999
2751 to 3000											1000	1000	999	999	999
3001 to 3250											1000	1000	1000	994	996
3251 to 3500												989	1000	1000	997
3501 to 3750												1000	989	996	994
3751 to 4000													1000	984	990
4001 to 4250														1000	1000
4251 to 4500														1000	1000
4501 to 4750															1000
4751 to 5000															1000
GT5															1000
Total	324	561	751	821	908	949	970	984	991	993	997	998	999	998	972

[a]The outcomes of 56,701 non-anomalous neonates born at, cared for in, and discharged from 234 hospitals in 28 states from 2005 to 2006. Minimum cell sample size was 20 patients. Data presented as survival per 1000 discharged patients. These numbers represent an estimate. The likelihood of a good outcome is influenced by many variables, only two of which are estimated gestational age and birth weight.

Source: Pediatrix-Obstetrix Outcomes Data: Survival without severe IVH or ROP by estimated gestational age (EGA) and birth weight. NATAL U Clinical Research Center (http://www.natalu.com/clinical_research_center.asp?log=1) 2008, Pediatrix Medical Group, Inc. Used with permission.

tables are especially valuable. The obvious advantages of reaching birth weight higher than 1000 g and EGA of 29 weeks and more is evident. At these levels, good survival exceeds 90%. Intentional resuscitation of infants of less than 24 weeks' gestation remains the subject of significant controversy. Families considering this option should be heavily counseled about the poor survival rates of infants born at less than 24 weeks' gestation and the poor long-term neurodevelopmental outcome of those that do survive.

■ SUMMARY

The most important resuscitation elements are understanding the capabilities and limitations of the facility, followed by temperature support, the provision of adequate ventilation and oxygenation, and reestablishing cardiovascular stability. Once these important technical aspects of perinatal resuscitation are understood and the organization and management of obstetrical and pediatric emergency services are in place, what remains are the ethical and legal concerns regarding the provision of life-sustaining support. The obstetrical provider is encouraged to seek out additional information regarding national- and institution-specific survival and morbidity data and state-specific statutes that govern perinatal care.

REFERENCE

1. National Vital Statistics Report. 57(19):1-6. (http://www.cdc.gov/nchs/data/nvsr/nvsr57/nvsr57_19.pdf), July 29, 2009.

SUGGESTED READING

American Heart Association/American Academy of Pediatrics. *Textbook of Neonatal Resuscitation.* 4th ed. Dallas, TX: American Heart Association National Center; 2000.

MacDorman MF, Minino AM, Strobino DM, Guyer B. Annual summary of vital statistics—2001. *Pediatrics.* 2002;110:1037.

Mychaliska GB, Bealer JF, Graf JL, et al. Operating on placental support: the ex utero intrapartum treatment procedure. *J Pediatr Surg.* 1997;32:227.

Thacker SB, Stroup DF, Peterson HB. Efficacy and safety of intrapartum electronic fetal monitoring: an update. *Obstet Gynecol.* 1995;86:613.

World Health Report. Geneva, Switzerland: World Health Organization, 1995.

CHAPTER 25

Fluid and Electrolyte Therapy in the Critically Ill Obstetric Patient

• *Cornelia R. Graves*

The ultimate goal of fluid and electrolyte therapy is to maintain a balance between the intracellular and extracellular compartments. This, easier said than done, means that fluid replacement and electrolyte balance become an afterthought of therapy instead of a goal. Many disease states in pregnancy can change the intracellular and extracellular compartments. Preeclampsia is a prime example of how changes in the dynamics of the intracellular and extra cellular compartments can affect overall fluid physiology. Common therapies used during pregnancy such as terbutaline or magnesium can change electrolyte balance. The purpose of this chapter is to explain basic fluid and electrolyte balance and to provide guidelines for initiating the therapy.

■ FLUID COMPARTMENTS

The human body is composed mostly of water. Approximately, 50% of total body weight in an average female is body water. [TBW (total body water) = 1/2 wt (kg)]. Given that, total blood volume increases by 50% during pregnancy with only 20% of that increase attributed to an increase in red cell mass, one can extrapolate that 60% to 65% of the total body weight in pregnancy can be attributed to TBW. The intracellular fluid compartment (ICF) contains 66% of TBW. The extracellular compartment is composed of 34% TBW. The extracellular fluid compartment (ECF) is composed of both intravascular and the interstitial components. Most of the extracellular fluid compartment is interstitial (26%), plasma composes

8% (Fig 25-1). Other examples of ECF include cerebrospinal fluid, synovial fluid, and secretions from the gastrointestinal tract. The fluid compartments are separated by semipermeable membranes. Water and smaller molecules may pass through the membranes; larger colloid substances and proteins are confined to the intravascular space. Hydrostatic pressure assists in maintaining an overall fluid balance as water moves by osmosis, from the area with the lowest concentration of plasma proteins (interstitial compartment) to the area with the highest concentration of plasma proteins (blood).

■ OSMOTIC ACTIVITY

Osmotic activity is the expression of the concentration of solute or the density of solute particles in a fluid. In the ECF, osmotic activity can be defined as the sum of the individual osmotic activities of each solute in the fluid. Plasma osmolality can be calculated using the following formula:

$$2\times[Na]+\frac{glucose}{18}+\frac{BUN}{28}$$

Colloid osmotic pressure (COP) is produced by serum albumin (60%-80%) with fibrinogen and the globulins accounting for the remainder. Normal COP is decreased in pregnancy. While COP can be measured with electronic equipment, the equation in Table 25-1 below can estimate COP by using total protein (TP) in g/dL (Table 25-1).

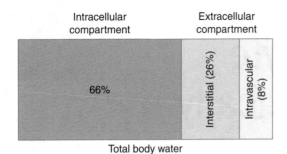

FIGURE 25-1. A breakdown of the human body fluid compartments.

■ TABLE 25-2. Signs of Hypovolemia	
Clinical	**Laboratory**
Pulse: weak, thready, and >120 bpm	Urine specific gravity >1.025
Orthostatic vital signs	Hemoconcentration
Dry mucous membranes	Urine Na >10 mEq/L
Poor skin turgor	BUN/creatinine >20
Prolonged capillary refill	

■ TABLE 25-1. Colloid Osmotic Pressure[a]		
	Normal pregnant (mm Hg)	**Preeclampsia (mm Hg)**
Antepartum COP	22	18
Postpartum COP	17	14

[a]Calculation of COP: COP = 2.1 (TP) + 0.16 (TP^2) + 0.009 (TP^3) mm Hg. Nonpregnant COP: 25-28 mm Hg.

■ TABLE 25-3. The Effect of Volume Replacement on Ventricular Filling Pressures
Measure hemodynamic parameters
Fluid bolus of 200-500 mL of isotonic fluid
Measure PAOP 30 min after fluid challenge
PAOP increase >7 mm Hg → no more fluid
PAOP increase 2-7 mm Hg (over baseline) → wait 10 min
If PAOP still >3 mm Hg → stop
If PAOP ≤3 mm Hg → continue fluid administration

■ EVALUATION OF VOLUME STATUS

In the obstetrical patient, depletion of intravascular volume can occur in two ways: overall fluid loss, eg, vomiting, diarrhea, perspiration, or by shifting of the intravascular volume to the interstitial space. Overall fluid loss may be manifested by a clinical examination that reveals orthostasis, poor skin turgor, dry mucous membranes, and a thready pulse. These clinical findings respond to rehydration (Table 25-2).

Shifting of intravascular fluid occurs in disease states such as preeclampsia. Evaluation of volume status in this subset of patients may be much more difficult. In critically ill patients, the evaluation of volume status can be obtained by the judicious use of central pressure catheters (Table 25-3). The central venous pressure (CVP) may be used to evaluate long-term trends in fluid status; however, in patients with cardiac disease or preeclampsia, the CVP may not reflect left ventricular filling. For acute management of the disease states previously mentioned, a pulmonary artery catheter can be more useful in guiding

therapy. The left ventricular end-diastolic pressure is best reflected by the pulmonary artery occlusion (wedge) pressure (PAOP). Numerous formulas have been used to evaluate the effect of volume replacement on ventricular filling pressures; we present the 7-3 rule as a handy guideline (Table 25-3).

■ INTRAVENOUS FLUID THERAPY

The majority of intravenous fluid therapy is directed at expanding the plasma component of the ECF. Some of the most common questions asked are: which fluid should I use, how much should I use, and when should I use it? The goal of this section is to review the pharmacology of the available colloid and crystalloid therapies and discuss their pros and cons.

Crystalloids

As sodium is the major cation and determinant of osmotic pressure in the ECF, it is not surprising that most crystalloid preparations contain mixtures of sodium chloride and other physiologically active solutes. As crystalloid fluids are designed to expand the interstitial space, only about 20% remain in the vascular space. Indications for the use of crystalloid include extracellular losses, as in dehydration, acute hemorrhage, and acute volume replacement.

Normal saline, 0.9%, is isotonic to normal body fluid, and, therefore, does not alter osmotic movement of water across the cell membrane. It is the most common fluid used for acute volume expansion. There are variations of this fluid such as one-half normal saline, 0.45%; however, these hypotonic fluids have no place in acute volume expansion. Infusing normal saline may produce a hyperchloremic metabolic acidosis; however, this occurrence is rare.

Ringer lactate is an isotonic fluid that may be used interchangeably with normal saline in the treatment of hypovolemia or shock. Ringer lactate is a balanced electrolyte solution that substitutes potassium and calcium for some of the sodium. Lactate is added as a buffer. The concern that acidosis may be worsened by the installation of Ringer lactate during shock is unfounded; however, it is recommended that extreme caution should be taken while using the fluid in patients with diabetes or renal failure.

Hypertonic sodium-containing solutions (600-2400 mOsm/L) may be used in patients in whom a large volume load is contraindicated. Some studies have noted that the infusion of a hypertonic solution may reduce interstitial edema as well as create a positive inotropic effect. Care should be taken to use a slow infusion rate and to monitor sodium regularly to avoid hypernatremia.

Plasmalyte is a highly buffered fluid that has a pH equivalent to plasma. Although theoretically its adjusted pH may be preferential to saline or Ringer lactate, there are no definitive studies that show a great difference in its effects on vascular volume.

Dextrose-Containing Solutions

Dextrose, 5% in water, is isotonic; but unlike normal saline, it penetrates the cell leaving behind the infused water. It provides a carbohydrate source during brief periods of fasting. One liter of a 5% solution contains approximately 170 kcal and a 10% solution contains 340 kcal. When dextrose is added to normal saline or to Ringer lactate, it raises the osmolality of the fluid to roughly twice that of plasma. This can promote significant changes in serum osmolality when large volumes of fluid are infused.

Colloid

Colloids are large molecular weight substances that do not pass readily across capillary walls. The rationale for the use of colloids is to expand the vascular volume and to decrease the amount of fluid that leaves the intravascular space A recent review in the Cochrane database does not support the routine use of colloid for volume resuscitation.

Human Serum Albumin

Albumin, which is synthesized in the liver, is the major oncotic protein of plasma. Responsible for about 80% of the colloid osmotic pressure of plasma, it also serves as the major transport protein for drugs and ions. The preparation is available as 5% (50 g/L) and 25% solution (250 g/L) in isotonic saline. The 5% solution has a colloid osmotic pressure (COP) of 20 mm Hg, which is equivalent to plasma (COP); the 25% solution has a COP of 70 mm Hg. An infusion of 100 mL of 25% albumin will expand the plasma volume to about 500 mL. The effect of the albumin infusion persists for 24 to 36 hours. Contrary to popular belief, albumin will eventually pass into the interstitial space. This may produce delayed pulmonary edema in patients at risk. Caution should also be exercised when using large volumes since dilutional coagulopathy can occur.

Hydroxyethyl Starch (Hespan)

Hetastarch is a synthetic colloid that closely resembles glycogen. It was introduced as a less expensive alternative to albumin. A 6% solution has a COP of 30 mm Hg, and the acute volume expansion is equivalent to that of albumin. Hetastarch has a longer half-life than albumin with 50% of the osmotic effect persisting for 24 hours. Coagulopathies are less common than albumin. The clinician should be aware that serum amylase may be elevated in patients receiving hetastarch as amylase is used to cleave polymers in order to facilitate renal excretion. This elevation usually persists 3 to 5 days after use.

Dextran

The dextrans are another group of synthetic colloids that are polysaccharides derived from the juice of sugar beets. The available preparations are dextran-40 (mean molecular weight—40,000) and dextran-70 (mean molecular weight—70,000). Dextran-40 is available as a 10% solution with a COP of 40 mm Hg. The acute volume expansion from dextran-40 is about twice the infused volume. However, more than 50% is cleared after 6 hours.

While an effective artificial colloid, significant side effects limit its use. Dextrans may inhibit platelet aggregation, decrease platelet factor 3, and produce an anticoagulation effect. Anaphylactic reactions can occur in up to 1% of patients. Dextrans coat the surface of red blood cells and interfere with the ability to crossmatch blood. Dextran-induced renal failure or an osmotic diuresis may interfere with the overall fluid status (Tables 25-4 and 25-5).

Crystalloid or Colloid

Much debate has raged over the use of cystalloid versus colloid solution. Colloids are much more expensive and associated with an increased risk of side effects. Champions of colloid use maintain that the cost and the side effects are outweighed by the benefit of colloid use. Proponents of crystalloid use point out that the infusion of crystalloid increases intravascular volume and that the shift in interstitial fluid is a result of the underlying pathological process. Pulmonary edema may occur with both types of fluid, although the edema associated with colloid use may be delayed. While judicious use of colloid may be useful in some clinical situations, it is the opinion of the author that crystalloid resuscitation is preferred in the obstetrical population.

■ ELECTROLYTE BALANCE AND ABNORMALITIES

As the major cation of the ECF and the major determinant of osmolality, sodium maintains the concentration and volume of the ECF. Normal sodium ranges from 135 to 145 mg/dL in most laboratories. Sodium maintains irritability and conduction in nerve and muscle tissue and assists in the regulation of acid-base balance. Since most diets have an excess of sodium, the kidney maintains normal levels through excretion of sodium and retention of free water.

Hypernatremia

Hypernatremia is defined as a sodium level greater than 145 mEq/L. It is a relative state of free water deficit and an increase in the solute concentration in all body fluids. The three major hypernatremic states result from loss of water, hypotonic fluid loss, and sodium retention.

Water Loss

Pure water loss usually occurs with increased insensible loss through the skin. Thermal burn injury is associated with the greatest risk of insensible water loss. Diabetes

insipidus, which results in massive amounts of dilute urine output, can be seen in patients with severe preeclampsia. Figure 25-2 offers a simple algorithm for the treatment of hypernatremia due to this cause.

Hypotonic Fluid Loss

Hypotonic fluid loss is the most common cause of hypernatremia. It is usually caused by dehydration due to gastroenteritis or an osmotic diuresis. Signs of ECF depletion may be present. Oliguria will be present unless the osmotic diuresis has been induced. Treatment is outlined in Fig 25-3.

Sodium Retention

Sodium retention is an uncommon phenomenon. It is usually seen only when hypertonic saline- or bicarbonate-containing solutions are being infused.

Hyponatremia

Hyponatremia is defined as a serum sodium level of 135 mEq/L or less. Three major categories of hyponatremia exist: isotonic (pseudohyponatremia), hypertonic, and hypotonic. Severe hyponatremia (less than 120 mEq/L) is a serious life-threatening condition. Mortality rate may exceed 50%; however, rapid correction of sodium may produce central pontine myelinolysis and cerebral edema which can be fatal.

Isotonic

Isotonic hyponatremia is characterized by a low serum sodium level but a normal plasma osmolality. Common causes include hyperproteinemic states and hyperlipidemic states. The management requires evaluation and correction of the underlying cause. The following correction factors may be used to assist in correcting the sodium concentration:

$$\text{Plasma triglycerides (g/L)} \times 0.002 = \text{mEq/L decrease in plasma Na}^+$$

$$\text{Plasma [protein] greater than 8 g/dL} \times 0.025 = \text{mEq/L decrease in plasma Na}^+$$

Hypertonic

Hypertonic hyponatremia is diagnosed by a low serum sodium and a plasma osmolality of greater than 290 mOsm/kg H_2O. The most common cause of this disorder is hyperglycemia seen in association with diabetic ketoacidosis

■ TABLE 25-4. Common Intravenous Fluids

Solution	Na$^+$ (mEq/L)	K$^+$ (mEq/L)	Cl$^-$ (mEq/L)	Mg^{2+} (mEq/L)	Ca^{2+} (mEq/L)	Lactate (mEq/L)	Other	Approx pH	Osmolality (mOsm/kg)
0.9 NaCl	154		154					4.2	308
Lactated Ringer	130	4.0	109		3.0	28		6.5	273
Hypertonic saline									
3%	513		513					5.0	
5%	855		855					5.6	
Plasmalyte	140	5.0	98	3.0			Acetate (27 mEq/L) Gluconate (23 mEq/L)	7.4	295
D$_5$W							Dextrose (5 g/dL)	5.0	278
Albumin 5%	145		145						
Hespan	154		154				Hetastarch (6 g/L)	5.5	
Dextran-70	154		154						

■ TABLE 25-5. Intravenous Fluids: A Comparison

Solution	Pros	Cons
Isotonic saline	Slightly hypertonic to plasma Minimizes fluid shifts	May produce hyperchloremic metabolic acidosis
Lactate Ringer	Relatively isotonic to plasma	Use with caution in patients with renal or adrenal disease. May interact with drugs due to calcium binding
Hypertonic saline	Less volume required May reduce the interstitial edema	May cause hypernatremia Rapid correction of sodium may increase risks of cerebra edema.
Plasmalyte	Isotonic to plasma	Theoretically, magnesium may interfere with compensatory vasoconstriction.
Dextrose	Provides substrate and caloric intake	Osmotic load Can fuel production of lactic acid especially in the CNS
Albumin	May help maintain colloid osmotic pressure and decrease interstitial edema	Coagulopathy Allergic reactions
Hespan	Equivalent to 5% albumin	Cleared entirely by the kidneys. May increase serum amylase.
Dextran	Volume expansion with small amounts	Reduction of Factor VIII, promotes fibrinolysis, anaphylactic reactions in 1% of pts. May interfere with the ability to crossmatch blood. Can cause acute renal failure.

(see Chap 11). Correction of hyponatremia requires addressing the underlying disorder and replacing the free water deficit (Fig 25-3).

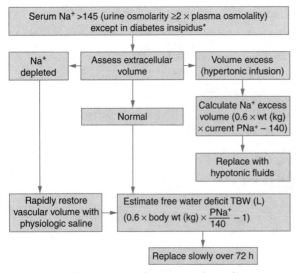

*Management of diabetes insipidus, vasopressin may be necessary 5-10 units aqueous dDAVP, sub q every 4°-6°

FIGURE 25-2. Hypernatremia.

Hypotonic

Hypotonic hyponatremia is characterized by a low serum sodium and plasma osmolality. It can be divided into three subtypes: isovolemic, hypervolemic, and hypovolemic. The clinician should address three major concerns. The patient's neurological status, volume status, and adrenal function.

Isovolemic hyponatremia is characterized by a small gain in free water. This may be related to inappropriate secretion of antidiuretic hormone or in rare instances

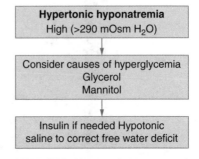

FIGURE 25-3. Hypertonic hyponatremia.

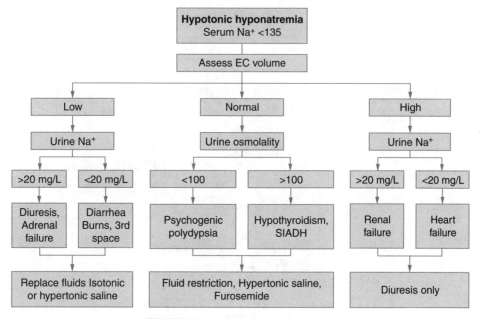

FIGURE 25-4. Hypotonic hyponatremia.

psychogenic polydipsia. Numerous drugs, including oxytocin, have been implicated in this disorder and they are listed as follows:

- Morphine
- Nonsteroidal anti-inflammatory drugs
- Carbamazepine
- Oxytocin

Hypovolemic hyponatremia is characterized by the loss of fluid that is isotonic to plasma combined with volume replacement using a hypotonic fluid. This results in a net sodium loss. The most common causes of this disorder are diuretics, adrenal insufficiency, or diarrhea. A urine sodium can help to identify the etiology (ie, renal or extrarenal) of the hyponatremia.

Hypervolemic hyponatremia occurs in patients in which there is excess water and sodium gain. Edema is common in this population. Causes include heart, renal, and liver failure. The evaluation and management of hypotonic hyponatremia is presented in Fig 25-4.

Potassium

Potassium is the major intracellular cation. The normal plasma potassium concentration is 3.5 to 5.0 mmol/L. Renal excretion is the major route of elimination of dietary or other sources of excess potassium. The clinician should keep in mind that serum potassium may be falsely elevated

in the presence of hemolysis or factitiously decreased when processing of a lab sample is delayed.

Hypokalemia

Hypokalemia is defined as a serum potassium concentration below 3.5 mEq/L. The causes of hypokalemia may be classified as transcellular shift, as in the use of beta agonist (ie, terbutaline), or from depletion. The major causes of the latter are renal loss, most commonly caused by diuretic therapy, or extrarenal, usually seen with excessive diarrhea. A number of drugs listed below are also associated with hypokalemia. Treatment is outlined in Fig 25-5.

- Laxatives
- Gentamycin-cephalexin combo
- Prostaglandin F2 alpha
- Steroids
- Furosemide
- Penicillins
- Lithium
- Beta agonists

Hyperkalemia

Hyperkalemia is defined as a serum potassium above 5.5 mEq/L. It is caused by the release of potassium into the extracelluar fluid such as in myonecrosis, or by reduced renal excretion.

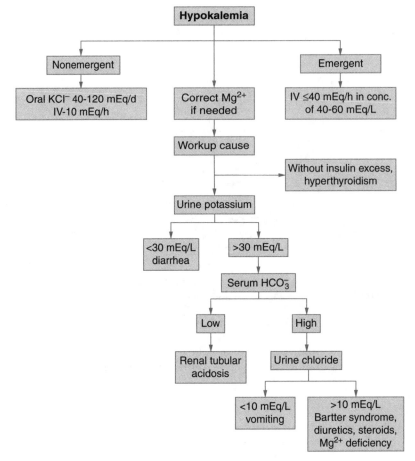

FIGURE 25-5. Hypokalemia.

Hyperkalemia can be associated with fatal cardiac arrythmias; therefore, it should be treated much more aggressively than hypokalemia (Fig 25-6).

Magnesium

Magnesium is not uniformly distributed in the body fluid compartments. Over half of the total body stores are located in the bone and less than 1% are distributed in plasma. This distribution creates a problem in diagnosing disturbances in magnesium balance. Magnesium levels are frequently overlooked in the critically ill patient and are not often replaced. For these reasons, magnesium may be the most common electrolyte abnormality in critically ill patients. In obstetrics, the use of magnesium for tocolysis and for neuroprophylaxis can further complicate the picture. The most common cause of magnesium depletion in our population is the use of diuretics.

The use of amnioglycosides can also lower magnesium levels. Alcoholism is a rare cause of magnesium depletion in obstetrical patients. Low levels of magnesium may potentiate cardiac arrythmias.

Hypermagnesemia is almost always associated with renal insufficiency, with excess magnesium intake, or in cases of diabetic ketoacidosis. Infusion of magnesium in patients with preeclampsia or other diseases that may be associated with renal insufficiency should be done with care. Hypotension can be seen with magnesium levels of 3.0 to 5.0 mEq/L. A level greater than 12 mEq/L can be associated with respiratory depression. Levels greater than 14 mEq/L can be associated with cardiac arrest. Treatment protocols are outlined in Table 25-6.

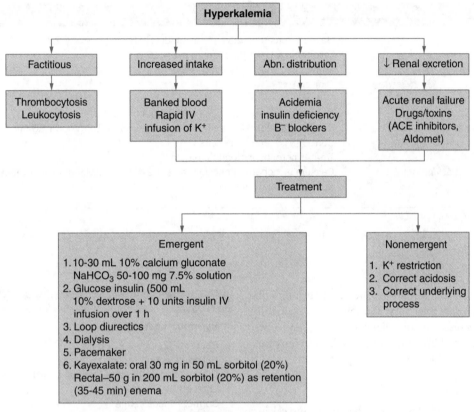

FIGURE 25-6. Hyperkalemia.

<table>
<tr><td colspan="1">

■ **TABLE 25-6.** Magnesium Disorders
</td></tr>
</table>

Hypomagnesemia

Oral magnesium oxide 500-2000 mg/d
$MgSO_4$ 1 mEq/kg for first 24 h; and 0.5 mEq/kg/c over 3 d
Severe, symptomatic[a]
2 g $MgSO_4$ over 1-2 min, follow with 5 g $MgSO_4$ over next 6 h
Continue 5 g $MgSO_4$ every 12 h (continuous infusion) for next 5 d

Hypermagnesemia

Discontinue magnesium infusion
20 mg 10% calcium gluconate over 5-10 min (if symptomatic)[b]
Infusion of D5.45NS with IV furosemide (40-80 mg IV every 1-2 h to enhance excretion)
Consider dialysis

[a]Care should be taken in patients with renal disease.
[b]May substitute calcium chloride.

Calcium and Phosphorus Balance

There are three fractions of calcium in the blood. About 50% of calcium is bound to serum proteins—with albumin accounting for 80% of protein binding. Five to ten percent of calcium is bound to anions like bicarbonate. The remainder of calcium is present as the free or "ionized" form of calcium. The interpretation of calcium levels must be adjusted for change in serum albumin. A correction factor, that increases the total calcium by 0.8 mg/dL for each 1 mg/dL decrease in albumin, should be used. Obtaining an ionized calcium may avoid using the above correction factor; however, changes in pH or other factors may also alter calcium levels.

Hypocalcemia

The most common cause in an acute care setting is magnesium depletion. Other causes such as hypoparathyroidism are usually not a concern in an acute setting. Massive transfusion, panacreatitis, and burns are other causes of decreased calcium level in this patient population.

■ **TABLE 25-7.** Treatment of Calcium Disorders

Hypercalcemia	Saline + forced diuresis (furosemide, 40-80 mg IV every 2 h)
	Calcitonin 4 U/kg IM or sub q every 12 h
	Mithracin 25 µg/kg IV every 2-3 d[a]
	Dialysis
Hypocalemia	
Severe	Calcium gluconate 10 mL of 10% solution over 10 min
Symptomatic	Calcium chloride 10 mL of 10% solution in 50 mL D_5W over 30 min
	Correct Mg^{2+} and K^+ deficits
	Treat hyperphosphatemia if needed
Nonemergent asymptomatic	Calcium gluconate or calcium lactate 2-4 g/d in divided doses every 6 h
	Supplemental vitamin D

[a]Pregnancy category X.

The clinical manifestations include neuromuscular excitability, which may vary, cardiovascular excitability including decreased myocardial contractility, and a prolonged QT interval. Treatment includes the infusion of calcium chloride or gluconate.

Hypercalcemia

Hypercalcemia should be treated when the serum calcium level approaches 13 mg/dL or higher. Causes of hypercalcemia include malignancy and hyper-parathyroidism. Mental status changes are the most common clinical symptoms and warrant immediate therapy. The aim of the therapy is to facilitate the excretion of calcium in the urine (Table 25-7).

Phosphorous

Like magnesium and potassium, phosphorous is predominately an intracellular ion. While phosphorous levels may show diurnal variation, severe hypophosphotemia (serum level below 0.5 mg/dL) is uncommon. The most common causes of hypophosphotemia in the obstetrical population are recovery from diabetic ketoacidosis, aluminum antacid use, or respiratory alkalosis. Phosphate deficiency reduces cardiac contractility, shifts the oxygen dissociation to the left, and may contribute to skeletal muscle weakness. Intravenous replacement is recommended (Table 25-8).

Hyperphosphatemia is seen in the face of renal failure or tissue destruction, such as rhabdomyolysis. Management is directed at correcting the underlying problem. Aluminum-containing antacids may also be administered (Table 25-8).

■ **TABLE 25-8.** Treatment of Phosphate Disorders

Hyperphosphatemia

Restrict PO_4 intake <200 mg/d
Saline infusion
Oral phosphate binders (aluminum hydroxide antacids)
Correct hypocalcemia
Dialysis

Hypophosphatemia

Profound depletion <1 mg/dL
Potassium or sodium phosphate (2.4-5.0 mg/kg/6 h)
Follow serum PO_4^-, Ca^{2+}, Mg^{2+}, K^+ every 12 h

Depletion

Neutra-phos (250 mg/tablet); 2 tablets every 8-12 h
Phospho-soda (129 mg/mL); give 5 mL every 8-12 h

■ SUMMARY

Caring for the critically ill obstetrical patient requires a coordinated effort involving the maternal-fetal medicine specialist, internist, neonatologist, and other members of the critical care team. Meticulous attention to fluid and electrolyte balance will enable the clinician to restore the altered physiology that results from the underlying pathological process.

SUGGESTED READINGS

Berl T, Robertson GL. Pathophysiology of water metabolism. In: Brenner BM, ed. *Brenners and Rectors, The Kidney.* 8th ed. Philadelphia, PA: W.B. Saunders; 2008:866-924.

Achinger SG, Ayus JC. Fluids and electrolytes. In: Civetta JM, Taylor RW, Kirby RR, eds. *Critical Care.* 4th ed. Philadelphia, PA: JB Lippincott; 2008.

Halperin ML, Kamel KS. Potassium. *Lancet.* 1998;352:135.

Miller RD. *Anesthesia.* 6th ed. New York, NY: Churchill Livingston; 2005.

Perel P, Roberts I. Colloids versus crystalloids for the fluid resuscitation in critically ill patients. *ACP J Club.* May 2008.

Verbalis JG. Adaptation to acute and chronic hyponatremia: implications for symptomatology, diagnosis and therapy. *Semin Nephrol.* 1998;18:3.

CHAPTER 26

Human Immunodeficiency Virus in Pregnancy

• *Linda R. Chambliss and Robert A. Myers*

Despite all we have learned about the HIV virus, HIV infection continues to ravage the world, particularly in underdeveloped nations. The United Nations estimates that worldwide over 35 million people are infected with the HIV virus and 16,000 new infections occur each day. In the United States, over 50,000 new infections occur each year. The care of HIV-infected pregnant women is more complex today than ever and pregnant women who are infected with the HIV virus present a challenge to even the most experienced clinician. Drug therapies have increased exponentially since the epidemic was first recognized. Obstetricians caring for HIV-infected women should only manage them in concert with clinicians who are fluent with current recommendation regarding drug therapies. HIV-infected patients should be managed by a team experienced in the medical, obstetrical, and psychosocial needs of these women.

It is important to remember that HIV seropositivity is not synonymous with AIDS. This is especially true today, as current HIV drug regimens have allowed many HIV seropositive patients to survive free from an AIDS defining condition for years. During the early period of the epidemic, most obstetricians had no experience treating an HIV-infected pregnant woman but with the dramatic increase in HIV infections in women, more and more obstetricians can expect to have an HIV-infected pregnant woman among their patients. The Centers for Disease Control estimates that women account for 25% of the >50,000 new cases of HIV infection acquired annually in the United States.

The vast majority of infected women are of reproductive age and overwhelmingly acquire HIV infection from high risk heterosexual contact. The epidemic continues to disproportionately affect women of color. Although African American and Hispanic women make up 24% of all women in the United States, they account for 82% of the total number of women with AIDS. African American women have four times the rate of HIV infection of Hispanic women and 15 times the rate of Caucasian women. In addition African American women are more likely to have AIDS. African American women have four times the rate of AIDS as compared to Hispanic women and 23 times the rate of Caucasian women. HIV infection is the leading cause of death for African American women ages 25-34 and the fifth leading cause of death for all women 35-44 years of age.

However, the good news is that the majority of HIV-infected patients who receive appropriate antiretroviral therapy can expect a much longer and healthier survival than those infected early in the epidemic. Likewise, the use of anti-retroviral drugs during pregnancy has drastically reduced the risk of perinatal transmission of HIV (see Fig 26-1).

■ PATHOGENESIS

HIV is an RNA retrovirus. There are two types of HIV virus, HIV-1 and HIV-2. In the United States, HIV-1 causes the vast majority of infections. The virus is composed of viral particles surrounded by a lipid membrane. The RNA retrovirus recognizes certain cell receptors and adheres to the CD4 lymphocyte cell wall. After adhering, the viral particles enter the host CD4 cell's cytoplasm. Once inside, the RNA virus is capable of using an enzyme called reverse transcriptase to make DNA using the HIV viral RNA. The viral DNA enters the cell's nucleus where it can begin to direct cell function. The viral DNA uses the

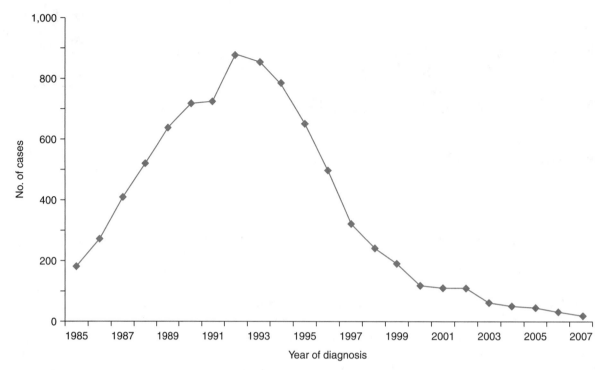

FIGURE 26-1. Estimated numbers of perinatally acquired AIDS cases, by year of diagnosis, 1985-2007—United States and dependent areas.

host cell to make viral products including more viral RNA. Billions of new HIV virions are made and released into the circulation each day and this cell-free HIV RNA can be measured by a test referred to as viral load. The consequences to the CD4 lymphocyte population are impaired functionality and a shortened half-life. In untreated patients, the number of CD4 lymphocytes falls over time and the patient becomes increasingly susceptible to HIV-related opportunistic complications. Viral production lasts for the life of the cell. New RNA viruses are shed into the body continuing the replication cycle. Many different types of cells and tissues are susceptible to HIV infection. These include B-lymphocytes, macrophages, the cervix, brain, myocardium, kidney, retina, colon, and liver among others. Since both T and B cells are affected, the HIV infection impacts both humoral and cellular immunity. Effective HIV antiretroviral therapy interrupts this life cycle. The result is a dramatic decrease in new virus production, an increase in the number of CD4 cells and improvement in immune function.

■ PRIMARY HIV INFECTION

Primary HIV infection can be asymptomatic, mildly symptomatic with a flu-like presentation, or severely symptomatic. Symptomatic primary HIV infection is called the acute retroviral syndrome and usually occurs within several weeks following HIV infection. Antibody to HIV may not be present at the time of the acute retroviral syndrome so an HIV antibody test will likely be nonreactive but HIV RNA (viral load) will be high. Both an HIV antibody test and viral load measurement should be obtained if primary HIV infection is being suspected. Symptoms usually begin within 5 to 30 days after infection with HIV occurs. Common findings are fever, rash, lymphadenopathy, pharyngitis, and myalgias. Neurologic symptoms may be present. The syndrome resembles mononucleosis and the correct diagnosis is often not considered. Patients recover and become asymptomatic but will develop progressive immunodeficiency if HIV infection is not diagnosed and treated. However, the course of HIV infection can vary depending upon the host's immune system, comorbid conditions, and the virulence of the virus. Some patients will show rapid progression of immune deficiency and on rare occasions a patient may have a fulminant course, rapidly progressing to AIDS.

■ TESTING FOR HIV INFECTION

It is wise to have a liberal policy with regard to offering any patient HIV testing and to offer HIV testing to *all* pregnant women. The Centers for Disease Control estimates that at least 1 in 5 people currently infected in the United States are unaware of their HIV seropositivity. It is crucial to remember that patients may not admit to risk behaviors or be unaware of their partners' activities. In addition a patient may have seroconverted since a previously negative test. The CDC has started a campaign, "One test, two Lives" to focus on the need for HIV testing in every pregnant woman. Testing pregnant patients becomes imperative since perinatal transmission rates drop from approximately 25% in the untreated HIV positive mother to 2% or less in a mother treated with antiretroviral drugs. Moreover, cesarean section before the onset of labor may offer an additional reduction in the risk of transmission in patients with high viral loads. Both the Institute of Medicine and the American College of Obstetrics and Gynecologist agree that HIV testing is part of routine obstetrical care. Both agree that pregnant women should "opt out" of testing, ie patients are counseled that testing is routine and it is done unless the patient refuses. Current guidelines advise a second HIV test before 36 weeks in women with ongoing risk behaviors. Testing at 36 weeks allows time to start antiretrovirals to reduce the risk of perinatal transmission. Patients who present in labor without a prior HIV test should be encouraged to have a rapid HIV test and be treated on the basis of the test results without waiting for the usual confirmatory western blot. Furthermore, if a patient has a positive rapid test it should be assumed that her viral load is greater than 1000 copies, since she has not had prior antiretroviral treatment. Rapid HIV tests can be performed in about 30 minutes.

In September 2006 the Centers for Disease Control issued revised recommendations for who should be tested for HIV infection. The guidelines recommend "opt-out" testing. This means that patients should be notified that HIV testing will be performed unless the patient declines. Laws governing the consent requirement for HIV testing are specific for each state and providers should be familiar with applicable regulations.

The CDC recommends HIV testing for

- All patients aged 13-64. Patients at high risk for HIV should be tested at least annually.
- All pregnant women.
- All patients initiating treatment for TB.
- All patients seeking treatment for STDs.

HIV testing consists of both a screening HIV test (ELISA) and a confirmatory test (Western blot) if the ELISA is repeatedly reactive. Both tests detect antibodies to HIV-1 proteins. Currently available rapid HIV tests are ELISAs and a reactive rapid test requires a confirmatory Western blot to establish a diagnosis of HIV infection. As with all testing, both false positive and false negative results occur. The incidence of these is related to the prevalence of the disease in the population. An ELISA is reported as either nonreactive or reactive. A nonreactive test does not require additional testing unless a patient continues to have risk behaviors, in which case testing should be reconsidered in 6 to 12 months. However, there are several conditions that rarely can result in a false positive ELISA. The lists of conditions that may cause a false positive ELISA are as follows:

- Autoimmune disease
- Alloantibodies resulting from transfusions
- Positive rapid plasma reagin (RPR)
- Recent influenza vaccination
- Pregnancy
- Malignancies
- Lab or clerical error

There are also conditions that can rarely result in a false negative ELISA. The list of conditions that may cause a false negative ELISA is as follows:

- Test done prior to seroconversion (patient has not yet made antibodies)
- Seroreversion (may occur in end stage disease)
- An atypical host response
- Agammaglobulinemia
- Infection with certain strains of HIV-2 virus
- Lab or clerical error

A positive ELISA makes it necessary to perform a confirmatory Western blot. A Western blot can be reported as negative, indeterminate, or positive. A reactive ELISA and a negative Western blot suggest a false positive ELISA. The patient is considered *not infected* and no further testing is required. An indeterminate Western blot means that the patient has antibodies to one or two bands on the Western blot.

It may be the result of recent infection and therefore, ongoing seroconversion, or may be a false positive test result. Approximately, 4% to 20% of Western blots are reported as indeterminate. Indeterminate Western blots appear to be more common during pregnancy. On the Western blot, anti-gp 160/120 antibodies appear first followed by anti-p24 antibody and anti-gp41 soon after. If the Western blot is indeterminate, measurement of HIV RNA viral load may help determine if the patient is HIV infected or not. The HIV RNA is not a diagnostic test, but may be helpful to determine if a Western blot is indicative of seroconversion. Alternatively, another option is the use of an immunofluorescent assay (IFA), as a confirmatory test. If that is negative, the patient should be considered negative. A patient is considered HIV infected if both the ELISA and the Western blot are positive. The Western blot has a 2% rate of false positives. Most patients will have positive HIV antibody test within 3 months of infection. A minority may not seroconvert until 6 months or later after the infection.

Other methods of testing are available but rarely used. In addition to blood, HIV tests can be performed on saliva, vaginal secretions, and urine. HIV testing of vaginal secretions can be helpful in cases of sexual assault. These tests are either serological or culture. These tests are not better than standard screening but may be helpful in difficult cases. Table 26-1 summarizes how to interpret serological testing.

■ INTERPRETING VIRAL LOADS AND CD4 COUNTS

The single best indicator of disease activity is the *quantitative* viral load, also known as HIV RNA. The viral load can be measured by the b-deoxyribonucleic acid assay (bDNA), the reverse transcription polymerase chain reaction assay (RT-PCR), or the nucleic acid sequence-based amplification assay (NABSA). A viral load is considered to be undetectable if the result is below the lower limit of detection of the test being used. Active infections and immunizations can artifactually increase viral loads; therefore, a viral load test should not be drawn until at least 4 to 6 weeks after an infection or a vaccination to avoid misinterpreting a spurious increase. The goal of effective antiretroviral therapy is an undetectable viral load; there can still be *viral blips* or small increases in the viral load that are usually 400 copies/mL or less. These blips do not appear to be clinically significant. The viral load should become and remain undetectable within the first 6 months after starting treatment. If it does not, adherence with antiretroviral therapy should be evaluated and HIV resistance testing obtained if the viral load is confirmed to be increased. The viral load should be repeated monthly in pregnancy until the virus is undetectable and then every 2 to 3 months thereafter. The CD4 (helper T lymphocyte) cell count is an important measure of the degree of immune deficiency. Certain opportunistic complications tend to occur below given CD4 counts. As a rule, CD4 counts should be repeated before any therapeutic decision is made since the trend of CD4 counts

■ TABLE 26-1. Interpretation of HIV Serological Testing			
Test	**Result**	**Interpretation**	**Further testing**
ELISA	Nonreactive	Not HIV infected	Not necessary Retest 6-12 mo if same risk factors Retest prior to 36 wk if pregnant and high risk
ELISA	Reactive	Possible HIV infection	Western blot
Western blot	Negative	Not HIV infected	Not necessary Retest 6-12 mo if same risk factors
Western blot	Indeterminate Reacts to bands gp41 + gp 120/160 or p24 + gp160	Seroconversion or false positive	RNA viral load or IFA or Repeat Western blot in 1 mo
Western blot	Positive	HIV infection	See Table 26-3

is probably more helpful than a single measurement. Multiple factors can depress the CD4 count and should be considered in the evaluation of a patient. In an asymptomatic patient antiretroviral treatment should be started when the CD4 count is below 500/mm^3. A CD4 count of <200/mm^3 constitutes a diagnosis of AIDS. If the asymptomatic patient is stable and does not require antiretroviral therapy, the count should be followed every 3 months. Some factors that may affect CD4 count are as follows:

- Recent corticosteroid use
- Intercurrent illness
- Diurnal variation (lowest at 12 PM and highest at 8 PM)
- Major surgery
- Intra/interassay variation
- Seasonal/monthly variation

■ RESISTANCE TESTING

The HIV virus can easily mutate because of the enormous amount of virus that is replicated on a daily basis, and the high rate of error in the reverse transcriptase enzyme. Mutations also can occur during treatment with antiretroviral medications. Mutations often lead to drug resistance, and it is possible for people to become infected with virus that is resistant to one or more antiretroviral drugs. Resistance testing should be done at the time of HIV diagnosis and before antiretroviral therapy is started. Resistance testing also is indicated if the viral load fails to become undetectable during treatment or if the viral load becomes measurable after being undetectable while on treatment. All HIV-infected pregnant patients should have a resistance test performed if they have measurable HIV RNA prior to starting or changing a treatment regimen. Resistance testing is done in one of two ways: genotypic or phenotypic. Genotype testing uses point mutations in the viral genome structure to predict which therapies the virus would be sensitive to. Phenotype testing has been likened to *culture and sensitivity* and predicts viral susceptibility based on the ability of the virus to grow in various concentrations of antiretrovirals. Results are reported as the amount of drug needed to reduce viral production at different concentrations of the drugs being tested. Genotype testing is generally more widely available, less expensive, and faster to obtain. The interpretation of both tests is complex and each test has its limitations. Some point mutations may mean increased resistance to a given drug, but enhanced sensitivity to another. Only clinicians with significant expertise in treating HIV patients should interpret the result. The tests

■ TABLE 26-2. Genotype versus Phenotype Testing

Genotype	Phenotype
Uses point mutations or structural changes	Uses ability of virus to grow in varying in viral genome to concentrations drug(s) predict drug sensitivity to predict sensitivity
Cheaper	More expensive
More widely available	Less widely available
Faster	Slower (requires virus to grow in culture)

are more helpful in deciding which drugs should not be used rather than deciding which drugs should be used. Table 26-2 compares the two types of testing.

■ IMMUNE SYSTEM CHANGES IN PREGNANCY

There are conflicting data as to the immune changes in pregnancy. Some studies have suggested pregnancy may result in less Th1 (cellular immunity) but more Th2 (antibody and humoral) immunity. Cytokines that produce antibodies increase while those that are cytotoxic decrease. It is not entirely clear how these changes could be mediated but both the placenta and the hormones of pregnancy are thought to play a role. Activated T cells have receptors for progesterone. In addition, in vitro studies progesterone, for example, can cause a shift from cell-mediated immunity to humoral immunity. Cell-mediated immunity appears to change so as to allow tolerance for the foreign fetus. There are reports of reduced maternal response to a variety of both viral and bacterial organisms including varicella, cytomegalovirus, polio, influenza, hepatitis, salmonella, leprosy, coccidioidomycosis, streptococcus, and malaria. However, pregnant women are able to respond to vaccination and can mount a delayed hypersensitivity response. Some women with autoimmune diseases, which are thought to be cell mediated, improve. Although there is improved antibody-mediated immunity, B lymphocytes do not increase, complement levels are normal to slightly increased and levels of IgG decline. The peripheral white blood cell count rises during gestation and also rises again in labor. In labor, the WBC count can approach 30,000/mm^3. The increased white count is primarily due to increased segmented neutrophils. White blood cells not only increase in number, they undergo metabolic changes as well resulting in what has been termed an "activated leukocyte." Local immunity may be changed as some studies have shown that white cells within the reproductive tract are less responsive. In general pregnant women are able to respond to infections normally.

■ PREGNANCY AND HIV INFECTION

Early, in the HIV epidemic, there were concerns that pregnancy would hasten the progression of HIV infection since there are changes in cell-mediated immunity in pregnancy. However, in controlled studies of HIV-infected pregnant women who were compared to asymptomatic HIV-infected nonpregnant women, pregnancy had no effect on disease progression. Pregnancy does not make HIV infection worse. The initial evaluation of a pregnant woman with HIV infection is given in Table 26-3.

■ ANTIRETROVIRAL THERAPY

In a national study the CDC found that fewer women were prescribed the most effective medications for HIV infection in comparison to the treatment men received. The decision to initiate antiretroviral therapy in pregnant women may

■ TABLE 26-3. Initial Assessment of an HIV-Infected Pregnant Woman

History

Complete prior medical and surgical history with attention to prior AIDS defining diagnosis(es)
Current and past medications, especially prior antiretroviral use
Immunization status
Prior or current sexually transmitted disease including dysplasia, hepatitis B and C, syphilis, gonorrhea, and Chlamydia
Substance abuse history including alcohol use and smoking
Mental health history: depression, domestic violence, and dementia
Availability of support systems
Postpartum contraception plans

Physical examination

Weight
Vital signs (particularly temperature and respiratory rate)
Skin: abscesses, dermatitis, rashes, vesicles, violaceous macules, evidence of prior SQ or IV injection drug use
Lymph nodes: lymphadenopathy
HEENT: dentition, funduscopic examination and visual fields, oral thrush or ulcers
Pulmonary: breath sounds, cough, sputum, dyspnea
Cardiac: cardiomegaly, murmurs, rubs
Abdomen: hepatosplenomegaly, fundal height, fetal heart tones
Genitourinary: vaginal discharge, genital lesions
Neurological: mental status, confusion, ability to concentrate, memory deficits, focal neurological deficits or neuropathy, weakness
Psychiatric: affect, mood, evidence of psychosis, support systems

Laboratory

Appropriate prenatal laboratories, baseline assessment of hematological, renal, and liver function, hepatitis A, B, and C serology, CMV and toxoplasmosis serologies, CD4 count, HIV-1 RNA viral load, HIV resistance testing, TB skin test, RPR, screening for gonorrhea and Chlamydia

Radiological

Ultrasound to determine gestational age and evaluate fetal anatomy

Miscellaneous

Nutritional assessment
Reduction of transmission (abstinence or safe sex practices, and prohibition against breast-feeding)

not be an easy one, but antiretroviral therapy clearly reduces the risk of vertical transmission. The clinician and the patient need to consider a number of factors including whether the treatment is being given for the sake of the mother or to prevent vertical transmission. Generally, antiretroviral therapy should be initiated after the first trimester to avoid potential teratogenic effects *unless* the mother requires it for her own health in which case treatment should be started immediately. Under current guidelines antiretroviral therapy is started in asymptomatic patients if the CD4 count is less than 350. There is no perfect combination of drugs or a standard regimen that can be given to all patients. As with any therapeutic decision, there are risks and benefits of antiretroviral therapy. The benefits are a longer disease-free interval due to preservation of immune function and less risk of transmission of the virus to others. Antiretrovirals have toxicities, both short term and long term for which we have incomplete understanding. The patient must adhere to complex medication schedules making compliance difficult. Noncompliance can quickly result in viral resistance making future therapy much more difficult and generally less effective. It may be difficult to tolerate medication due to hyperemesis. Additionally, one must consider the risks of teratogenicity of various medications and often there may be very little data to guide the clinicians. There are significant fetal implications for infections such as CMV or toxoplasmosis which are more common in immune-suppressed patients. Table 26-4 lists several considerations that need to be addressed before initiating antiretroviral therapy.

There are five major classes of antiretroviral drugs: nucleos(t)ide reverse transcriptase inhibitors, non-nucleoside reverse transcriptase inhibitors, protease inhibitors, integrase inhibitors, and entry inhibitors. Table 26-5 outlines the available drugs and their class. Treatment regimens are complex and should only be undertaken in consultation with an expert in HIV therapy. Doses may need to be altered depending upon the combinations used and the circumstances. For example, if a patient is taking antepartum d4T, this should not be continued while she is intrapartum as it antagonizes zidovudine. The d4T should be discontinued in favor of the zidovudine.

The US Public Health Task Force 2009 recommendations (*available at http://aidsinfo.nih.gov/ContentFiles/ PerinatalGL.pdf*) are that patients who have been taking antiretrovirals continue taking them while intrapartum *regardless of route of delivery*. In addition, the Task Force recommends an initial intravenous loading dose of zidovudine at 2 mg/kg followed by a continuous infusion at 1 mg/kg/h until delivery. Zidovudine should be used even if a woman has not received it antenatally because of known or suspected resistance and/or toxicity unless the patient has demonstrated a hypersensitivity reaction. Patients who are scheduled for cesarean sections should have zidovudine started 3 hours before surgery. Some women who receive antiretroviral therapy during pregnancy, but who otherwise do not meet current guidelines for antiretroviral therapy, may elect to discontinue treatment after delivery.

Heath care providers are advised to report instances of prenatal exposure to antiretroviral drugs to the Antiretroviral

---

■ **TABLE 26-4. Considerations in Starting Antiretroviral Therapy**

Does the patient meet criteria for treatment?
   Patients coinfected with hepatitis B requiring treatment for hepatitis B
   Pregnancy
   Patients with HIV-associated nephropathy
   Patients with symptomatic HIV infection or AIDS
   Asymptomatic patients with CD4 count <500/mm^3
   Rapidly declining CD4 count (consider)
   High viral load (consider)
   Acute retroviral syndrome (consider)
Is the patient willing to continue long-term treatment?
Does the patient understand the importance of compliance?
Does the patient have the resources to continue treatment?
   Funds to pay for treatment, stable living situation, absence of psychosis, severe depression, dementia, substance abuse
What is known about the medication in pregnancy?

■ TABLE 26-5. Antiretroviral Therapy

Generic	Trade name	Common side effects
Nucleos(t)ide reverse transcriptase inhibitors		
Zidovudine (AZT)	Retrovir	Anemia, nausea, headaches
Didanosine (ddI)	Videx	Pancreatitis especially in alcoholics
		Peripheral neuropathy
		Avoid using with d4T in pregnancy
Dideoxycytidine (ddc)	Hivid	Peripheral neuropathy
Stavudine (d4T)	Zerit	Peripheral neuropathy, Pancreatitis
		Avoid using with ddI in pregnancy
Lamivudine	Epivir	Rare hepatic dysfunction
Abacavir	Ziagen	Hypersensitivity reaction that can be fatal if treatment is continued or restarted after an interruption in dosing
Emtricitabine	Emtriva	Headache, diarrhea, nausea, rash
Tenofovir	Viread	Renal dysfunction, Fanconi syndrome
Non-nucleoside reverse transcriptase inhibitors		
Nevirapine	Viramune	Rash, toxic hepatitis (especially in women with CD4 >250 or men with CD4 >400)
Delavirdine	Rescriptor	Rash, headaches
Efavirenz	Sustiva	Avoid in pregnancy especially during the first trimester
Etravirine	Intelence	Rash, hepatitis
Integrase inhibitors		
Raltegravir	Isentress	Diarrhea, nausea, headache
Protease inhibitors		
Indinavir	Crixivan	Renal stones, hyperbilirubinemia,
Fosamprenavir	Lexiva	GI intolerance
Lopinavir/ritonavir	Kaletra	GI complaints, Pancreatitis, hyperlipidemia, hyperglycemia
Saquinavir	Invirase, Fortovase	GI intolerance, rash
Nelfinavir	Viacept	Diarrhea, hepatic dysfunction, drug interactions, lipodystrophies, diabetes
Ritonavir	Norvir	Perioral paresthesia, diarrhea, liver dysfunction, hyperglycemia, drug interaction, diabetes, lipodystrophies
Atazanavir	Reyataz	Hyperbilirubinemia
Darunavir	Prezista	GI symptoms
Tipranavir	Aptivus	Hepatotoxicity, GI intolerance, ? risk of intracranial hemorrhage
Entry inhibitors		
Enfuvirtide (T-20)	Fuzeon	Injection site reactions
Maraviroc	Selzentry	Hepatotoxicity, cardiac events

Pregnancy Registry that was formed to assess the potential teratogenicity of these drugs. Phone number: 1-800-8001052.

In addition, pregnant women should receive antimicrobial prophylaxis to prevent opportunistic infections according to the guidelines published by the US Public Health Service.

■ PREVENTION OF VERTICAL TRANSMISSION

The cornerstone of preventing vertical transmission of the HIV virus is to recognize which pregnant women are infected and to use antiretroviral therapy to reduce the viral load in both blood and genital secretions. In general there is strong correlation between the viral load in the blood and genital secretions but different levels have been reported. The longer in pregnancy a woman takes medication, the better the effect is. Current guidelines suggest antiretroviral therapy should be started by 28 weeks' gestation. If a HIV-infected patient has not taken antepartum antiretrovirals, she should receive intrapartum treatment in conjunction with infant prophylaxis. If a pregnant women who is HIV infected does not receive antenatal or intrapartum medication, the infant should be treated with zidovudine for the first 6 weeks of life. Reducing viral load is far and away the most important factor in reducing vertical transmission. However, perinatal transmission has been confirmed even with undetectable blood levels of viral RNA. Therefore, RNA levels are not the sole indication for treatment with antiretrovirals. There are other measures that may help to reduce perinatal transmission. Table 26-6 outlines these measures. About 70% of perinatal transmission occurs at delivery and 30% occurs in utero. About two-thirds of the in-utero transmissions are thought to occur within the last 14 days before delivery. If the patient has a viral load of >1000 copies/mL, the American College of Obstetricians and Gynecologists recommends that she be offered an elective cesarean section at 38 weeks before the onset of labor to reduce her chances of vertical transmission. The estimated gestational age should be based on as much clinical data as are available, but amniocentesis to document fetal lung maturity presents an unknown risk of transmitting HIV infection to the fetus and is *not* recommended. Cesarean section offers a reduction in vertical transmission, especially if the mother has a high viral load and has not had prolonged rupture of membranes. However, the benefits of cesarean section are not as pronounced once labor has started or if ruptured

■ **TABLE 26-6. Measures to Reduce the Risk of Vertical Transmission**

- Keep the mother's viral load at 50 copies or less (undetectable).
- Cesarean section at week 38 of gestation and before rupture of membranes for women with viral loads of 1000 or more. Individualize if PROM or PPROM.
- Administer progesterone 250 mg IM from 16-36 wk if the patient has had a prior preterm birth and consider measuring transvaginal cervical length to detect early cervical shortening.
- Treat vitamin A deficiency.
- Avoid invasive fetal procedures such as chorionic villus sampling, amniocentesis, percutaneous fetal blood samples.
- Avoid scalp electrodes, fetal scalp sampling, artificial rupture of membranes, operative vaginal deliveries.
- Avoid episiotomies.
- Wash the infant in an antimicrobial bath as soon as possible and immediately *before* administering parenteral medication or obtaining blood.
- Avoid breast-feeding where formula is inexpensive and readily available.

membranes are present. If the patient has ruptured membranes before 37 weeks the decision regarding delivery is a complex one involving the estimated gestational age, the viral load, whether or not the patient has had medication and if there are other factors such as advanced cervical dilation, bleeding, non-reassuring fetal status or chorioamnionitis. The decision about the timing and route of delivery should be individualized and there are not clear data to direct care for every patient scenario. Cesarean sections are not without risk, particularly if the mother's viral load is high. The higher is the maternal viral load, the greater is the risk of postpartum infectious morbidity. Table 26-7 summarizes current recommendations.

Unfortunately, about 15% of HIV-infected women do not receive prenatal care and have not had antenatal antiretroviral therapy. The list of drugs that are recommended by the Public Health Task Force for treating HIV positive women in labor who have not had antepartum antiretroviral therapy is as follows:

- Zidovudine
- Nevirapine
- Zidovudine-lamivudine
- Nevirapine and zidovudine

■ TABLE 26-7. Intrapartum Management

HIV	PROM	Viral load	Prior HAART	Management
+	No	<1000 copies	Yes	Continue HAART. ZDV 2 mg/kg loading dose over 1 h. ZDV 1 mg/kg/h continuous infusion until delivery. C-section for obstetrical indications. Prophylactic antibiotics if C/S is done. Some argue mother may elect C/S with unknown but possible benefit to reduce infant risk. Counsel re-increased maternal risks of C/S in HIV positive women. Avoid AROM, invasive fetal procedures, forceps, vacuum. Notify nursery for infant treatment.
+	Yes	<1000 copies	Yes	Same as above
+	No	>1000 copies	Yes	Continue HAART. ZVD 2 mg/kg loading dose over 1 h and 3 h before C/S, if possible. ZVD 1 mg/kg/h continuous infusion until delivery. Counsel benefit of C/S for less perinatal transmission but higher risk of maternal complications with C/S in HIV positive patients. C/S prophylactic antibiotics. Notify nursery for infant treatment.
+	No	<1000 copies	No	Consult with HIV specialist as to whether or not to begin HAART. Some use single dose nevirapine +/− 3TC. Some would use ZVD alone. Should do resistance testing *before* starting therapy. ZVD 2 mg/kg loading dose over 1 h and 3 h before C/S, if possible. ZVD 1 mg/kg/h continuous infusion until delivery. Individualize route of delivery. No clear data. Counsel benefit of C/S for less perinatal transmission but higher risk of maternal complications. C/S prophylactic antibiotics. Notify nursery for infant treatment.
+	Yes	<1000 copies	No	Consult with HIV specialist as to whether or not to begin HAART. Some use single dose nevirapine +/− 3TC. Some would use ZVD alone. Should do resistance testing *before* starting therapy. ZVD 2 mg/kg loading dose over 1 h and 3 h before C/S, if possible. ZVD 1 mg/kg/h continuous infusion until delivery. Individualize route of delivery. No clear data. Counsel benefit of C/S for less perinatal transmission but higher risk of maternal complications. C/S prophylactic antibiotics. Notify nursery for infant treatment.

HIV	PROM	Viral load	Prior HAART	Management
+	Yes	>1000 copies	Yes	Continue HAART. ZVD 2 mg/kg loading dose over 1 h and 3 h before C/S, if possible. ZVD 1 mg/kg/h continuous infusion until delivery. Counsel benefit of C/S for less perinatal transmission but higher risk of maternal complications with C/S in HIV positive patients. C/S may be warranted if unfavorable cervix and long labor is anticipated. C/S prophylactic antibiotics. Notify nursery for infant treatment.
+	No	>1000 copies	No	Begin HAART. ZVD 2 mg/kg loading dose over 1 h and 3 h before C/S, if possible. ZVD 1 mg/kg/h continuous infusion until delivery. Counsel benefit of C/S for less perinatal transmission but higher risk of maternal complications. C/S prophylactic antibiotics. Notify nursery for infant treatment.
+	No	Unknown	Yes	Continue HAART. ZVD 2 mg/kg loading dose over 1 h and 3 h before C/S, if possible. ZVD 1 mg/kg/h continuous infusion until delivery. Most would counsel for C/S if viral load is unknown and no PPROM. Counsel mother about higher risk of maternal complications with C/S in HIV positive patients. C/S prophylactic antibiotics. Notify nursery for infant treatment.
+	Yes	Unknown	Yes	Continue HAART. ZVD 2 mg/kg loading dose over 1 h and 3 h before C/S, if possible. ZVD 1 mg/kg/h continuous infusion until delivery. Individualize route of delivery. No data regarding neonatal benefit of C/S if PROM. Counsel mother about higher risk of maternal complications with C/S in HIV positive patients. C/S prophylactic antibiotics. Notify nursery for infant treatment.
+	No	Unknown	No	Begin HAART. ZVD 2 mg/kg loading dose over 1 h and 3 h before C/S, if possible. ZVD 1 mg/kg/h continuous infusion until delivery. Most would counsel for C/S if viral load is unknown and no PPROM. C/S prophylactic antibiotics. Notify nursery for infant treatment.

(continued)

■ TABLE 26-7. Intrapartum Management (continued)

HIV	PROM	Viral load	Prior HAART	Management
+	Yes	Unknown	No	Continue HAART. ZVD 2 mg/kg loading dose over 1 h and 3 h before C/S, if possible. ZVD 1 mg/kg/h continuous infusion until delivery. Individualize route of delivery. No data regarding neonatal benefit of C/S if PROM. C/S prophylactic antibiotics. Notify nursery for infant treatment.
Rapid test +	No	Unknown	No	Begin HAART. ZVD 2 mg/kg loading dose over 1 h and 3 h before C/S, if possible. ZVD 1 mg/kg/h continuous infusion until delivery. Most would counsel for C/S if viral load is unknown and no PPROM and no prior HAART. C/S prophylactic antibiotics. Notify nursery for infant treatment.
Rapid test +	PROM	Unknown	No	Begin HAART. ZVD 2 mg/kg loading dose over 1 h and 3 h before C/S, if possible. ZVD 1 mg/kg/h continuous infusion until delivery. Individualize route of delivery. No data regarding neonatal benefit of C/S if PROM. C/S prophylactic antibiotics. Notify nursery for infant treatment.

■ OTHER CONSIDERATIONS IN PREGNANCY

HIV affects humoral immunity and B-cell function. As a result, HIV-infected patients may produce a range of antibodies including antiphospholipid antibodies. These are not associated with an increased risk of thrombosis.

Breast-feeding increases the risk of vertical transmission and is not recommended in the United States.

Protease inhibitors have been associated with carbohydrate intolerance in pregnancy. However, the development of gestational diabetes is not a contraindication to their continued use. Gestational diabetes should be managed in a conventional manner. Postpartum hemorrhage in an HIV positive patient needs to be managed differently. Methergine is contraindicated if a patient is concurrently taking either some protease inhibitor or nonnucleoside reverse transcriptase that are CYP3A4 enzyme inhibitors. The combination has resulted in severe vasoconstriction. Methergine should only be used if there is a serious

hemorrhage and other methods to control bleeding are not available. If a patient requires a transfusion she should receive CMV negative blood if possible.

The combination of stavudine and didanosine should be avoided in pregnancy, as there have been reports of fatal lactic acidosis when they have been used concurrently.

Postpartum Concerns

The postpartum patient who is HIV positive requires careful consideration, particularly if the infection was first diagnosed when the patient presented in labor. If a rapid test is positive, the patient needs a confirmatory Western blot. The postpartum period may also be a time when a patient can undergo treatment for substance abuse. The postpartum period may be a time when a patient can undergo treatment for substance abuse. It is estimated that breast-feeding accounts for about 15% of HIV infection in infants. Breast-feeding is contraindicated in developed countries such as the United States, where formula is inexpensive and readily available. Breast engorgement can be treated with ice packs, binders, and analgesia but bromocripton, a drug used previously, is not FDA approved and has been associated with serious side effects. Patients should avoid breast stimulation including warm showers which can cause a reflex let down. Some patients who do not have another indication for antiretrovirals may elect to discontinue treatment. The decision to stop antiretrovirals should be made on the basis of a number of factors including the ability of the patient to comply with a complex schedule, the viral load, the CD4 count, symptoms or an AIDS defining illness. Patients should be screened for postpartum depression and substance abuse and assessed for support in caring for the infant as this may impact their ability to comply with a demanding medication regime and follow-up care.

In addition the postpartum care should include updating immunizations, obtaining Pap smears, and treating cervical neoplasms as well as a discussion of available contraception. There are several aspects to consider when counseling patients regarding contraception. Some forms of contraception such as barrier methods pose little risk in terms of interaction with medications but are less effective. Some may be reluctant to use IUDs in an immunocompromised patient, but infection usually occurs at the time of insertion and prophylactic antibiotics may help to reduce the risk. Most authors do not consider HIV infection to be a contraindication to IUD placement. Oral contraceptives may interact with antiretrovirals and some antiretrovirals are known to induce liver enzymes resulting in a change in either steroid or antiretroviral concentration.

■ SAFETY PRECAUTIONS FOR THE LABOR AND DELIVERY TEAM

Caring for obstetrical patients presents a risk of exposure to body fluids for healthcare workers (HCW). The Centers for Disease Control and Prevention established universal precautions in 1987. Table 26-8 lists these universal precautions. At least one blood exposure can be documented in over 30% of surgical procedures, most (75%) of which may have been preventable. Suggestions to reduce exposure with needles or sharp instruments are as follows:

- Observe universal precautions.
- Do not recap needles.
- Wear double gloves.
- Place sharps boxes near where sharps are used.

■ TABLE 26-8. Body Fluids and Universal Precautions

Universal precautions necessary	Universal precautions not necessary unless contaminated with blood
Blood	Breast milk
Semen	Urine
Vaginal secretions	Sputum
Tissue	Sweat
Fluids	Vomitus
Amniotic	Feces
Peritoneal	Nasal secretions
Pericardial	Tears
Pleural	Saliva
Synovial	
Cerebrospinal	

- Announce all sharp instruments prior to passing them.
- Pass sharp instruments in an emesis basin.
- Use instruments to load needles.
- "One wound, one surgeon."
- Check hourly for disruptions of protective barriers.

The overall risk of HIV transmission to an HCW depends upon the type of exposure, the volume of the blood, the patient's viral load, and possibly, the immune response of the HCW. The risk of HIV infection with a percutaneous exposure is 0.3%, while the risk with a mucous membrane exposure is much less, about 0.09%. There appears to be minimal risk with exposure to intact skin. The risks are higher with large bore needles, deep intramuscular injections, larger volumes of blood, and higher viral loads. The risks after exposure to other body fluids have not been well defined.

If exposure occurs, the contact area should be washed immediately with soap and water. Other solutions such as betadine are not superior. Eyes should be flushed with sterile normal saline. The exposed HCW should be evaluated as soon as possible for postexposure prophylaxis.

Figures 26-2 and 26-3 provide the current CDC recommendations for postexposure prophylaxis (PEP) in an HCW. It is always important to seek expert opinion after HCW exposure, particularly in special circumstances such as pregnancy in the HCW or exposure with a drug-resistant virus. Animal studies have shown that early initiation of PEP and small inoculums of blood are the most predictive of successful PEP.

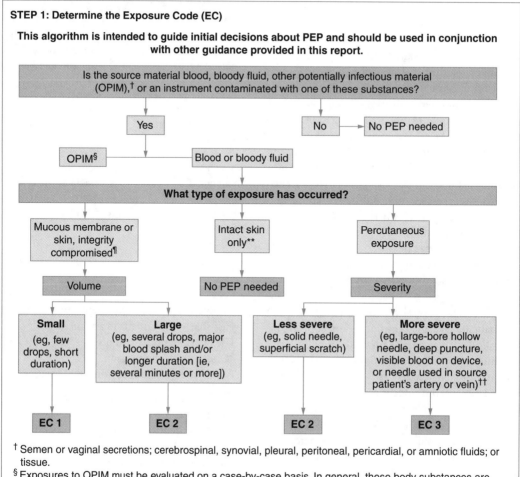

STEP 1: Determine the Exposure Code (EC)

This algorithm is intended to guide initial decisions about PEP and should be used in conjunction with other guidance provided in this report.

Is the source material blood, bloody fluid, other potentially infectious material (OPIM),[†] or an instrument contaminated with one of these substances?

Yes → OPIM[§] / Blood or bloody fluid

No → No PEP needed

What type of exposure has occurred?

- Mucous membrane or skin, integrity compromised[¶] → Volume
- Intact skin only[**] → No PEP needed
- Percutaneous exposure → Severity

Volume:
- **Small** (eg, few drops, short duration) → EC 1
- **Large** (eg, several drops, major blood splash and/or longer duration [ie, several minutes or more]) → EC 2

Severity:
- **Less severe** (eg, solid needle, superficial scratch) → EC 2
- **More severe** (eg, large-bore hollow needle, deep puncture, visible blood on device, or needle used in source patient's artery or vein)[††] → EC 3

[†] Semen or vaginal secretions; cerebrospinal, synovial, pleural, peritoneal, pericardial, or amniotic fluids; or tissue.

[§] Exposures to OPIM must be evaluated on a case-by-case basis. In general, these body substances are considered a low risk for transmission in health-care settings. Any unprotected contact to concentrated HIV in a research laboratory or production facility is considered an occupational exposure that requires clinical evaluation to determine the need for PEP.

[¶] Skin integrity is considered compromised if there is evidence of chapped skin, dermatitis, abrasion, or open wound.

[**] Contact with intact skin is not normally considered a risk for HIV transmission. However, if the exposure was to blood, and the circumstance suggests a higher volume exposure (eg, an extensive area of skin was exposed or there was prolonged contact with blood), the risk for HIV transmission should be considered.

[††] The combination of these severity factors (eg, large-bore hollow needle **and** deep puncture) contribute to an elevated risk for transmission if the source person is HIV positive.

FIGURE 26-2. Determining the need for HIV postexposure prophylaxis (PEP) after an occupational exposure (Step 1).

■ SUMMARY

The care of HIV-infected pregnant women is challenging and constantly evolving as new therapies arise. Unfortunately, since this epidemic continues, many obstetricians can expect to care for an HIV-infected patient at some point. Fortunately, new therapies, especially the protease inhibitors, have markedly reduced the risk of perinatal transmission and have significantly increased the life expectancy of HIV-infected women. It is crucial for obstetricians to continue to alert patients to the risks of HIV, to screen all pregnant women for the infection, and to consult with experts in HIV therapy to appropriately manage antiretroviral therapy and HIV-related complications.

STEP 2: Determine the HIV Status Code (HIV SC)

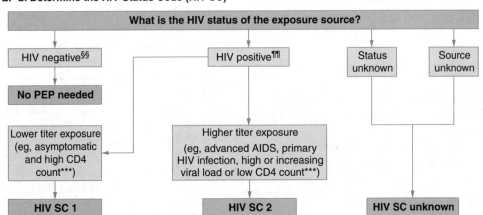

§§ A source is considered negative for HIV infection if there is laboratory documentation of a negative HIV antibody. HIV polymerase chain reaction (PCR), or HIV p24 antigen test result from a specimen collected at or near the time of exposure and there is no clinical evidence of recent retroviral-like illness.

¶¶ A source is considered infected with HIV (HIV positive) if there has been a positive laboratory result for HIV antibody, HIV PCR, or HIV p24 antigen or physician-diagnosed AIDS.

***Examples are used as surrogates to estimate the HIV titer in an exposure source for purposes of considering PEP regimens and do not reflect all clinical situations that may be observed. Although a high HIV titer (HIV SC 2) in an exposure source has been associated with an increased risk for transmission, the possibility of transmission from a source with a low HIV titer also must be considered.

STEP 3: Determine the PEP Recommendation

EC	HIV SC	PEP recommendation
1	1	**PEP may not be warranted.** Exposure type does not pose a known risk for HIV transmission. Whether the risk for drug toxicity outweights the benefit of PEP should be decided by the exposed HCW and treating clinician.
1	2	**Consider basic regimen.**††† Exposure type poses a negligible risk for HIV transmission. A high HIV titer in the source may justify consideration of PEP. Whether the risk for drug toxicity outweights the benefit of PEP should be decided by the exposed HCW and treating clinician.
2	1	**Recommend basic regimen.** Most HIV exposures are in this category; no increased risk for HIV transmission has been observed but use of PEP is appropriate.
2	2	**Recommend expanded regimen.**§§§ Exposure type represents an increased HIV transmission risk.
3	1 or 2	**Recommend expanded regimen.** Exposure type represents an increased HIV transmission risk.
Unknown		If the source or, in the case of an unknown source, the setting where the exposure occurred suggests a possible risk for HIV exposure and the EC is 2 or 3, consider PEP basic regimen.

†††Basic regimen is four weeks of zidovudine, 600 mg per day in two or three divided doses, **and** lamivudine, 150 mg twice daily.

§§§Expanded regimen is the basic regimen plus **either** indinavir, 800 mg every 8 hours, **or** nelfinavir, 750 mg three times a day.

FIGURE 26-3. Determining the need for HIV postexposure prophylaxis (PEP) after an occupational exposure (Steps 2 and 3).

■ APPENDIX: AIDS DEFINING CONDITIONS (CENTERS FOR DISEASE CONTROL AND PREVENTION) revised December 5, 2008

CD4 <200

- *Candida* infection of esophagus, trachea, bronchi, or lungs
- Invasive cervical cancer
- Coccidiomycosis, disseminated or extrapulmonary
- Cryptococcosis, extrapulmonary
- Cryptosporidiosis with diarrhea >1 month
- Cytomegalovirus of any organ except the liver, spleen, or lymph nodes

Encephalopathy, HIV related

- Herpes simplex with mucocutaneous ulcer >1 month or bronchitis, pneumonitis, or esophagitis

Histoplasmosis, disseminated or extrapulmonary

- HIV wasting
- Isosporiasis with diarrhea >1 month
- Kaposi sarcoma
- Lymphoma of the brain
- Lymphoma, Burkitt or immunoblastic
- *Mycobacterium avium* or *Mycobacterium kansasii*, disseminated or extrapulmonary
- *Mycobacterium tuberculosis* or any site
- *Mycobacterium*, other species, disseminated or extrapulmonary
- *Pneumocystis jirovecii* pneumonia

Progressive multifocal leukoencephalopathy

- Recurrent pneumonia
- *Salmonella* septicemia, recurrent
- Toxoplasmosis of brain

SUGGESTED READINGS

AIDS*info*. Web site updated recommendations for HIV management. http://AIDSinfo.nih.gov. Accessed September 1, 2009.

American College of Obstetricians and Gynecologists. ACOG Committee Opinion No. 234: Scheduled cesarean delivery and the prevention of vertical transmission of HIV infection. Washington, DC: American College of Obstetricians and Gynecologists; 2000.

American College of Obstetricians and Gynecologists. ACOG Committee Opinion No. 344: Human papilloma vaccination. Washington, DC: American College of Obstetricians and Gynecologists; September, 2006.

American College of Obstetricians and Gynecologists. ACOG Committee Opinion No. 389: Human immunodeficiency virus. Washington, DC: American College of Obstetricians and Gynecologists; December, 2007.

American College of Obstetricians and Gynecologists. ACOG Committee Opinion No. 417: Addressing health risks of noncoital sexual activity. Washington, DC: American College of Obstetricians and Gynecologists; September, 2008.

American College of Obstetricians and Gynecologists. ACOG Committee Opinion No. 422: At risk drinking and illicit drug use: ethical issues in obstetrics and gynecology practice. Washington, DC: American College of Obstetricians and Gynecologists; December, 2008.

Gabbe S, Niebyl J, Simpson JL. *Obstetrics: Normal and Problem Pregnancies*. 5th ed. New York, NY: Churchill Livingston; 2007.

Guidelines for Prevention and Treatment of Opportunistic Infections in HIV-Infected Adults and Adolescents. Recommendations from the CDC, the National Institutes of Health, and the HIV Medicine Association of the Infectious Diseases Society of America. http://www.cdc.gov/mmwr/preview/mmwrhtml/rr5804a1.htm. Accessed September 1, 2009.

National HIV/AIDS Clinicians' Consultation Center. http://www.nccc.ucsf.edu/hivcntr. Accessed September 1, 2009.

National Institute for Occupation Health and Safety. Bloodborne infectious diseases HIV/AIDS, hepatitis B virus, and hepatitis C virus. http://www.cdc.gov/niosh/topics/bbp/. Accessed September 1, 2009.

Public Health Service Guidelines for the Management of Health-Care Worker Exposures to HIV and Recommendations for Postexposure Prophylaxis. *MMWR*. May 15, 1998.

Public Health Service Task Force. Recommendations for use of antiretroviral drugs in pregnant HIV-infected women for maternal health and interventions to reduce perinatal HIV transmission in the United States. Available at http://aidsinfo.nih.gov/ContentFiles/PerinatalGL.pdf. Accessed April 29, 2009.

Recom for Partner Services Programs for HIV Infection, Syphilis, Gonorrhea, and Chlamydial Infection. http://www.cdc.gov/mmwr/preview/mmwrhtml/rr5709a1.htm. Accessed September 1, 2009.

CHAPTER 27

Systemic Lupus Erythematosus in the Pregnant Patient

• *Bob Silver*

Systemic lupus erythematosus (SLE) is a multisystemic chronic inflammatory disease that affects patients in many different ways over a varying course of time. The disease is typically characterized by periods of remission and relapse, although the causes of exacerbation remain uncertain. SLE, like most autoimmune diseases, has a clear predilection for women. Indeed, women are affected seven times more frequently than men. The disorder may be diagnosed between the ages of 15 and 50 years, although it is most often detected in women in their twenties. Therefore, SLE is the most commonly encountered autoimmune disease in pregnancy. Although no specific gene mutation for SLE has been identified, the disease likely has a genetic component.[1] Approximately 10% of affected patients have a relative with SLE and monozygotic twin studies demonstrate that 50% of affected twins are concordant for the disease. It is estimated that about 2% of children born to mothers with SLE will develop the disease themselves.[2] The symptoms of SLE are extremely heterogeneous which can make the diagnosis difficult. The disease may affect joints, skin, kidneys, lung, nervous system, and other organs. The most common presenting complaints are extreme fatigue, arthralgias, fever, and rash (Table 27-1).

In 1982, the American Rheumatism Association (ARA) revised previously set criteria for the diagnosis of SLE[3] (Table 27-2). According to the ARA, a person must have had at least 4 of the 11 specific criteria in order to carry the diagnosis of SLE. However, many patients have less than four clinical or laboratory features of SLE and do not meet strict diagnostic criteria. These patients should not be considered to have SLE, but are often referred to as having lupus-like disease. Such individuals may benefit from therapies for SLE and some will ultimately develop the clinical syndrome.

■ LUPUS IN PREGNANCY

The Effect of Pregnancy on SLE

Fertility

Typically, patients with SLE do not have impaired infertility. However, patients on high dose steroids may become amenorrheic or anovulatory. Women with end-stage lupus nephritis requiring dialysis also are frequently amenorrheic. In addition, depending on the cumulative dose of medication and the age of the patient, 10% to 60% of patients who have been treated with cyclophosphamide become permanently amenorrheic. Patients with mild-moderate disease have fertility rates comparable to the general population and should be counseled appropriately about contraception unless they desire to become pregnant. Estrogen-containing oral contraceptives (and other forms of contraception) are considered safe to use in women with SLE as long as they do not have comorbidities such as thrombosis or hypertension.

Maternal Complications

A recent study using a database including detailed information regarding about 20% of all (not necessarily pregnancy related) hospitalizations in the United States estimated a 20-fold increased risk in mortality in women

TABLE 27-1. Frequency of Clinical Symptoms in Patients with SLE

Clinical symptoms	Frequency (%)
Fatigue	80-100
Fever	80-100
Arthritis	95
Myalgia	70
Weight loss	60
Photosensitivity	60
Malar rash	50
Nephritis	50
Pleurisy	50
Lymphadenopathy	50
Pericarditis	30
Neuropsychiatric	20

TABLE 27-3. Studies on the Frequency of Lupus Flares during Pregnancy

Author	Pregnancies (n)	Results
Lockshin et al[10]	33	No difference
Lockshin[9]	80	No difference
Mintz et al[8]	102	No difference
Urowitz (1993)[11]	79	No difference
Tandon et al[7]	78	No difference
Nossent (1990)[12]	39	Increased
Wong (1991)[13]	29	Increased
Petri et al[6]	40	Increased
Ruiz-Irastorza (1996)[14]	78	Increased

with SLE.[4] There was a three- to sevenfold increase in the risk for thrombosis, infection, thrombocytopenia, and the need for blood transfusion. Women with SLE also are more likely to have comorbid conditions such as diabetes and hypertension that are associated with adverse maternal (and fetal) outcomes.

Lupus Flares

There is an association between estrogen and SLE, as evidenced by the female predilection for the disorder.[5] Thus, conditions such as pregnancy that are associated with high

TABLE 27-2. American Rheumatic Association Criteria for the Diagnosis and Classification of SLE

Malar rash
Discoid rash
Photosensitivity
Oral ulcers
Arthritis
Serositis
Nephritis (proteinuria ≥500 mg/d or cellular casts)
Neurologic disorder (seizures, psychosis, stroke)
Hematologic disorder (hemolytic anemia, thrombocytopenia, leukopenia, lymphopenia)
Immunologic disorder (anti-dsDNA, anti-Sm, positive LE, false positive RPR)
Antinuclear antibodies

Note: Patient must have four of these criteria either serially or simultaneously.

estrogen levels have the potential to exacerbate SLE. The reported incidence of flares during pregnancy ranges between 15% and 63%. Several retrospective, uncontrolled studies performed prior to 1985 suggest that pregnancy exacerbates lupus flares. Table 27-3 reviews multiple studies on the frequency of lupus flares during pregnancy.[2,6-14] It is difficult to interpret available data because control groups were often unmatched, and the SLE cohorts among studies vary greatly regarding patient characteristics, severity of disease, and the definition of lupus flares. Furthermore, normal physiologic changes of pregnancy such as palmar erythema, facial blushing, proteinuria, and alopecia can be misinterpreted as lupus flares.

Doria and colleagues investigated the relationship of steroid hormone levels in pregnancy to SLE activity.[15] The group prospectively studied 17 women with lupus during pregnancy and matched them to eight healthy pregnant controls. They reported that women with SLE had significantly lower serum levels of estradiol and progesterone than controls. Furthermore, the highest levels of estrogen and progesterone occurred in the third trimester, when patients with SLE had both the lowest disease activity and serum immunoglobulin levels. These data challenge previous work that supports the association between increased levels of steroid hormones and lupus activity, and raise the question of whether or not estrogens and progesterones suppress humoral immune responses and therefore disease activity.

Regardless of whether or not the rate of SLE flares increase during pregnancy, flares are common and may occur in any trimester, or in the postpartum period. In general lupus flares during pregnancy are mild and easily treated. Furthermore, it has been demonstrated that active disease at the time of conception, active nephritis, a systemic lupus erythematosus disease activity index (SLEDAI) score of five or more, and abruptly stopping hydroxychloroquine therapy are significant risk factors for lupus flares. Approximately, 50% of patients with active disease at the time of conception experience flares during pregnancy compared to 20% of patients who are in remission when they conceive. Conversely, patients who have been in remission for 6 to 12 months prior to conception have a lower risk of lupus flares and do better than those with active disease.

Preexisting Renal Disease

Approximately, 50% of patients with lupus will develop renal disease. Lupus nephritis is a result of immune complex deposition, complement activation, and inflammation in the kidney. Several reports have emphasized the potential for a permanent decrease in renal function after pregnancy in women with lupus nephritis. On the other hand, more recent series indicate excellent outcome for most women with mild renal disease.[16-18] Burkett reviewed several retrospective reports including 242 pregnancies in 156 women with lupus nephritis.[19] He demonstrated that 59% of patients had no change in their renal function, 30% experienced transient renal impairment, and 7% had permanent renal insufficiency. Similar results were noted in a recent cohort of 113 pregnancies in 81 women in Italy.[20] Most patients with prior nephritis had successful pregnancies and flares were predicted by renal status (remission decreases the risk) at conception.

It is clear that there is a strong correlation between renal insufficiency prior to conception and the risk of deterioration during and after pregnancy. Women with a serum creatinine level greater than 1.5 mg/dL have a significantly increased risk of deterioration in renal function. Conversely, patients with serum creatinine levels less than 1.5 mg/dL can be reassured that pregnancy will not increase the rate of deterioration of renal function. The specific type of renal disease as demonstrated by histologic studies does not appear to influence pregnancy outcome or postnatal renal function.

Preeclampsia

Preeclampsia is among the most common pregnancy complications in patients with SLE. The incidence ranges between 20% and 35%. The cause of the increased incidence of preeclampsia in women with SLE is not clear, but may be due to unrecognized renal disease that is likely present in many patients with SLE. Renal disease, hypertension, and antiphospholipid syndrome all increase a patient's risk for developing preeclampsia. In the prospective study of Lockshin et al,[10] 8 of 11 (72%) patients with lupus nephritis developed preeclampsia compared to 12 of 53 (22%) women who did not have nephritis. In some cases, it is difficult to distinguish preeclampsia from a lupus flare manifesting as lupus nephritis. Both disorders may be characterized by increased proteinuria, hypertension, and fetal growth restriction. Table 27-4 lists several features that may aid in the distinction of preeclampsia from nephritis. Despite these parameters, it is often difficult to distinguish between the two, and in some cases a renal biopsy may be required to differentiate between the conditions. For example, confirmation of lupus nephritis may

---

■ **TABLE 27-4. Laboratory Tests That May Be Used to Distinguish Preeclampsia from a Lupus Flare**

Test	Preeclampsia	SLE
Decreased complement levels	+	+++
Increased anti-dsDNA	–	+++
Antithrombin III defiency	++	+/–
Microangiopathic hemolytic anemia	++	–
Coombs postitve hemolytic anemia	–	++
Thrombocytopenia	++	++
Leukopenia	–	++
Hematuria	+	+++
Cellular casts	–	+++
Increased serum creatinine	+/–	++
Hypocalciuria	++	+/–
Increased liver transaminases	++	+/–

prevent unnecessary iatrogenic preterm birth in an attempt to treat preeclampsia. Although there is a theoretical increased risk of complications from the procedure, it has been performed safely during pregnancy. Preeclampsia and lupus nephrits may also coexist and a definitive diagnosis cannot always be made.

Fetal Complications

Pregnancy Loss

Patients with SLE have an overall increased risk of pregnancy loss. The rate of first trimester spontaneous miscarriage is as high as 35%. The risk of fetal death is also increased and approaches 22% in some series. Several factors have been associated with pregnancy loss in women with SLE including antiphospholipid syndrome (see below), renal disease (especially Class III-IV glomerulonephritis), active disease during pregnancy, a history of fetal loss, and African American and Hispanic race/ethnicity.[21-23] However, in the absence of these, SLE patients have pregnancy loss rates that are similar to the general population.

Preterm Delivery

There is a higher incidence of preterm birth in patients with lupus than in healthy women. Preterm delivery <37 weeks has been reported in as few as 3% and as many as 73% of SLE pregnancies (median 30%). The variation in preterm birth in these studies may be due, in part, to the tendency of some obstetricians to intentionally deliver patients with SLE in order to avoid fetal morbidity. However, a well-designed cohort study by Johnson et al[24] including careful obstetric detail, reported a 50% rate of preterm birth in patients with SLE. Preterm delivery typically occurs because of preeclampsia, fetal growth impairment, abnormal fetal testing, and preterm premature rupture of membranes.[24] Increased disease activity, chronic hypertension, and antiphospholipid antibodies are all associated with an increased risk for both medically indicated and spontaneous preterm delivery.

Neonatal Lupus Erythematosus

Neonatal lupus erythematosus (NLE) is a rare condition that occurs in approximately 1:20,000 live births. The disease is characterized by neonatal or fetal heart block, skin lesions, or less commonly, anemia, thrombocytopenia, and hepatitis. Approximately, 50% of fetuses with NLE have skin lesions, 50% have heart block, and 10% have both. NLE is an immune-mediated disease and is a result of transplacental passage of maternal autoantibodies. Most cases are associated with antibodies to the cytoplasmic ribonucleo-proteins SSA (Ro), more specifically the five anti-SS2-kDa epitope of SSA. SSB (La) antibodies are also detected in 50% to 75% of these women. However, NLE is rarely associated with isolated antibodies to SSB.

Typical skin lesions associated with NLE are erythematous, scaling plaques usually seen on the scalp or face of the infant. The lesions appear within the first weeks after delivery and last only for a few months. Skin biopsies of the lesions show changes typical of cutaneous lupus in adults. The hematologic abnormalities of NLE also resolve within a few months, coinciding with the disappearance of maternal autoantibodies.

Cardiac lesions associated with NLE are heart block and endocardial fibroelastosis.[25,26] The anti-SSA (most specifically anti-SSA-52), binds to myocardial tissue. Histologic analysis of affected fetal hearts demonstrates mononuclear cell infiltration, fibrin deposition, calcification of the conduction system (specifically the AV and SA nodes), and diffuse fibroelastosis throughout the myocardium. It is hypothesized that the earliest effect of the antibody-mediated disease is global pancarditis with subsequent fibrosis of the conduction system. Congenital heart block is usually detected as fetal bradycardia with a rate between 60 and 80 beats/min between 16 and 25 weeks' gestation. Fetal echocardiography demonstrates a structurally normal heart with AV dissociation. In some cases, fetal hydrops develops in utero.

The presence of autoantibodies alone is insufficient to cause NLE. This is demonstrated by the fact that approximately 30% of patients with SLE have anti-SSA antibodies, and 15% to 20% of patients have anti-SSB autoantibodies. However, prospective studies indicate that the incidence of congenital heart block in infants born to women with SLE is only 2%. Also, the recurrence risk ranges between 15% and 20% and there are reports of twins who are discordant for NLE. Thus, anti-SSA alone does not always lead to NLE. It is also important to recognize that maternal SLE is not a prerequisite for NLE. In fact, up to 50% of cases occur in the offspring of healthy women with circulating autoantibodies. Some, but not all of these women eventually develop connective-tissue disorders. Prospective studies of women with anti-SSA or anti-SSB antibodies (regardless of SLE status) have confirmed that about 2% will have a child with NLE.

The clinical course of NLE is highly variable. Cutaneous and hematologic abnormalities resolve by 6 months of age. However, heart block is a permanent condition that is associated with significant morbidity and even mortality. Approximately, 15% to 20% of fetuses affected with heart block die within 3 years of age due to a fatal cardiomyopathy. Up to 60% of neonates require pacing during the neonatal period and most affected children eventually require permanent pacemakers before adulthood. There are few data regarding long-term outcomes. However, preliminary reports suggest that anti-SSA may be associated with an increased risk of dyslexia. Thus, long-term neuropsychological evaluation may be useful.

Whether treatment of heart block detected in utero is beneficial is not clear. Many clinicians advocate the use of flourinated corticosteroids since they cross the placenta. The rationale for steroid treatment is based on the fact that the cardiac histology of fetuses with CHB demonstrates diffuse inflammation, IgG, fibrin, and complement deposition. Initially, improvement in myocardial function was reported by some investigators. However, it is now clear that once heart block is complete it is irreversible even with steroid treatment. Thus, steroids should not be routinely used once heart block is complete. Some authorities advocate their use in cases of myocarditis, heart failure, or mild hydrops but efficacy is uncertain.[26]

It is even more controversial as to whether screening for first or second degree heart block and treating such patients with steroids can reduce progression to complete heart block. A cohort of pregnancies in women with anti-SSA and anti-SSB antibodies was prospectively followed with serial fetal echocardiograms (PRIDE study). The investigators noted rapid progression from normal sinus rhythm to complete heart block without a graded progression through early stage heart block. In some cases steroids appeared to reverse a prolonged PR interval. However, spontaneous reversal may also occur. Thus, the benefit of screening for and/or treating prolonged PR intervals in women with anti-SSA or anti-SSB remains unproven.[27,28]

Importantly, there are significant maternal and fetal risks to treatment with high dose, chronic fluorinated corticosteroids including osteoporosis, glucose intolerance, adrenal suppression, fetal growth restriction, decreased brain growth, learning disabilities, and developmental delay. Therefore, steroid therapy in the treatment of congenital heart block diagnosed *in utero should* be considered experimental and used with extreme caution. Ongoing studies are evaluating the potential efficacy of intravenous immune globulin as a prophylactic or therapeutic agent for the prevention of congenital heart block in at-risk pregnancies.

The Management of Pregnancies Complicated by SLE

Table 27-5 summarizes the management of a patient with SLE during pregnancy. Ideally, women with SLE should have preconceptual counseling to discuss both medical and obstetric risks including lupus flares, preeclampsia, fetal growth restriction, pregnancy loss, and preterm delivery. Patients should also be made aware of the risk of NLE and the clinical implications of the disease. All patients with SLE should have an assessment of their renal function in the form of a serum creatinine level and a 24-hour urine analysis for protein and creatinine clearance. In addition, a hematocrit and platelet count should be determined to exclude hematologic abnormalities associated with SLE. Finally, all patients should be tested for antiphospholipid antibodies (see below in lupus and antiphospholipid syndrome). A number of studies have demonstrated that active lupus at the time of conception is associated with a higher risk of lupus flares, preeclampsia, and fetal loss. Thus, the optimal timing of conception in SLE patients is after a patient has been in remission for 6 months. In addition, nonsteroidal anti-inflammatory drugs (NSAIDs) and cytotoxic agents should be stopped prior to conception (see below in medications).

During pregnancy, patients with the disease should be comanaged by an obstetrician and a rheumatologist. Obstetric visits should be as frequent as every 2 weeks during the first and second trimesters, and weekly during the third. Blood pressure, urinalysis, and symptoms of lupus flare should be assessed at each visit. Serial ultrasounds should be preformed to screen for fetal growth restriction. Nonstress testing and evaluation of the amniotic fluid volume should begin at 32 weeks' gestation or sooner if IUGR is suspected or other complications, such as preeclampsia occur.

Routine testing for ANA titers and complement levels do not improve obstetric outcome and are unnecessary. Some physicians advocate routine testing for anti-SSA and SSB antibodies in all patients with SLE. However, these tests are not cost effective, since one would neither advise a patient against a pregnancy, nor institute a specific treatment if the serum titers were positive.

Medications

The medical management of SLE includes four categories of drugs: NSAIDs, antimalarials, corticosteroids, and cytotoxic agents (Table 27-6).

Nonsteroidal Anti-inflammatory Drugs NSAIDs are the most common anti-inflammatory agents used in the treatment of SLE. Unfortunately, their use during pregnancy is

■ **TABLE 27-5. Management Protocol for Patients with Systemic Lupus Erythematosus**

I. Priorities

A. Avoid medications that are harmful to the fetus
B. Prompt detection of preeclampsia and uteroplacental insufficiency
C. Discern between lupus exacerbations and preeclampsia
D. Appropriate detection and treatment of lupus flares

II. Management

A. Preconception counseling

1. Discuss potential pregnancy complications including preeclampsia, preterm labor, miscarriage, fetal death, fetal growth restriction, and neonatal lupus.
2. Clinically evaluate lupus activity. Delay pregnancy until remission f 6-12 months.
3. Evaluate patient for nephritis, hematologic abnormalities, and antiphospholipid antibodies.
4. Discontinue NSAIDs and cytotoxic agents.

B. Antenatal care

1. Frequent visits to assess SLE status and to screen for hypertension.
2. Serial ultrasounds to evaluate interval fetal growth.
3. Antenatal surveillance at 32 wk or earlier if indicated.

C. Treatment of SLE exacerbations

1. Mild to moderate exacerbations
   a. If the patient is taking glucocorticoids, increase the dose to at least 20-30 mg/d.
   b. If the patient is not taking glucocorticoids, start 15-20 mg prednisone daily. Alternatively, intravenous methylprednisolone (1000 mg daily) for 3 d may avoid the need for daily maintenance doses of steroids.
   c. If the patient is not taking hydroxychloroquine, initiate 200 mg twice daily.
2. Severe exacerbations without renal or CNS manifestations
   a. Rheumatology consult and consider hospitalization.
   b. Glucocorticoid treatment 1.0-1.5 mg/kg. Expect clinical improvement in 5-10 d.
   c. Taper the glucocorticoids once the patient demonstrates clinical improvement.
   d. If the patient cannot be tapered off high doses of glucocorticoids, consider starting cyclosporine or azathioprine.
3. Severe exacerbations with renal or CNS involvement
   a. Hospitalization and rheumatology consult.
   b. Initiate intravenous glucocorticoid treatment, 10-30 mg/kg/d of methylprednisolone for 3-6 d.
   c. Maintain patient on 1.0-1.5 mg/kg of oral prednisone.
   d. When the patient responds, taper the glucocorticoid.
   e. For unresponsive patients, consider plasmapheresis.

associated with significant fetal morbidity. NSAIDs readily cross the placenta and can block prostaglandin synthesis in fetal tissue. The use of NSAIDs during pregnancy is associated with premature closure of the ductus arteriosus, fetal pulmonary hypertension, necrotizing enterocolitis, and fetal renal insufficiency. There was speculation that selective COX-II inhibitors might cause fewer fetal side effects than nonselective inhibitors. However, untoward fetal effects occur even with selective COX-II inhibitors. Aspirin crosses the placenta and may adversely affect fetal platelet function. The use of aspirin in the third trimester is associated with intracranial fetal hemorrhage. Aspirin should be avoided in pregnancy.

Glucocorticoids Glucocorticoids are the first line of treatment for SLE in pregnancy.[29] They are not considered to be human teratogens. Hydrocortisone, prednisone, and prednisolone are the steroids of choice since these agents are inactivated by 11-beta hydroxysteroid in the placenta,

■ TABLE 27-6. Medications Used for the Treatment of SLE in Pregnancy

Medication	Pregnancy category	Recommendations
NSAIDs	B	Avoid, especially in the third trimester.
Hydroxychloroquine	C	Appears to be safe during pregnancy. Teratogenicity based on older studies of other antimalarial agents: chloroquine. Stopping hydroxychloroquine is associated with an increased risk of SLE flares. Therefore, recommend continuing if needed to control SLE.
Glucocorticoids	B	Avoid fluorinated glucocorticoids because they cross the placenta. High doses associated with significant maternal side effects and subsequent fetal side effects. Avoid empiric treatment.
Cyclosporine A	C	Extensive experience with the use of cyclosporine in pregnant renal transplant patients. Not an animal teratogen. Appears safe in humans. Long-term follow-up studies are limited.
Azathioprine	D	Teratogenic in animals. Appears safe in humans.
Cyclophosphamide	D	Associated with cleft palate and skeletal abnormalities. Avoid if possible.
Mycophenolate Mofetil	D	Associated with facial clefts, and facial and ear abnormalities. Avoid if possible.
Methotrexate	X	Avoid. The drug is embryolethal. Also associated with multiple types of congenital anomalies.

allowing less than 10% of active drug to reach the fetus. The incidence of fetal adrenal suppression after maternal gucocorticoid use is extremely low.

There are severe maternal side effects from glucocorticoid use including osteoporosis, glucose intolerance, sodium and water retention, infection, hypertension, and avascular necrosis. There is also an increased risk of obstetric complications such as gestational diabetes, preeclampsia, preterm premature ruptured membranes, and fetal growth restriction. Typically, the benefits of glucocorticoid use for controlling lupus flares in pregnancy outweigh the risks. However, patients should be maintained on the lowest possible dose and weaned off if symptoms permit. Patients receiving chronic steroids (20 mg or more of prednisone for a duration of ≥3 weeks during the last 6 months) should receive stress doses in labor.

Antimalarials Chloroquine has been associated with congenital anomalies raising concern for the safety of using antimalarial medications during pregnancy. However, hydroxychloroquine is not associated with an increased risk for fetal malformations and is considered *safe* during

pregnancy. In fact, a prospective study by Cortes-Hernandez and colleagues demonstrated that stopping hydroxychloroquine treatment during pregnancy was associated with a significant increase in the risk of lupus flares.[23] Therefore, if a patient requires this medication to control her disease, stopping the drug is ill adversed.

Cytotoxic Agents Cyclosporine is a pregnancy category C drug. There is abundant data obtained from transplant patients regarding the use of cyclosporine in pregnancy. The use of this medication appears to be safe, but long-term follow-up studies are limited. Azathioprine does not appear to be a teratogen in humans. However, its use in pregnancy has been associated with fetal growth restriction. In severe cases of SLE in pregnancy requiring chronic high doses of glucocorticoids, either cyclosporine or azathioprine may be added to help control symptoms and to lower the dose of steroids used. Cyclophosphamide is an alkylating agent and is the drug of choice in nonpregnant patients for the treatment of proliferative lupus nephritis. However, this drug is known to cross the placenta and is associated with fetal cleft palate and skeletal abnormalities. It should be used only with extreme caution in pregnancy. Methotrexate, an antimetabolite, is sometimes used in SLE patients. It is embryolethal in early pregnancy and is also a known human teratogen when used later in gestation. It is pregnancy category X and is absolutely contraindicated in the treatment of pregnant women with SLE.

Treatment of Lupus Flares

Lupus flares in pregnancy are usually mild, and most commonly are manifested by skin lesions or joint pain. However, patients may present with severe nephritis, stroke, seizures, or psychosis as a result of a lupus exacerbation. Treatment of lupus flares depends on the severity of the patient's symptoms, and with few exceptions can be controlled with NSAIDs, hydroxychloroquine, and glucocorticoids.

Lupus Nephritis Patients with severe nephritis may present with acute renal insufficiency. As discussed above, the differential diagnosis includes preeclampsia and in transplant patients, acute rejection. Interestingly, there are only rare case reports of recurrent lupus nephritis in transplanted kidneys. Therefore, acute renal insufficiency in transplant patients is likely due to transplant rejection or preeclampsia. However, the distinction between rejection, nephritis, and preeclampsia is often difficult and may require a renal biopsy.

Patients frequently respond well to glucocorticoids. However, patients with proliferative nephritis may require cyclophosphamide. A recent study comparing low-dose to high-dose cyclophosphamide for the treatment of proliferative nephritis demonstrated that low doses were as effective as high doses and associated with fewer maternal side effects. Patients who do not respond to medical therapy, and who have serum creatinine levels >3.5 mg/dL should be started on dialysis in order to optimize pregnancy outcome.

Neuropsychiatric SLE There are many different central nervous system manifestations of SLE, making the treatment of neuropsychiatric SLE complex. These include peripheral neuropathy, headaches, seizures, chorea, stroke, mood disorders, and psychosis. It is also essential to exclude other causes of neurologic symptoms such as metabolic abnormalities, infection, and intracranial lesions. Infection is especially common in SLE patients with chronic steroid use. Thus, a complete evaluation for infection including cerebral spinal fluid analysis is required. In addition, brain imaging and EEG are often helpful in excluding other causes of neurologic abnormalities.

Unfortunately, there are no randomized-controlled studies regarding the appropriate treatment of lupus cerebritis. As such, treatment is empiric. Patients presenting with recurrent psychosis, mood changes, or delirium do not readily respond to mood stabilizing medications, but instead typically respond to high-dose steroids. Cyclophosphamide may be added, if needed, to help lower the dose of steroids required to control symptoms. Patients with mild neuropsychiatric symptoms (infrequent seizures, mild depression, headaches, peripheral neuropathy) and no other manifestations of systemic disease may be treated symptomatically. Lupus patients presenting with a thrombotic stroke often also have antiphospholipid antibodies. The primary treatment for these women is anticoagulation with heparin.

In general, with the exception of methotrexate, cyclophosphamide, and NSAIDs, the benefits of medical therapy for the treatment of severe lupus flares far exceed the risks. Although these medications should be used prudently, there are circumstances wherein they are indicated in pregnancy.

■ LUPUS AND ANTIPHOSPHOLIPID SYNDROME

Antiphospholipid syndrome (APS) is an autoimmune disorder defined by distinct clinical and laboratory features[30] including the presence of antiphospholipid antibodies (aPL) (Table 27-7). aPL are a heterogeneous group of autoantibodies that bind phospholipids, proteins, or a phospholipid-protein complex. Approximately, 30% of patients with SLE also have antiphospholipid antibodies. Individuals with SLE and APS are considered to have secondary APS, while those with APS and no other connective tissue disorders have primary APS.

Although several aPL have been described, lupus anticoagulant, anticardiolipin antibodies, and anti-beta-2-glycoprotein-I antibodies are the three best characterized, and are recommended for clinical use.[31] Lupus anticoagulant is a misnomer because patients may not have SLE and they are hypercoagulable as opposed to anticoagulated. It is also an unusual name for an antibody. Lupus anticoagulant is detected in plasma using one of several phospholipid-dependent clotting tests (eg, activated partial thromboplastin time or dilute Russel viper venom time). If the autoantibody is present, it will interfere with clotting, thus prolonging the clotting time. Confirmatory tests are then performed to exclude other reasons for prolongation of

■ **TABLE 27-7. Criteria for the Classification of the Antiphospholipid Syndrome**

Clinical criteria

1. Vascular thrombosis: One or more episodes of arterial, venous, or small vessel thrombosis in any tissue or organ confirmed by imaging, Doppler studies, or histopathology. Superficial venous thromboses are excluded.
2. Pregnancy morbidity:
   a. One or more unexplained deaths of a morphologic normal fetus at or beyond the 10th week of gestation, with normal morphology documented by ultrasound or direct examination of the fetus OR
   b. One or more premature births of a morphologically normal neonate prior to 34 weeks' gestation because of severe preeclampsia, eclampsia, or severe placental insufficiency OR
   c. Three or more unexplained consecutive spontaneous miscarriages prior to the 10th week of gestation, with maternal anatomic or hormonal abnormalities, and paternal and maternal chromosome causes excluded.

Laboratory criteria

1. Lupus anticoagulant present in plasma on two or more occasions at least 12 wk apart, detected according to the guidelines of the International Society on Thrombosis and Hemostasis.
2. Anticardiolipin of IgG and/or IgM isotype in blood present in medium or high titer (>40 GPL or MPL, or >99%) on two or more occasions at least 12 wk apart, measured by standardized ELISA.
3. Anti-beta-2-glycoprotein-I antibody of IgG and/or IgM isotype in blood (titer >99%) on two or more occasions at least 12 wk apart, measured by standardized ELISA.

Note: Definite antiphospholipid syndrome is present if a patient meets at least one of the clinical criteria and one of the laboratory criteria.

clotting assays (such as clotting factor deficiency). Clinicians may order a *lupus anticoagulant screen* in a *blue top tube* which is reported as either present or absent.

Anticardiolipin antibodies are detected in a more traditional fashion via immunoassay. Results are reported in a semiquantitative manner and the assay is standardized using standard sera. Medium-high titers of the IgG isotype are most strongly associated with the clinical features of APS. Low-positive results and isolated IgM or IgA antibodies are common, nonspecific, and are of questionable clinical relevance. They are not considered diagnostic criteria for APS.

Over the past decade, medium to high titers of IgG or IgM antibodies against beta-2-glycoprotein-I also have become accepted as criteria for APS. As with anticardiolipin antibodies, anti-beta-2-glycoprotein-I antibodies are detected by a standardized immunoassay and reported in a semiquantitative fashion.

Several other autoantibodies have been associated with APS. Some are aPL such as the false positive serologic test for syphilis and antiphosphatidylserine antibodies. Although these antibodies may eventually prove to be clinically useful, they are not recommended for routine testing in the absence of further study.

APS is associated with significant medical problems including arterial and venous thrombosis, recurrent pregnancy loss, and autoimmune thrombocytopenia. Pregnancies resulting in live births are often complicated by obstetric disorders associated with uteroplacental insufficiency such as preeclampsia, fetal growth restriction, and abnormal antenatal testing.[32,33] Preeclampsia has been reported in one-fourth to one-half of women with well-characterized APS. It is often severe and occurs prior to 34 weeks' gestation. Although women with APS are at increased risk for preeclampsia, most women with preeclampsia do not have APS. This is not surprising given the relative frequency of preeclampsia compared to APS.

In utero fetal growth restriction is also associated with antiphospholipid antibodies, occurring in 15% to 30% of women with APS. It appears that fetal growth restriction is more likely in patients with higher levels of IgG anticardiolipin antibodies. Abnormal fetal heart rate tracings indicative of uteroplacental insufficiency are also more common in APS patients. In a large cohort study of women with APS, 50% of patients had abnormal antenatal testing which ultimately prompted obstetric intervention and delivery. Placental insufficiency, manifested by abnormal fetal heart rate tracings, may occur as early as the second trimester.

The increased incidence of preeclampsia, fetal growth restriction, and abnormal fetal heart rate tracings all contribute to iatrogenic preterm birth in women with APS. Preterm birth occurs in up to one-third of women with APS. Delivery prior to 34 weeks is most likely in women with strict clinical and laboratory criteria for APS.

Treatment for APS

Initially, high-dose prednisone (40 mg daily or greater) in combination with low-dose aspirin was the accepted treatment for antiphospholipid syndrome in pregnancy. This regimen resulted in a 60% to 70% successful pregnancy rate. Subsequently, the use of heparin in the treatment of antiphospholipid syndrome was proposed. Several case series demonstrated a success rate comparable to that of high-dose prednisone. A small randomized trial comparing heparin and prednisone demonstrated that heparin and prednisone are equally efficacious. However, patients treated with prednisone had a higher rate of adverse obstetric events including preeclampsia, preterm premature rupture of membranes, and preterm labor. Success with heparin has been confirmed by other studies.[34] Thus, heparin (or low molecular weight heparin [LMWH; see below in this section]) is the treatment of choice for APS in pregnancy. Intravenous immune globulin has been used as adjunctive therapy in patient's refractory to heparin. It is not recommended for use as primary therapy due to cost and a lack of improved efficacy compared to heparin alone.[35] Heparin is also potentially useful for the treatment of APS during pregnancy due to an increased risk of thrombosis, even in women without history of thromboembolism. Patients without a prior history of thrombosis should be treated with thromboprophylactic doses of heparin (10,000-20,000 units of unfractionated heparin daily). Patients with a history of thrombosis should receive a dose of heparin that will provide full anticoagulation. The goal of therapy is to maintain the activated partial thromboplastin time (aPTT) 1.5 to 2.5 times the normal value. Patients with no history of thrombosis should continue anticoagulation therapy until 6 weeks postpartum. Individuals with APS and prior thromboses should be anticoagulated for life. Heparin may be exchanged for sodium warfarin in the postpartum period. Despite initial concerns about transfer through breast milk, it is safe to take warfarin while breast-feeding.

It is important to remember that the lupus anticoagulant causes a prolongation of the activated partial thromboplastin time. Therefore, this test cannot be used to monitor anticoagulation in patients who test positive for the lupus anticoagulant. Rather, antifactor Xa levels can be followed. To achieve full anticoagulation using unfractionated heparin, antifactor Xa levels should fall between 0.4 and 0.7 U/mL.

Side effects of heparin are uncommon but potentially serious and include bleeding, osteopenia, and thrombocytopenia. Heparin-induced osteoporosis with fractures occurs in 1% to 2% of women treated during pregnancy with unfractionated heparin. Patients should therefore be encouraged to engage in weight-bearing exercise and take calcium supplements. In addition, heparin causes an immune-mediated thrombocytopenia in up to 5% of patients. Thrombocytopenia is detected within 10 days after the initiation of therapy. Accordingly, platelet counts should be checked serially for the first 10 days of therapy.

Low-molecular-weight heparin (LMWH) has been used with increasing frequency in pregnancy. Initially it was thought that LMWH might cross the placenta and cause fetal hemorrhage. However, several studies have shown that this does not occur and LMWH is safe in pregnancy. In order to achieve full anticoagulation, the recommended dose of enoxaparin is 1 mg/kg, administered subcutaneously in two equal doses 12 hours apart. However, due to the increased plasma volume and renal blood flow in the pregnant patient, the pharmacokinetics of enoxaparin is altered by pregnancy. It is necessary to monitor antifactor Xa levels in order to ensure adequate dosing. The target antifactor Xa level for full anticoagulation using LMWH is 0.5 to 1.1 U/mL. LMWH appears to have less risk for osteopenia and thrombocytopenia than unfractionated heparin. However, it is more expensive and has a longer half life, making it less convenient for intrapartum anticoagulation. The advantages of LMWH are usually worth the downside in women who require full anticoagulation. However, unfractionated heparin may be preferable in women taking only prophylactic doses. In women taking LMWH, it is often useful to switch to unfractionated heparin at 34 to 36 weeks' gestation. The shorter half life of unfractionated heparin increases the chances that neuraxial anesthesia mat be safely administered if the patient spontaneously labors of ruptures membranes. Table 27-8 summarizes the management of pregnant women with APS.

Catastrophic APS

A majority of patients with APS experience single large vessel thrombotic events. In patients with recurrent

■ **TABLE 27-8. Management Protocol for Patients with Antiphospholipid Syndrome**

I. Goals of therapy

A. Embryonic and fetal survival
B. Prompt detection of uteroplacental insufficiency and preeclampsia
C. Prevention of thrombosis

II. Management

1. Preconception counseling

  a. Review pregnancy risks such as miscarriage, fetal death, preeclampsia, fetal growth restriction, uteroplacental insufficiency, and preterm birth.
  b. Evaluate the accuracy of the diagnosis. Confirm the presence of antiphospholipid antibodies if necessary.

2. Antenatal care

  a. When a live embryo is detected, start subcutaneous unfractionated heparin 10,000-20,000 U/d in divided doses or the equivalent dose of LMWH (prophylactic). Higher doses (therapeutic) should be used in patients with prior thrombosis.
  b. Calcium supplementation and weight bearing exercise.
  c. Frequent assessment for the development of preeclampsia.
  d. Serial ultrasounds to evaluate interval fetal growth.
  e. Fetal surveillance starting at 32 wk or earlier if complications arise.
  f. If a patient has a history of a thromboembolic event, or suffers an acute episode during pregnancy, start therapeutic doses of heparin to maintain the PTT 1.5-2.5 times normal, or enoxaparin, 1 mg/kg twice a day.
  g. If using low molecular weight heparin, antifactor Xa levels should be checked every trimester in order to maintain levels of 0.5-1.1 U/mL.

thrombosis, the subsequent event typically occurs months to years after the initial episode. In 1992, Asherson et al described a small subset of patients with APS who presented with what has been described as *catastrophic APS*.[36] Unlike the majority of patients with APS, those with catastrophic APS suffer microvascular thromboses in multiple organs, most commonly the kidneys, lungs, and gastrointestinal tract. The heart, brain, liver, and adrenal glands are less frequently involved. Catastrophic APS has a 50% to 65% mortality rate.

In a retrospective review of 50 patients with catastrophic APS, Asherson found that 78% presented with renal involvement which typically resulted in concurrent malignant hypertension. Renal biopsies in these patients demonstrated frank microangiopathy and occasional renal infarctions. Sixty-six percent of patients demonstrated pulmonary involvement. The most common presenting symptom was severe dyspnea. Approximately, half of patients with pulmonary involvement developed ARDS and 25% had pulmonary embolism. In this series, 56% of patients had central nervous system involvement. Symptoms were

highly variable and included confusion, drowsiness, stupor, seizures, and infarction of either large or small vessels. Half of the patients had myocardial involvement and 38% had gastrointestinal involvement. The most common symptom of patients with gastrointestinal involvement is severe abdominal pain. Occlusion of the mesenteric vessels (both arterial and venous) was frequently noted. Other organs that were less commonly affected were liver (35%), adrenal (26%), spleen (20%), and pancreas (1%). Up to 50% of patients had skin involvement manifested as superficial necrosis and gangrene, splinter hemorrhages, and purpura.

Diagnosis

The diagnosis of catastrophic APS can be difficult, and the differential diagnosis includes DIC, TTP, and SLE nephritis. Furthermore, Drenkard and colleagues[37] reported a decrease in anticardiolipin antibody titer at the time of thrombosis in six patients with previously high antibody titers. The authors speculate that acute thrombosis may cause transient antibody consumption, which could complicate the diagnosis of APS at the time of the acute event.

The laboratory diagnosis of catastrophic APS can be made by the presence of lupus anticoagulant and high titers of anticardiolipin IgG antibodies, both of which are detected in approximately 95% of patients. Patients may also demonstrate thrombocytopenia and anti-ds DNA if they also carry a diagnosis of SLE. There may also be evidence of hemolytic anemia and laboratory values consistent with DIC.

Treatment

There is no standard treatment for catastrophic APS. Patients often are critically ill and require admission to intensive care units. Supportive treatment depends on presenting symptoms, and may include aggressive antihypertensive therapy, assisted ventilation, dialysis, and vasopressors. Plasmapheresis has been recommended by some. However, others report improved outcome in patients who are treated with a combination of anticoagulation, steroids, and either intravenous immunoglobins or plasmapheresis in order to rapidly decrease the titer of antiphospholipid antibodies.

REFERENCES

1. Arnett FC, Reveille JD, Wilson RW, et al. Systemic lupus erythematosus: current state of the genetic hypothesis. *Semin Arthritis Rheum.* 1984;14:24-35.

2. Doria A, Tincani A, Lockshin M. Challenges of lupus pregnancies. *Rheumatology.* 2008;47:iii9-iii12.

3. Tan EM, Cohen AS, Fries JF, et al. The 1982 revised criteria for the classification of systemic lupus erythematosus. *Arthritis Rheum.* 1982;25:1271-1277.

4. Clowe MEB, Jamison M, Myers E, James AH. A national study of the complications of lupus in pregnancy. *Am J Obstet Gynecol.* 2008;199:127.e1-127.e6.

5. Petri M. Sex hormones and systemic lupus erythematosus. *Lupus.* 2008;17:412-415.

6. Petri M, Howard D, Repke J. Frequency of lupus flare in pregnancy. The Hopkins Lupus Pregnancy Center experience. *Arthritis Rheum.* 1991;34:1538-1545.

7. Tandon A, Ibanez D, Gladman DD, Urowitz MB. The effect of pregnancy on lupus nephritis. *Arthritis Rheum.* 2004;50:3941-3946.

8. Mintz G, Niz J, Gutierrez G, et al. Prospective study of pregnancy in systemic lupus erythematosus. Results of a multidisciplinary approach. *J Rheumatol.* 1986;13:732-739.

9. Lockshin MD. Pregnancy does not cause systemic lupus erythematosus to worsen. *Arthritis Rheum.* 1989;32:665-670.

10. Lockshin MD, Reinitz E, Druzin ML, et al. Lupus pregnancy. Case-control prospective study demonstrating absence of lupus exacerbation during or after pregnancy. *Am J Med.* 1984;77:893-898.

11. Urowitz MB, Gladman DD, Farewell VT, Stewart J, McDonald J. Lupus and pregnancy studies. *Arthritis Rheum.* 1993;36:1392-7.

12. Nossent HC, Swaak TJ. Systemic lupus erythematosus. VI. Analysis of the interrelationship with pregnancy. *J Rheumatol.* 1990;17:771-6.

13. Wong KL, Chan FY, Lee CP. Outcome of pregnancy in patients with systemic lupus erythematosus: a prospective study. *Arch Intern Med.* 1991;15:269-73.

14. Ruiz-Irastorza G, Lima F, Alves J, Khamashta MA, Simpson J, Hughes GR, Buchanan NM. *Br J Rheumatol.* 1996;35:133-8.

15. Doria A, Cutolo M, Ghirardello A, et al. Steroid hormones and disease activity during pregnancy in systemic lupus erythematosus. *Arthritis Rheum.* 2002;47:202-209.

16. Wagner SJ, Craici I, Reed D, et al. Maternal and fetal outcomes in pregnant patients with active lupus nephritis. *Lupus.* 2009;18:342-347.

17. Packham DK, Lam SS, Nicholls K, et al. Lupus nephritis and pregnancy. *Q J Med.* 1992;83:315-324.

18. Day CJ, Lipkin GW, Savage COS. Lupus nephritis and pregnancy in the 21st century. *Nephrol Dial Transplant.* 2009;24:344-7.15.

19. Burkett G. Lupus nephropathy and pregnancy. *Clin Obstet Gynecol.* 1985;28:310-323.

20. Imbasciati E, Tincani A, Gregorini G, et al. Pregnancy in women with pre-existing lupus nephritis: predictors of fetal and maternal outcome. *Nephrol Dial Transplant.* 2009;24:519-525.

21. Ambrosio P, Lermann R, Cordeiro A, Borges A, Nogueira I, Serrano F. Lupus and pregnancy—15 years of experience in a tertiary center. *Clinic Rev Allerg Immunol.* 2009;Epub ahead of print.

22. Andrade R, Sanchez ML, Alarcon GS, et al. Adverse pregnancy outcomes in women with systemic lupus erythematosus from a multiethnic US cohort: LUMINA (LVI). *Clin Experimental Rheumatol.* 2008;26:268-274.

23. Cortes-Hernandez J, Ordi-Ros J, Paredes F, et al. Clinical predictors of fetal and maternal outcome in systemic lupus erythematosus: a prospective study of 103 pregnancies. *Rheumatology (Oxford).* 2002;41:643-650.

24. Johnson MJ, Petri M, Witter FR, et al. Evaluation of preterm delivery in a systemic lupus erythematosus pregnancy clinic. *Obstet Gynecol.* 1995;86:396-339.

25. Waltuck J, Buyon JP. Autoantibody-associated congenital heart block: outcome in mothers and children. *Ann Intern Med.* 1994;120:544-551.

26. Buyon JP, Clancy RM, Friedman DM. Cardiac manifestations of neonatal lupus erythematosus: guidelines to management, integrating clinical clues from the bench and bedside. Nature clinical practice. *Rheumatology.* 2009;5:139-148.

27. Friedman DM, Kim MY, Copel JA, et al; for the PRIDE investigators. Utility of cardiac monitoring in fetuses at risk for congenital heart block. The PR interval and dexamethasone evaluation (PRIDE) prospective study. *Circulation.* 2008;117:485-493.

28. Friedman DM, Kim MY, Copel JA, Llanos C, Davis C, Buyon JP. Prospective evaluation of fetuses with autoimmune-associated congenital heart block followed in the PR interval and dexamethasone evaluation (PRIDE) study. *Am J Cardiol.* 2009;103:1102-1106.

29. Meehan RT, Dorsey JK. Pregnancy among patients with systemic lupus erythematosus receiving immunosuppressive therapy. *J Rheumatol.* 1987;14:252-258.

30. Miyakis S, Lockshin MD, Atsumi D, et al. International consensus statement on an update of the classification criteria for definite antiphospholipid syndrome (APS). *J Thromb Haemost.* 2006;4:295-306.

31. Branch DW, Khamashta MA. Antiphospholipid syndrome: obstetric diagnosis, management, and controversies. *Obstet Gynecol.* 2003;101:1333-1344.

32. Branch DW, Silver RM, Blackwell JL, et al. Outcome of treated pregnancies in women with antiphospholipid syndrome: an update of the Utah experience. *Obstet Gynecol.* 1992; 80:614-620.

33. Lima F, Khamashta MA, Buchanan NM, et al. A study of sixty pregnancies in patients with the antiphospholipid syndrome. *Clin Exp Rheumatol.* 1996;14:131-136.

34. Kutteh WH. Antiphospholipid antibody-associated recurrent pregnancy loss: treatment with heparin and low-dose aspirin is superior to low-dose aspirin alone. *Am J Obstet Gynecol.* 1996;174:1584-1589.

35. Branch DW, Peaceman AM, Druzin M, et al. A multicenter, placebo-controlled pilot study of intravenous immune globulin treatment of antiphospholipid syndrome during pregnancy. The Pregnancy Loss Study Group. *Am J Obstet Gynecol.* 2000;182:122-127.

36. Asherson RA, Cervera R, Piette JC, et al. Catastrophic antiphospholipid syndrome. Clinical and laboratory features of 50 patients. *Medicine (Baltimore).* 1998;77:195-207.

37. Drenkard C, Sanchez-Guerrero J, Alarcon-Segovia D. Fall in antiphospholipid antibody at time of thromboocclusive episodes in systemic lupus erythematosus. *J Rheumatol.* 1989;16:614-7.

Index

Note: Page numbers referencing figures are followed by an *f*; page numbers referencing tables are followed by a *t*; page numbers referencing boxes are followed by a *b*.